# Topics in Cognitive Rehabilitation in the TBI Post-Hospital Phase

Renato Anghinah • Wellingson Paiva
Linamara Rizzo Battistella • Robson Amorim
Editors

# Topics in Cognitive Rehabilitation in the TBI Post-Hospital Phase

Springer

*Editors*
Renato Anghinah
University of São Paulo
São Paulo, SP, Brazil

Linamara Rizzo Battistella
University of São Paulo
São Paulo, SP, Brazil

Wellingson Paiva
University of São Paulo
São Paulo, SP, Brazil

Robson Amorim
University of São Paulo
São Paulo, SP, Brazil

ISBN 978-3-319-95374-8 ISBN 978-3-319-95376-2 (eBook)
https://doi.org/10.1007/978-3-319-95376-2

Library of Congress Control Number: 2018959862



This Springer imprint is published by the registered company Springer Nature Switzerland AG
The registered company address is: Gewerbestrasse 11, 6330 Cham, Switzerland

# Preface

Traumatic brain injury (TBI) is a nondegenerative, noncongenital insult to the brain from an external mechanical force, possibly leading to permanent or temporary impairment of cognitive, physical, and psychosocial functions, with an associated diminished or altered state of consciousness. There are many possible causes, including road traffic accidents, assaults, falls, and accidents at home or at work.

The term "silent epidemic" is used to characterize the incidence of TBI worldwide, because many cases are not recognized and are excluded from official statistics. Despite being the leading cause of death and disability worldwide, especially among young adults, there is still so much we don't know about TBI.

The subject of TBI is of extreme importance. We need to take care of these patients. We need to disseminate the information so that the multidisciplinary teams can give to these subjects the assistance they need.

This book serves as an impetus for more research in the area to take place and works as a guide to show researchers in the field. We do not intend to exhaust the subject about TBI, because this is very vast, but we want to spread knowledge and help health professionals to better understand this health problem that affects so many people.

We aim to assist survivors of traumatic brain injury and family members so they can better adjust and cope with life post injury. Brain injury rehabilitation focuses on restoring the best possible level of physical, cognitive, and behavioral function; improvement for a return to home, school, or work; training and adaptation for long-term limitations; and maximizing function and independence to help patients achieve their fullest potential after a TBI. Our final goal is the community reintegration of people who suffered a TBI.

After a TBI, seeking support and knowledge can help individuals with TBI and their families to increase their awareness about brain injury issues.

São Paulo, SP, Brazil

Renato Anghinah

# Contents

# Contributors

**Sonia-Luz Albarracin, PhD** Nutrition and Biochemistry Department – Pontifical Xavierian University, Bogotá, Colombia

**Robson Luis Oliveira de Amorim, MD, PhD** Department of Neurology – Neurosurgery – Clinics Hospital – School of Medicine – University of São Paulo, São Paulo, Brazil

Department of Neurology – Neurosurgery – Amazonas State University, Amazonas, Brazil

**Celi Santos Andrade, MD, PhD** Department of Radiology and Oncology, School of Medicine – University of São Paulo, São Paulo, Brazil

**Danielle M. Andrade, MD, FRCPC** Division of Neurology, Department of Medicine, University of Toronto, Toronto, ON, Canada

Krembil Neuroscience Collaborative Program, Toronto Western Hospital, University Health Network, Toronto, ON, Canada

Krembil Neurosciences Epilepsy Genetics Program, Toronto Western Hospital, University of Toronto, Toronto, ON, Canada

Krembil Research Institute, University Health Network, Toronto, ON, Canada

**Christian Henrique de Andrade Freitas, MD** Movement Disorders Unit, Department of Neurology, Clinics Hospital – School of Medicine – University of São Paulo, São Paulo, Brazil

**Tatiana de Andrade Jardim Rodriguez, PhD** Department of Physical Therapy, Speech Therapy and Occupational Therapy – School of Medicine – University of São Paulo, São Paulo, Brazil

**Renato Anghinah, MD, PhD** Department of Neurology – Cognitive Rehabilitation after TBI, Clinics Hospital – School of Medicine – University of São Paulo, São Paulo, Brazil

Center of Excellence in Neurology – Americas Serviços Médicos, São Paulo, Brazil

**Renata Areza-Fegyveres, MD, PhD** University of São Paulo, School of Medicine – University of São Paulo, São Paulo, Brazil

**Egberto Reis Barbosa, MD, PhD** Movement Disorders Unit, Department of Neurology, Clinics Hospital – School of Medicine – University of São Paulo, São Paulo, Brazil

**Linamara Rizzo Battistella, MD, PhD** Legal Medicine, Medical Ethics, Social and Occupational Medicine and Physical and Rehabilitation Medicine Institute, Clinics Hospital – School of Medicine – University of São Paulo, São Paulo, Brazil

**Christina May Moran de Brito, MD, PhD** Rehabilitation Department, Institute of Cancer of São Paulo, Clinics Hospital – School of Medicine – University of São Paulo, São Paulo, Brazil

**Carlos Alberto Buchpiguel, MD, PhD** Department of Radiology and Oncology, School of Medicine – University of São Paulo, São Paulo, Brazil

**Sara Carvalho Barbosa Casagrande, MD** Movement Disorders Unit, Department of Neurology, Clinics Hospital – School of Medicine – University of São Paulo, São Paulo, Brazil

**Rebeca Boltes Cecatto, MD, PhD** Rehabilitation Department, Institute of Cancer of São Paulo, Clinics Hospital – School of Medicine – University of São Paulo, São Paulo, Brazil

**Fernanda Coelho, MSc** Department of Neurology – Cognitive Rehabilitation after TBI, Clinics Hospital – School of Medicine – University of São Paulo, São Paulo, Brazil

**Claudia da Costa Leite, MD, PhD** Department of Radiology and Oncology, School of Medicine – University of São Paulo, São Paulo, Brazil

LIM 44-Laboratory of Magnetic Resonance Imaging in Neuroradiology, São Paulo, Brazil

**Fabio Rios Freire, BSc** Department of Neurology – Cognitive Rehabilitation after TBI, Clinics Hospital – School of Medicine – University of São Paulo, São Paulo, Brazil

**André Luiz Nunes Gobatto, MD, PhD** Internal Medicine, Hospital São Rafael, Salvador, Brazil

Intensive Care Unit, Hospital da Cidade, Salvador, Brazil

Internal Medicine Department, Salvador University, Salvador, Brazil

**Maria Lúcia Costacurta Guarita, MD** Institute of Cancer of São Paulo – Rehabilitation Department, São Paulo, São Paulo, Brazil

**Jéssica Natuline Ianof, MSc** Department of Neurology – Cognitive Rehabilitation after TBI, Clinics Hospital – School of Medicine – University of São Paulo, São Paulo, Brazil

**Selma Lancman, PhD** Department of Physical Therapy, Speech Therapy and Occupational Therapy – School of Medicine – University of São Paulo, São Paulo, Brazil

**Leandro Tavares Lucato, MD, PhD** Department of Radiology and Oncology, School of Medicine – University of São Paulo, São Paulo, Brazil

LIM 44-Laboratory of Magnetic Resonance Imaging in Neuroradiology, São Paulo, Brazil

**Patricia De Lucia Nadruz, BSc** Department of Neurology – Cognitive Rehabilitation after TBI, Clinics Hospital – School of Medicine – University of São Paulo, São Paulo, Brazil

**Bruno Prata Martinez, PhD** Physiotherapy Department, Federal University of Bahia (UFBA), Salvador, Brazil

Bahia State University (UNEB), Salvador, Brazil

**Marcia Mitie Nagumo, MSc** Department of Neurology – Neurosurgery – Clinics Hospital – School of Medicine – University of São Paulo, São Paulo, Brazil

**Matheus Fernandes de Oliveira, MD, PhD** Division of Functional Neurosurgery of the Institute of Psychiatry, Clinics Hospital, University of São Paulo, São Paulo, Brazil

**Juliana de Oliveira Barros, PhD** Department of Physical Therapy, Speech Therapy and Occupational Therapy – School of Medicine – University of São Paulo, São Paulo, Brazil

**Fernando Campos Gomes Pinto, MD, PhD** Division of Functional Neurosurgery of the Institute of Psychiatry, Clinics Hospital, University of São Paulo, São Paulo, Brazil

**Aylin Reid, MD, PhD** Division of Neurology, Department of Medicine, University of Toronto, Toronto, ON, Canada

Krembil Neuroscience Collaborative Program, Toronto Western Hospital, University Health Network, Toronto, ON, Canada

Krembil Research Institute, University Health Network, Toronto, ON, Canada

**Arezoo Rezazadeh, MD** Division of Neurology, Department of Medicine, University of Toronto, Toronto, ON, Canada

Krembil Neuroscience Collaborative Program, Toronto Western Hospital, University Health Network, Toronto, ON, Canada

Krembil Neurosciences Epilepsy Genetics Program, Toronto Western Hospital, University of Toronto, Toronto, ON, Canada

**Andrea Toshye Sato, BSc** Department of Physical Therapy, Speech Therapy and Occupational Therapy – School of Medicine – University of São Paulo, São Paulo, Brazil

**Daniele Vieira da Silva, PhD** Nursing School – University of São Paulo, São Paulo, Brazil

**Leonardo Pamponet Simões, BSc** Intermediate Care Unit of Aliance Hospital, Salvador, Brazil

Physiotherapy Service of Woman Hospital, Salvador, Brazil

**Jhon-Jairo Sutachan, PhD** Nutrition and Biochemistry Department – Pontifical Xavierian University, Bogotá, Colombia

**Maria Carmela Tartaglia, MD, FRCPC** Institute of Medical Science, University of Toronto, Toronto, ON, Canada

Centre for Research in Neurodegenerative Diseases, University of Toronto, Toronto, ON, Canada

Division of Neurology, University Health Network, Toronto, ON, Canada

**Anna Vasilevskaya, BSc** Institute of Medical Science, University of Toronto, Toronto, ON, Canada

Centre for Research in Neurodegenerative Diseases, University of Toronto, Toronto, ON, Canada

# Spontaneous Recovery Mechanisms-Brain Reorganization

1

Sonia-Luz Albarracin and Jhon-Jairo Sutachan

## Introduction

Traumatic brain injury (TBI) is now considered a major cause of death and disability [1] For instance, in the United States, it has been estimated that 5.3 million people, who survived TBI, live with disability [2, 3]. This number is even higher in the European Union in which 7.7 million survived with TBI-related disability [3, 4]. The development of TBI is characterized by an initial phase in which the mechanical impact leads to the disruption of brain tissue. This stage is followed by a secondary injury that is associated with activation of astrocytes and microglia, production of lactate and reactive oxygen species (ROS), changes in cellular metabolism, and high levels of glutamate and calcium. Astrocytes and microglia activation also increases the production and release of pro-inflammatory cytokines that recruit immune cells from the periphery. Finally, in a search for homeostasis, the system begins a repair-regenerative stage that contributes to spontaneous neurological recovery [5].

Although the mechanisms involved in the spontaneous recovery and brain reorganization after TBI have not been fully established, it has been suggested that neurogenesis, reorganization of connectivity (synaptogenesis and plasticity), and angiogenesis play a key role. In this chapter, we will focus on the current knowledge about how neurogenesis is regulated during TBI, how plasticity can contribute to brain reorganization, and how they can be used as specific targets for further improving recovery after TBI.

## TBI and Neurogenesis

From a functional point of view, for brain reorganization and spontaneous recovery to be achieved after TBI, it is necessary either to reestablish new connections among survived neurons or to replace dead neurons with new neurons that can integrate and make new contacts with surviving ones. In the second scenario, it is plausible to think that incorporation of new neurons can help restore the full integrity, function, and neuronal field of the impaired circuit.

Several studies have found that neurogenesis can be induced after different kinds of brain injuries [6–9]. In the adult brain, two neurogenic niches have been identified: one in the subventricular zone of the lateral ventricles [10] and one in the subgranular zone of the hippocampal dentate gyrus [11]. The niche in the subventricular zone (SVZ) is characterized by the presence of type B cells that can be in a quiescent or active state. The transition of type B cells from quiescent to active state gives rise to neural progenitors type C cells that express nestin and divide symmetrically originating neuroblast (type A cells) that later migrate to integrate in circuits of the olfactory bulb [11, 12]. Similar to the SVZ, the subgranular zone (SGZ) of the hippocampus is characterized by the presence of type I cells (adult neural stem cells) that once are activated generate type IIa cells (neural progenitor) which in turn transform into type b cells (neuroblasts). Neuroblasts later mature in type III cells that later express NeuN and Calbindin and integrate by making connections with neurons of the entorhinal cortex and CA3 region of the hippocampus (Fig. 1.1).

Although the mechanisms underlying TBI-induced neurogenesis have not been fully established, it is thought that mitogenic and neurotrophic factors can regulate this process after a brain injury [13]. The source of these molecules has been associated with cells such as astrocytes and microglia that activate and respond during the secondary injury. For instance, astrocytes from postnatal hippocampus that are in close contact with neurogenic niches instruct stem cells to adopt a neuronal fate [14]. Interestingly, it has been found that an astrocytic-dependent regulation of neurogenesis can be influence by their site of origin. In vitro, astrocytes, isolated from the cortex and hippocampus, have a high capacity to induce differentiation of neural progenitor stem cells (NPSCs), while spinal cord astrocytes impair differentiation [15]. Activation

S.-L. Albarracin · J.-J. Sutachan (✉)
Nutrition and Biochemistry Department – Pontifical Xavierian University, Bogotá, Colombia
e-mail: albarra@javeriana.edu.co



R. Anghinah et al. (eds.), *Topics in Cognitive Rehabilitation in the TBI Post-Hospital Phase*,
https://doi.org/10.1007/978-3-319-95376-2_1

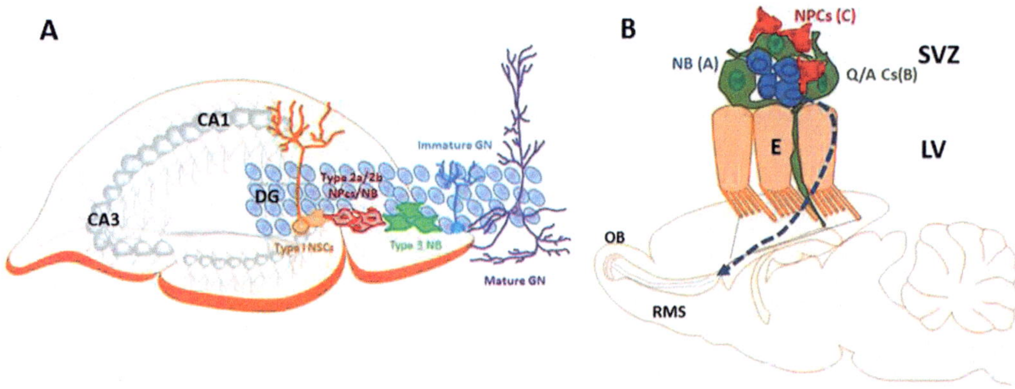


**Fig. 1.1** Adult neurogenic niches. (**a**) Neurogenesis process in the subgranular zone of the hippocampal dentate gyrus. (**b**) Neurogenesis process in the subventricular zone of the lateral ventricule. *NSCs*: neural stem cells, *NPCs*: neural progenitor cells, *NB*: neuroblast, *GN*: granular neurons, *Q/A cells*: quiescent/activated cells, *SVZ*: subventricular zone, *LV*: lateral ventricule, *OB*: olfactory bulb, *RMS*: rostral migratory stream. Illustration were designed using the Motifolio Neuroscience Toolkit

of signaling pathways like Notch, Wnt, Sonic hedgehog (Shh), and Eph/ephrin has been implicated in the astrocytic-dependent regulation of neurogenesis [16, 17].

## Notch Signaling Pathway

Notch works as a cell-cell mediator system of cell communication that regulates cell fate, proliferation, and death [18]. To date, four Notch receptors have been identified (Notch 1–4). These receptors are activated by a series of ligands such as jagged1 and jagged2; Delta-like 1, 3, and 4; and Delta-like homologue 1 and 2. It has been shown that astrocytes trough the activation of the Notch signaling pathway can regulate neurogenesis by maintaining the pool of undifferentiated neural progenitor cells (NPCs) [19, 20]. In addition, the Notch signaling pathway promotes progenitor cell differentiation into glial cells and decreases neuronal differentiation and proliferation [21, 22]. During TBI, reactive astrocytes upregulate the expression of the intermediate filaments, glial fibrillary acid protein (GFAP), and vimentin. Astrocytic-dependent inhibition of NPSCs is mediated by jagged1-mediated Notch signaling in which jagged1 activity is regulated by the GFAP and vimentin. This has been further corroborated in GFAP and vimentin knockout mice where hippocampal neurogenesis is further increased in basal conditions and after trauma. A recent study has found that astrocytes are a heterogeneous population with regard to their Notch signaling competence. For instance, few astrocytes are competent to activate Notch signaling, while the grand majority can activate Notch signaling independently of the GFAP and vimentin expression [23]. In stroke, it has been reported that astrocytes have a decrease in Notch signaling that triggers these cells to active a neurogenic program [23]. These results have been further corroborated in other models of injury in which it has been found that there is an increase in the population of incompetent astrocytes that can lead to the generation of neurons from these incompetent cells.

## Wnt Signaling Pathway

Intravenous administration of bone marrow-derived mesenchymal stem cells has shown a significant improvement effect in cognition after TBI. This effect is mediated by the release of soluble factors that not only impact in the survival of neural stem cells but also stimulate hippocampal neurogenesis (proliferation and differentiation). Further characterization of the released factor leads to the identification of high levels of Wnt3a in serum. High levels of Wnt3a were parallel to the activation of the Wnt/β-catenin signaling in the hippocampus [24]. Wnt is produced and secreted by mature astrocytes. For instance, the release of Wnt-3 promotes both neuroblast proliferation and neuronal commitment by inducing the activation of NeuroD1, a well-known transcription factor that is required for the survival and maturation of adult-born neurons [25, 26]. NeuroD1 works by a complex mechanism that includes reprogramming of transcription factor landscape, conversion of heterochromatin to euchromatin, and increased chromatin accessibility [27].

## Sonic Hedgehog Signaling Pathway (Shh)

Shh is a morphogen that plays a role in the development of the nervous system. For instance, gradients in Shh have been shown to be fundamental for the patterning of the spinal cord and development of the ventral CNS [28]. Shh binds to patched receptors which leads to the release of Smoothened (Smo) inhibition. Smo translocation to the cilium then regulates the processing of GLI2 and GLI3 and the activation of GLI2A and GLI2/3, which regulates the expression of *Gli1*. Initial studies found that Shh regulates the behavior of stem cells in the developing embryonic neocortex and that SVZ cells express Shh and *Gli1* [29]. Moreover, inhibition of hedgehog downregulates the expression of *Gli1* and reduces the proliferation of SVZ cells, while the addition of Shh increases proliferation and neurons number. This suggests that Shh plays a key role in the maintenance of stem cell lineages and neurogenesis in the adult brain [30]. After a brain injury, Shh expression is upregulated, suggesting that activation of this signaling pathway is important not only for maintaining neural stem cell populations but also for the generation of neuroblast and oligodendrocyte progenitors [29].

## Ephrins and Their Receptors (Eph)

Eph are well-known regulators of cell migration, pattern formation, and synaptogenesis. During development, ephrin-A/EphA signaling regulates the size of the mouse cerebral cortex by regulating apoptosis of cortical progenitor cells. The ephrin-A/EphA-induced apoptosis led to an early depletion of neuronal progenitors [31]. Additionally, it has been reported that astrocytes from areas outside of the SGZ and SVZ negatively regulate neuronal progenitor cell growth by a mechanism that involves ephrin-A2/A3 [32]. Although these results suggest an inhibiting role of ephrins and their receptors in neurogenesis, recent studies have found that hippocampal-derived astrocytes can promote neuronal differentiation of adult NSCs in vivo through Ephrin-B2. Activation of EphB4 receptors in NSCs by ephrin-B2 induces the activation of β-catenin. This Wnt-independent activation of β-catenin induces differentiation of progenitors cells into neurons in the SGZ [33]. Although so far there are no studies evaluating Ephrin-B2/EphB4 signaling after TBI, the results obtained from ephrins studies strongly suggest the importance of activation of specific signaling languages in the neurogenesis process after TBI as it has been shown for neuronal patterning.

## Neurotrophins (NTs)

NTs are a family of closely related proteins that were initially identified as survival, growth, and differentiation factors for sensory and sympathetic neurons [34]. Neurotrophins signal through a family of three receptor tyrosine kinases (Trk). Nerve growth factor (NGF) binds preferentially to tyrosine receptor kinase A (TrkA), brain-derived neurotrophic factor (BDNF) and neurotrophin-4 (NT4) to tyrosine receptor kinase B (TrkB), and neurotrophin-3 (NT3) to tyrosine receptor kinase C (TrkC) [35]. Additionally, each of the neurotrophins can bind to the p75 neurotrophin receptor (p75NTR). Moreover, it has been established that dimerization between Trk and p75NR can happen and increase the affinity of Trk receptors for neurotrophins [35].

Neurotrophins expression has not only been found in neurogenic niches but also in areas that are in contact with NPCs [36]. While at the neurogenic niches BDNF expression is low and it is mainly expressed by astrocytes [11], in the rostral migratory stream (RMS) and in the olfactory bulb, BDNF levels are high [37, 38]. The source of BDNF at the RMS is endothelial cells that through the release of BDNF guide newborn neurons to their final destination at the olfactory bulb where BDNF release is assumed by local and long projection neurons [38, 39]. Although NT3 and NT4 have not been found at the neurogenic niches, these neurotrophins are also released by endothelial cells of the choroid plexus to the cerebrospinal fluid that is in contact with NPCs [11, 40, 41]. Neurotrophin receptor expression is dominated by the full-length TrkB and the truncated form of TrkB-T1 in ependymal cells and type B cells [40, 42, 43]. Both isoforms are also expressed by maturing neuroblasts in the RMS and olfactory bulb [37–39]. In addition, TrkC is also expressed in type B NSCs [41]. Surprisingly, the p75NTR is also expressed mainly in type C cells and neuroblasts [40].

Due to the importance of neurotrophins in learning and memory, especial attention has been paid to the role of BDNF/TrkB in neurogenesis at the SGZ. Gain and loss experiments have found that BDNF/TrkB signaling mediates neurogenesis in this area by regulating proliferation [44, 45]. Interestingly, if TrkB function is impaired by overexpressing TrkB-T1, survival is affected, suggesting that BDNF signaling may be regulating both processes [46]. However, a recent study evaluating the role of p75NTR has found that activation of this receptor is more important that TrkB for survival of neuroblasts and newborn neurons [47]. While activation of TrkB and p75NTR can be important for proliferation and survival, TrkC activation by NT3 is essential for maturation. In mice lacking the expression of NT3, there is a misbalance between $NeuN^+$ granule neurons and cells expressing differentiation markers [48].

Microglia are immune cells of the nervous system that similar to astrocytes are in close contact with neuronal progenitor cells. It is thought that microglia phagocyte newborn neurons that fail to integrate or survive during the neurogenesis process [6]. Like astrocytes, microglia is also activated after a brain injury. Microglia activation lead to the production of cytokines and chemokines that can either induce pro- and anti-inflammatory responses [6]. Both cytokines and chemokines have been implicated in neurogenesis by regulating different processes such as neuronal differentiation, migration, and integration of newborn neurons.

## Interleukin-1β

IL-1β, IL-6, and TNF-α have been implicated in memory and neurogenesis. IL-1β, released by neurons, microglia, astrocytes, and immune cells, can affect proliferation, differentiation, and NSC survival. Binding of IL-1β to IL-1R1-type receptor leads to the activation of the mitogen-activated protein kinases and the nuclear factor kappa B (NF-kB) [49]. In development and adulthood, it has been shown both in vitro and in vivo that activation of IL-1R1 impairs proliferation of NSCs by impairing the cell cycle [50, 51].

Although the mechanism by which IL-1β can induce cell cycle arrest in NSCs has not been fully established. A recent study found that the suppressor protein p53, which has a role in apoptosis and cell cycle, is involved in the IL-1β-dependent regulation of NSC survival. IL-1β activates p53, which in turn activates the cyclin-dependent kinase inhibitor p21 and the pro-apoptotic Bcl-2, Puma, and Noxa by a mechanism involving oxidative stress. Furthermore, activation of Puma leads to the activation of Bax-mediated mitochondrial apoptotic pathway in NSCs [49].

## Interleukin-6

IL-6 is expressed by microglia, astrocytes, and neurons, and IL-6 levels are rapidly upregulated and maintained after TBI for several weeks [52]. IL-6 action is mediated either by a classic or trans-signaling mode. The classic signaling involves the activation of the specific transmembrane IL-6Rα, while the trans-signaling mode involves activation of a soluble form of IL-6Rα (sIL-6R) that is generated either by cleavage or by alternative splicing. Activation of IL-6Rα or sIL-6R triggers the oligomerization of the ubiquitous transmembrane protein gp130, which results in activation of the JAK/STAT pathway [53]. IL-6 regulates the proliferation and survival of bone marrow progenitors suggesting that this cytokine can promote survival, differentiation, and growth of neurons. Mice overexpressing IL-6 in astrocytes show a decrease in neurogenesis. Although the mechanism by which IL-6 impairs neurogenesis has not been fully established, it is thought that IL-6 can indirectly affect neurogenesis by regulating circulating glucocorticoids or by acting directly on progenitors or neighboring cells through the release of paracrine factors [54]. For instance, IL-6 released from microglia induces the differentiation of NSPCs to astrocytes through the activation of the JAK/STAT and MAPK pathways [55]. Additionally, activation of sIL-6R can also induce neurogenesis through the activation of the MAPK pathway in vitro [56]. Although these results go in opposite direction to the IL-6 impairment effect also observed in neurogenesis, it will be possible that activation of the canonical mode can impair neurogenesis, while activation of the trans-signaling mode can instead induce neurogenesis [56].

## Tumor Necrosis Factor-Alpha (TNF-α)

TNF-α is a pro-inflammatory cytokine that is produced and released by activated microglia and astrocytes. Action of TNF-α is achieved by the binding to TNF-R1 (p55) and TNF-R2 (p75) receptors that can mediate antagonistic effects such as neuronal damage or neuroprotection [57]. Experimental models have shown that TNF is upregulated early in TBI and participates in the activation of several cascades that involves other cytokines and growth factors [57–59].

Recent studies have shown that TNF-α affects the survival of hippocampal progenitor cell lines in vitro [60], inhibits the proliferation of neural progenitors in neurospheres derived from neonatal rat striatum [61], and also stimulates the number of striatal and hippocampal neuroblasts generated after brain injury [57, 62]. Although, these results seem to be in some way contradictory, experimental evidence during basal and pathological conditions has shown that signaling through p55 receptor suppresses neural progenitor proliferation and neurogenesis in the adult brain. In contrast, p75 receptor does not have any affect in basal conditions, but it influences proliferation in pathological conditions [63]. In this regard, Iosif et al. [57] suggest that the effect of TNF-α can depend on the availability of this cytokine and on the affinity and relative expression of the p55 and p75 receptor in progenitor cells [57]. In agreement, with this hypothesis, mice engineered to lack of either p55 or p75 receptors have different outcomes after TBI. For instance, p55−/− mice showed a marked improvement in sensorimotor behavior and cognitive performance up to 4 weeks after injury when compared with wild type and p75−/− mice. In contrast, p75 gene deletion worsened post-traumatic sensorimotor and cognitive dysfunction. These results strongly suggest that after TBI, p55 activation mediates early deleterious effects of TNF-alpha, while activation of p75 can be important for long-term events involved in TBI recovery [58]. In neurogenesis, activation of p55 by TNF may inhibit proliferation early after TBI, while activation of p75 can stimulate other factors beyond proliferation like survival and incorporation of newly born neurons [57, 63]. The mechanism by which the differential activation of p55 and p75 receptors by TNF can lead to antagonistic effects on neurogenesis has not been fully established; however, it is thought that kinetics of activation of NF-kB may play a role. While the activation of p55 gives rise to transient activation of NF-kB, P75 receptor activation induces long-lasting activation of this factor throughout phosphatidylinositol 3-kinase [57].

During TBI, pro-inflammatory cytokines regulation is mediated by the production and release of anti-inflammatory cytokines like interleukin-10 (IL-10). For instance, IL-10 inhibits the production of TNF, IL-1β, IL-6, and among others [52]. IL-10 binds to IL-10R1 and IL-10R2 receptors and activates the JAK/STAT signaling pathway. IL-10 activates STAT1, STAT3, and not always STAT5, and it has been shown that STAT1 and STAT3 are critical for IL-10 function and regulation of pro-inflammatory cytokines [64].

## Interleukin-10 (IL-10)

IL-10 is expressed in Nestin-positive progenitors (NPG) restricted to the dorsal SVZ, and its receptor IL-10R1 while not expressed in the ventral NPG in the SVZ is highly expressed in all dorsal NPG that are ready to enter the RMS. The IL-10R1 profile expression in these PNG suggests a role of IL-10 in regulating SVZ neuronal differentiation. Loss- and gain-of-function experiments have indeed demonstrated that IL-10 balances the neuronal differentiation in the adult neurogenic niche by promoting an undifferentiating state of the neural progenitors by inducing the expression of nestin, sox1, sox2, and Mash1 and maintaining them in an active cell-cycling state [65].

As mentioned before, activation of IL-10R1 induces a JAK1-mediated phosphorylation of STAT3, which mediates the anti-inflammatory action of IL-10. Similarly, in vitro preparations of SVZ have shown that IL-10 induces rapidly phosphorylation of STAT3 on Ser727 in Nestin+ progenitors. STAT3 can be activated independently of JAK by other kinases such as AKT, mTOR, and MAPK. In NPG, IL-10 induces activation of STAT3 throughout the activation of ERK1/2 that induces NPG cells to stay in a undifferentiated state reducing the number of newly born neurons in the olfactory bulb [66].

## Transforming Growth Factor Beta (TGF-β)

TGF-β was originally identified as a potent chemotactic cytokine that participates in inflammation. However, studies using in TGF-β1 knockout mice demonstrated that this cytokine is mainly an immune suppressor [67]. It has been found that TGF-β1 levels are high in TBI at early time points; however, as time passes, TGF-β1 levels decrease, although they remain above normal levels [68].

TGFβ1 signaling involves binding to a serine/threonine kinase receptor type 2 (R2) that induces the recruitment of the receptor type 1 (R1) to finally activate members of the Smad family of proteins [69]. Due to the role of TGFβ1 in proliferation of different cells, it has been hypothesized that this cytokine can regulate adult neural stem and progenitor cell biology [70].

In vitro studies using spheres of undifferentiated neural stem cell and progenitor cells have found that TGF-β1 receptors R1, R2, and R3 are expressed in neuroprogenitor cells under proliferation conditions. Specifically, TGFβ1-R2 is predominantly expressed on nestin-positive neural stem and progenitor cells. Addition of TGF-β1 but not of TGF-β2 decreases the proliferation rate of NPG cells, suggesting that TGF-β1 acts by arresting the cell cycle in NPG. In agreement with these results, TGF-β1 does not affect the self-renewal or the differentiation of these cells. Importantly, TGF-β1 seems to affect more neural stem cells than progenitor or precursor cells [70]. In conclusion, these results suggests that TGF-β1 can be deleterious for neurogenesis early in TBI, but its downregulation during late phases of TBI can be beneficial for proliferation of NPC.

## TBI and Reorganization of Connectivity

Neurogenesis per se implies that immature neurons migrate from their place of origin to the circuits in which they will incorporate as functional neurons. As it was seen, neurogenesis after TBI is a complex process that involves signaling molecules, growth factors, and pro-and anti-inflammatory cytokines among others that should work synergistically not only to prevent cell death but also to guide and position newborn neurons to the right place.

TBI can cause cell death in both the cortex and hippocampus [71, 72]. This cell death has been associated with impairments in cognitive, sensory, and motor functions. Although, TBI induces neurogenesis, it can also induce cell death of immature neurons by a mechanism that involves necrosis [71]. This mechanism significantly affects the number of newly born neurons that can migrate; however, the few surviving are able to migrate although to a high price. Comparing to normal neurogenesis, after TBI there is an increased redistribution of immature granular neurons, suggesting that these immature neurons have an aberrant migration process. The extension of this aberrant migration process correlates with the TBI severity, being higher in the most dramatic injuries [71]. This implies that spontaneous recovery mediated by neurogenesis can be reduced by the misplacement of these granular neurons. Aberrant migration led to the innervation of inappropriate targets and to the impairment in dendritic development that can induce performing abnormal functions that further contribute to the development of epilepsy, dyslexia, and schizophrenia [71, 73].

The molecules involve in guiding the migration of neurons during adult neurogenesis have not been fully characterized. However, recent studies have found that Slit guide newly born neurons migrating from the SVZ to the olfactory bulb [71, 74], while disrupted-in-schizophrenia I (DISC-1) is required

**Table 1.1** TBI-inducing molecules that affect neurogenesis, guidance, and position of newly born neurons

| Signaling molecule | Cellular effect | References |
|---|---|---|
| Notch | Maintain neural progenitor cells undifferentiated<br>Promote cell differentiation into glial cells<br>Decreases neuronal differentiation and proliferation | [18, 19] |
| Wnt | Promotes neuroblast proliferation and neuronal commitment | [25, 26] |
| Sonic hedgehog | Increases proliferation and neurons number | [29, 30] |
| Ephrins | Negatively regulate neuronal progenitor cell growth<br>Promote neural differentiation of neural stem cells | [32, 33] |
| Neurotrophins | Regulate proliferation and survival in neurogenesis | [44, 45, 47] |
| IL-1β | Impairs proliferation of neural stem cells | [50, 51] |
| IL-6 | Impairs neurogenesis by affecting progenitor cells | [54, 56] |
| TNF-α | Inhibits the proliferation of neural progenitors<br>Survival of newly born neurons | [63] |
| IL-10 | Maintain neural progenitor cells undifferentiated | [65] |
| TGF-β | Decreases the proliferation rate of NPG cells | [70] |
| Slit | Guide newly born neurons migrating from the SVZ to the olfactory bulb | [71, 74] |
| DISC-1 | Required for relaying positional signals of newly born neurons | [75] |

for relaying positional signals [71, 75]. Although the role of pro- and anti-inflammatory cytokines has been established in neurogenesis, it is not known if these molecules can also alter the migration and positioning of newly born neurons.

Beyond neurogenesis, spontaneous recovery, after TBI, can be also achieved by processes of local and distant rewiring [71]. Although the cellular mechanisms that mediate these rewiring processes have not been fully established, this recovery may be due to behavioral compensation (BC) [76]. In BC, there is not a true recovery, but instead there is a second behavior in intact circuits that overtake the original function, producing shifts in map topography. In other words, one part of the brain substitutes the function of another [76]. For instance, in peri-infarct cortex, there is a significant increase in neurite outgrowth that later is followed by a period of arteriolar and capillary growth and synaptogenesis [76, 77]. Interestingly, this compensatory mechanism not only involves local circuits but also distant ones. After an initial period of depressed metabolism and blood flow, cortico-striatal efferent fibers that usually innervate the ipsilateral striatum now sprout and innervate the contralateral striatum in the side of the lesion [76].

## Final Remarks

After traumatic brain injury, there is a big effort of the system to recuperate homeostasis by activating mechanisms that regulate metabolic processes, neurogenesis, and synaptogenesis and plasticity. The way by which the system achieves homeostasis is by using molecules that are produced by activated cells such as microglia and astrocytes. Therefore understanding how these molecules impact in spontaneous recovery should led to the development of new therapies or the improvement of previous one. Special attention then should be paid to how pro- and anti-inflammatory cytokines together with growth factors like neurotrophins and ephrins in conjunction with signaling molecules such as Notch, Shh, and Wnt work together to induce neurogenesis, incorporation of newborn neurons, and structural and functional plasticity (Table 1.1). Once we understand this cross talk, we will pave the road to improve targeted therapies after TBI.

## Acknowledgments

This chapter was funded by Grant 4800 "BDNF-TrkB signaling regulation of GABAergic neurotransmission" from Vicerrectoria de Investigaciones at Pontificia Universidad Javeriana.

## References

1. Hyder AA, Wunderlich CA, Puvanachandra P, Gururaj G, Kobusingye OC. The impact of traumatic brain injuries: a global perspective. NeuroRehabilitation. 2007;22(5):341–53.
2. Langlois JA, Sattin RW. Traumatic brain injury in the United States: research and programs of the Centers for Disease Control and Prevention (CDC). J Head Trauma Rehabil. 2005;20(3):187–8.
3. Roozenbeek B, Maas AI, Menon DK. Changing patterns in the epidemiology of traumatic brain injury. Nat Rev Neurol. 2013;9(4):231–6.
4. Tagliaferri F, Compagnone C, Korsic M, Servadei F, Kraus J. A systematic review of brain injury epidemiology in Europe. Acta Neurochir. 2006;148(3):255–68; discussion 68.
5. Ray SK, Dixon CE, Banik NL. Molecular mechanisms in the pathogenesis of traumatic brain injury. Histol Histopathol. 2002;17(4):1137–52.
6. Yu TS, Washington PM, Kernie SG. Injury-induced neurogenesis: mechanisms and relevance. Neuroscientist. 2016;22(1):61–71.
7. Jin K, Wang X, Xie L, Mao XO, Zhu W, Wang Y, et al. Evidence for stroke-induced neurogenesis in the human brain. Proc Natl Acad Sci U S A. 2006;103(35):13198–202.
8. Li D, Ma S, Guo D, Cheng T, Li H, Tian Y, et al. Environmental circadian disruption worsens neurologic impairment and inhibits hippocampal neurogenesis in adult rats after traumatic brain injury. Cell Mol Neurobiol. 2016;36:1045.
9. Sun D, Daniels TE, Rolfe A, Waters M, Hamm R. Inhibition of injury-induced cell proliferation in the dentate gyrus of the hippocampus impairs spontaneous cognitive recovery after traumatic brain injury. J Neurotrauma. 2015;32(7):495–505.

10. Doetsch F, García-Verdugo JM, Alvarez-Buylla A. Cellular composition and three-dimensional organization of the subventricular germinal zone in the adult mammalian brain. J Neurosci. 1997;17(13):5046–61.
11. Reznikov KI. Local proliferation of cells of the granular layer of the dentate gyrus of the mouse hippocampus during postnatal ontogenesis and following brain injury. Ontogenez. 1975;6(3):242–50.
12. García-Verdugo JM, Doetsch F, Wichterle H, Lim DA, Alvarez-Buylla A. Architecture and cell types of the adult subventricular zone: in search of the stem cells. J Neurobiol. 1998;36(2):234–48.
13. Kleindienst A, McGinn MJ, Harvey HB, Colello RJ, Hamm RJ, Bullock MR. Enhanced hippocampal neurogenesis by intraventricular S100B infusion is associated with improved cognitive recovery after traumatic brain injury. J Neurotrauma. 2005;22(6):645–55.
14. Song H, Stevens CF, Gage FH. Astroglia induce neurogenesis from adult neural stem cells. Nature. 2002;417(6884):39–44.
15. Oh J, McCloskey MA, Blong CC, Bendickson L, Nilsen-Hamilton M, Sakaguchi DS. Astrocyte-derived interleukin-6 promotes specific neuronal differentiation of neural progenitor cells from adult hippocampus. J Neurosci Res. 2010;88(13):2798–809.
16. Tao Y, Ma L, Liao Z, Le Q, Yu J, Liu X, et al. Astroglial β-Arrestin1-mediated nuclear signaling regulates the expansion of neural precursor cells in adult hippocampus. Sci Rep. 2015;5:15506.
17. Horgusluoglu E, Nudelman K, Nho K, Saykin AJ. Adult neurogenesis and neurodegenerative diseases: a systems biology perspective. Am J Med Genet B Neuropsychiatr Genet. 2016;174(1):93–112.
18. Kopan R, Ilagan MX. The canonical Notch signaling pathway: unfolding the activation mechanism. Cell. 2009;137(2):216–33.
19. Ables JL, Decarolis NA, Johnson MA, Rivera PD, Gao Z, Cooper DC, et al. Notch1 is required for maintenance of the reservoir of adult hippocampal stem cells. J Neurosci. 2010;30(31):10484–92.
20. Imayoshi I, Sakamoto M, Yamaguchi M, Mori K, Kageyama R. Essential roles of Notch signaling in maintenance of neural stem cells in developing and adult brains. J Neurosci. 2010;30(9):3489–98.
21. Givogri MI, de Planell M, Galbiati F, Superchi D, Gritti A, Vescovi A, et al. Notch signaling in astrocytes and neuroblasts of the adult subventricular zone in health and after cortical injury. Dev Neurosci. 2006;28(1–2):81–91.
22. Chambers CB, Peng Y, Nguyen H, Gaiano N, Fishell G, Nye JS. Spatiotemporal selectivity of response to Notch1 signals in mammalian forebrain precursors. Development. 2001;128(5):689–702.
23. Lebkuechner I, Wilhelmsson U, Möllerström E, Pekna M, Pekny M. Heterogeneity of Notch signaling in astrocytes and the effects of GFAP and vimentin deficiency. J Neurochem. 2015;135(2):234–48.
24. Zhao Y, Gibb SL, Zhao J, Moore AN, Hylin MJ, Menge T, et al. Wnt3a, a protein secreted by mesenchymal stem cells is neuroprotective and promotes neurocognitive recovery following traumatic brain injury. Stem Cells. 2016;34(5):1263–72.
25. Gao Z, Ure K, Ables JL, Lagace DC, Nave KA, Goebbels S, et al. Neurod1 is essential for the survival and maturation of adult-born neurons. Nat Neurosci. 2009;12(9):1090–2.
26. Kuwabara T, Hsieh J, Muotri A, Yeo G, Warashina M, Lie DC, et al. Wnt-mediated activation of NeuroD1 and retro-elements during adult neurogenesis. Nat Neurosci. 2009;12(9):1097–105.
27. Pataskar A, Jung J, Smialowski P, Noack F, Calegari F, Straub T, et al. NeuroD1 reprograms chromatin and transcription factor landscapes to induce the neuronal program. EMBO J. 2016;35(1):24–45.
28. Araújo GL, Araújo JA, Schroeder T, Tort AB, Costa MR. Sonic hedgehog signaling regulates mode of cell division of early cerebral cortex progenitors and increases astrogliogenesis. Front Cell Neurosci. 2014;8:77.
29. Mierzwa AJ, Sullivan GM, Beer LA, Ahn S, Armstrong RC. Comparison of cortical and white matter traumatic brain injury models reveals differential effects in the subventricular zone and divergent Sonic hedgehog signaling pathways in neuroblasts and oligodendrocyte progenitors. ASN Neuro. 2014;6(5):175909141455178.
30. Palma V, Lim DA, Dahmane N, Sánchez P, Brionne TC, Herzberg CD, et al. Sonic hedgehog controls stem cell behavior in the postnatal and adult brain. Development. 2005;132(2):335–44.
31. Depaepe V, Suarez-Gonzalez N, Dufour A, Passante L, Gorski JA, Jones KR, et al. Ephrin signalling controls brain size by regulating apoptosis of neural progenitors. Nature. 2005;435(7046):1244–50.
32. Jiao JW, Feldheim DA, Chen DF. Ephrins as negative regulators of adult neurogenesis in diverse regions of the central nervous system. Proc Natl Acad Sci U S A. 2008;105(25):8778–83.
33. Ashton RS, Conway A, Pangarkar C, Bergen J, Lim KI, Shah P, et al. Astrocytes regulate adult hippocampal neurogenesis through ephrin-B signaling. Nat Neurosci. 2012;15(10):1399–406.
34. Reichardt LF. Neurotrophin-regulated signalling pathways. Philos Trans R Soc Lond Ser B Biol Sci. 2006;361(1473):1545–64.
35. Chao MV. Neurotrophins and their receptors: a convergence point for many signalling pathways. Nat Rev Neurosci. 2003;4(4):299–309.
36. Vilar M, Mira H. Regulation of neurogenesis by neurotrophins during adulthood: expected and unexpected roles. Front Neurosci. 2016;10:26.
37. Bagley JA, Belluscio L. Dynamic imaging reveals that brain-derived neurotrophic factor can independently regulate motility and direction of neuroblasts within the rostral migratory stream. Neuroscience. 2010;169(3):1449–61.
38. Snapyan M, Lemasson M, Brill MS, Blais M, Massouh M, Ninkovic J, et al. Vasculature guides migrating neuronal precursors in the adult mammalian forebrain via brain-derived neurotrophic factor signaling. J Neurosci. 2009;29(13):4172–88.
39. Bergami M, Vignoli B, Motori E, Pifferi S, Zuccaro E, Menini A, et al. TrkB signaling directs the incorporation of newly generated periglomerular cells in the adult olfactory bulb. J Neurosci. 2013;33(28):11464–78.
40. Galvão RP, Garcia-Verdugo JM, Alvarez-Buylla A. Brain-derived neurotrophic factor signaling does not stimulate subventricular zone neurogenesis in adult mice and rats. J Neurosci. 2008;28(50):13368–83.
41. Delgado AC, Ferrón SR, Vicente D, Porlan E, Perez-Villalba A, Trujillo CM, et al. Endothelial NT-3 delivered by vasculature and CSF promotes quiescence of subependymal neural stem cells through nitric oxide induction. Neuron. 2014;83(3):572–85.
42. Chiaramello S, Dalmasso G, Bezin L, Marcel D, Jourdan F, Peretto P, et al. BDNF/ TrkB interaction regulates migration of SVZ precursor cells via PI3-K and MAP-K signalling pathways. Eur J Neurosci. 2007;26(7):1780–90.
43. Bath KG, Mandairon N, Jing D, Rajagopal R, Kapoor R, Chen ZY, et al. Variant brain-derived neurotrophic factor (Val66Met) alters adult olfactory bulb neurogenesis and spontaneous olfactory discrimination. J Neurosci. 2008;28(10):2383–93.
44. Taliaz D, Stall N, Dar DE, Zangen A. Knockdown of brain-derived neurotrophic factor in specific brain sites precipitates behaviors associated with depression and reduces neurogenesis. Mol Psychiatry. 2010;15(1):80–92.
45. Scharfman H, Goodman J, Macleod A, Phani S, Antonelli C, Croll S. Increased neurogenesis and the ectopic granule cells after intrahippocampal BDNF infusion in adult rats. Exp Neurol. 2005;192(2):348–56.
46. Lee J, Seroogy KB, Mattson MP. Dietary restriction enhances neurotrophin expression and neurogenesis in the hippocampus of adult mice. J Neurochem. 2002;80(3):539–47.
47. Catts VS, Al-Menhali N, Burne TH, Colditz MJ, Coulson EJ. The p75 neurotrophin receptor regulates hippocampal neurogenesis and related behaviours. Eur J Neurosci. 2008;28(5):883–92.
48. Shimazu K, Zhao M, Sakata K, Akbarian S, Bates B, Jaenisch R, et al. NT-3 facilitates hippocampal plasticity and learning and memory by regulating neurogenesis. Learn Mem. 2006;13(3):307–15.

49. Guadagno J, Swan P, Shaikh R, Cregan SP. Microglia-derived IL-1β triggers p53-mediated cell cycle arrest and apoptosis in neural precursor cells. Cell Death Dis. 2015;6:e1779.
50. Ryan SM, O'Keeffe GW, O'Connor C, Keeshan K, Nolan YM. Negative regulation of TLX by IL-1β correlates with an inhibition of adult hippocampal neural precursor cell proliferation. Brain Behav Immun. 2013;33:7–13.
51. Green HF, Treacy E, Keohane AK, Sullivan AM, O'Keeffe GW, Nolan YM. A role for interleukin-1β in determining the lineage fate of embryonic rat hippocampal neural precursor cells. Mol Cell Neurosci. 2012;49(3):311–21.
52. Woodcock T, Morganti-Kossmann MC. The role of markers of inflammation in traumatic brain injury. Front Neurol. 2013;4:18.
53. Campbell IL, Erta M, Lim SL, Frausto R, May U, Rose-John S, et al. Trans-signaling is a dominant mechanism for the pathogenic actions of interleukin-6 in the brain. J Neurosci. 2014;34(7):2503–13.
54. Vallières L, Campbell IL, Gage FH, Sawchenko PE. Reduced hippocampal neurogenesis in adult transgenic mice with chronic astrocytic production of interleukin-6. J Neurosci. 2002;22(2):486–92.
55. Nakanishi M, Niidome T, Matsuda S, Akaike A, Kihara T, Sugimoto H. Microglia-derived interleukin-6 and leukaemia inhibitory factor promote astrocytic differentiation of neural stem/progenitor cells. Eur J Neurosci. 2007;25(3):649–58.
56. Islam O, Gong X, Rose-John S, Heese K. Interleukin-6 and neural stem cells: more than gliogenesis. Mol Biol Cell. 2009;20(1):188–99.
57. Iosif RE, Ekdahl CT, Ahlenius H, Pronk CJ, Bonde S, Kokaia Z, et al. Tumor necrosis factor receptor 1 is a negative regulator of progenitor proliferation in adult hippocampal neurogenesis. J Neurosci. 2006;26(38):9703–12.
58. Longhi L, Perego C, Ortolano F, Aresi S, Fumagalli S, Zanier ER, et al. Tumor necrosis factor in traumatic brain injury: effects of genetic deletion of p55 or p75 receptor. J Cereb Blood Flow Metab. 2013;33(8):1182–9.
59. Scherbel U, Raghupathi R, Nakamura M, Saatman KE, Trojanowski JQ, Neugebauer E, et al. Differential acute and chronic responses of tumor necrosis factor-deficient mice to experimental brain injury. Proc Natl Acad Sci U S A. 1999;96(15):8721–6.
60. Cacci E, Claasen JH, Kokaia Z. Microglia-derived tumor necrosis factor-alpha exaggerates death of newborn hippocampal progenitor cells in vitro. J Neurosci Res. 2005;80(6):789–97.
61. Ben-Hur T, Ben-Menachem O, Furer V, Einstein O, Mizrachi-Kol R, Grigoriadis N. Effects of proinflammatory cytokines on the growth, fate, and motility of multipotential neural precursor cells. Mol Cell Neurosci. 2003;24(3):623–31.
62. Heldmann U, Thored P, Claasen JH, Arvidsson A, Kokaia Z, Lindvall O. TNF-alpha antibody infusion impairs survival of stroke-generated neuroblasts in adult rat brain. Exp Neurol. 2005;196(1):204–8.
63. Chen Z, Palmer TD. Differential roles of TNFR1 and TNFR2 signaling in adult hippocampal neurogenesis. Brain Behav Immun. 2013;30:45–53.
64. Ouyang W, Rutz S, Crellin NK, Valdez PA, Hymowitz SG. Regulation and functions of the IL-10 family of cytokines in inflammation and disease. Annu Rev Immunol. 2011;29:71–109.
65. Perez-Asensio FJ, Perpiñá U, Planas AM, Pozas E. Interleukin-10 regulates progenitor differentiation and modulates neurogenesis in adult brain. J Cell Sci. 2013;126(Pt 18):4208–19.
66. Pereira L, Font-Nieves M, Van den Haute C, Baekelandt V, Planas AM, Pozas E. IL-10 regulates adult neurogenesis by modulating ERK and STAT3 activity. Front Cell Neurosci. 2015;9:57.
67. Han G, Li F, Singh TP, Wolf P, Wang XJ. The pro-inflammatory role of TGFβ1: a paradox? Int J Biol Sci. 2012;8(2):228–35.
68. Morganti-Kossmann MC, Hans VH, Lenzlinger PM, Dubs R, Ludwig E, Trentz O, et al. TGF-beta is elevated in the CSF of patients with severe traumatic brain injuries and parallels blood-brain barrier function. J Neurotrauma. 1999;16(7):617–28.
69. Attisano L, Cárcamo J, Ventura F, Weis FM, Massagué J, Wrana JL. Identification of human activin and TGF beta type I receptors that form heteromeric kinase complexes with type II receptors. Cell. 1993;75(4):671–80.
70. Wachs FP, Winner B, Couillard-Despres S, Schiller T, Aigner R, Winkler J, et al. Transforming growth factor-beta1 is a negative modulator of adult neurogenesis. J Neuropathol Exp Neurol. 2006;65(4):358–70.
71. Ibrahim S, Hu W, Wang X, Gao X, He C, Chen J. Traumatic brain injury causes aberrant migration of adult-born neurons in the Hippocampus. Sci Rep. 2016;6:21793.
72. Lighthall JW. Controlled cortical impact: a new experimental brain injury model. J Neurotrauma. 1988;5(1):1–15.
73. Marín O, Rubenstein JL. Cell migration in the forebrain. Annu Rev Neurosci. 2003;26:441–83.
74. Wu W, Wong K, Chen J, Jiang Z, Dupuis S, Wu JY, et al. Directional guidance of neuronal migration in the olfactory system by the protein Slit. Nature. 1999;400(6742):331–6.
75. Duan X, Chang JH, Ge S, Faulkner RL, Kim JY, Kitabatake Y, et al. Disrupted-in-schizophrenia 1 regulates integration of newly generated neurons in the adult brain. Cell. 2007;130(6):1146–58.
76. Nudo RJ. Recovery after brain injury: mechanisms and principles. Front Hum Neurosci. 2013;7:887.
77. Stroemer RP, Kent TA, Hulsebosch CE. Neocortical neural sprouting, synaptogenesis, and behavioral recovery after neocortical infarction in rats. Stroke. 1995;26(11):2135–44.

# 2 Respiratory Rehabilitation

André Luiz Nunes Gobatto, Leonardo Pamponet Simões, and Bruno Prata Martinez

## Introduction

Patients with traumatic brain injury (TBI) may present several respiratory complications during the acute and subacute phases. These complications may become chronic, depending on the extent of the injury.

One of the main problems that patients in a more severe condition can exhibit is the need for invasive mechanical ventilation (MV), which may be required for a long period. MV can induce further complications, such as a higher risk of ventilator-associated pneumonia (VAP), an increased accumulation of secretions and an inability to eliminate them, ventilator-induced diaphragmatic dysfunction, and ventilator-induced lung injury, especially in patients with other pulmonary diseases. For ventilated patients with signs of intracranial hypertension (ICH), the main actions performed are the adjustments of the initial mechanical ventilator settings for a normoventilation, aimed at maintaining $PaCO_2$ levels in the lower normal ranges (close to 35 mmHg).

Examples of physiotherapeutic interventions related to respiratory function are measures to prevent VAP, bronchial hygiene therapy, spontaneous breathing test and follow-up of the ventilator weaning process, alveolar recruitment, and early mobilization. These interventions are not standard for all patients, and their indication and employment will depend on the patient's condition.

After MV withdrawal, some respiratory alterations justify the need for specific physiotherapeutic interventions, such as pulmonary expansion therapy and bronchial hygiene maneuvers, respiratory muscle training, and mobilization.

## Interventions for Patients on Mechanical Ventilation

One of the key steps for respiratory rehabilitation of TBI patients under MV is the success of the ventilator weaning process, which should occur as quickly as possible. Weaning can be classified into three types: (1) simple weaning for patients extubated without difficulty after the first spontaneous breathing trial (SBT); (2) difficult weaning for patients who require up to three attempts of SBT and/or up to 7 days for a successful weaning; and (3) prolonged weaning for patients who require more than three attempts of SBT and/or more than 7 days after the first SBT for a successful weaning [1] (Table 2.1). When TBI patients have a major neurological impairment, with reduced consciousness levels and a greater inability to remove secretions, they usually have prolonged weaning, increasing the risk of acquiring respiratory infections and the chances of morbidity and mortality. This group of patients may benefit from receiving early tracheostomy, with procedures performed within 10 days of intubation. A systematic review has shown that early tracheostomy in this patient profile is associated with a reduction in long-term mortality, weaning time from MV, the length of stay in the ICU, and a lower rate of respiratory infections [2].

As previously mentioned, patients who require MV, and especially those who are ventilated for more than 48 h, accumulate secretions, which may promote an increased risk of respiratory infections as well as deficits in oxygenation.

A. L. N. Gobatto (✉)
Internal Medicine, Hospital São Rafael, Salvador, Brazil

Intensive Care Unit, Hospital da Cidade, Salvador, Brazil

Internal Medicine Department, Salvador University, Salvador, Brazil

L. P. Simões
Intermediate Care Unit of Aliance Hospital, Salvador, Brazil

Physiotherapy Service of Woman Hospital, Salvador, Brazil

B. P. Martinez
Physiotherapy Department, Federal University of Bahia (UFBA), Salvador, Brazil

Bahia State University (UNEB), Salvador, Brazil


R. Anghinah et al. (eds.), *Topics in Cognitive Rehabilitation in the TBI Post-Hospital Phase*,
https://doi.org/10.1007/978-3-319-95376-2_2

**Table 2.1** Classification of patients according to the weaning process

| Group/category | Definition |
|---|---|
| Simple weaning | Patients who succeed the first weaning trial and are extubated without difficulty |
| Difficult weaning | Patients who fail the first weaning trial and require up to three spontaneous breathing trials or 7 days to achieve successful weaning |
| Prolonged weaning | Patients who require more than 7 days of weaning after the first weaning trial |

One of the techniques performed on these patients is the transient ventilator hyperinflation, which is based on the increase of air volume offered to the patient to promote a greater elastic recoil with consequent acceleration of the expiratory flow and displacement of secretions from distal airways to proximal airways [3].

Some randomized crossover trials have shown positive results with the use of hyperinflation, such as increased removal of secretions, static compliance of the respiratory system, and oxygenation [3–5]. Despite the lack of scientific evidence demonstrating positive results in mortality outcomes, a randomized clinical trial reported a reduction in MV time by testing manual hyperinflation combined with chest compressions [6, 7]. It is important to note that ventilator hyperinflation is relatively equivalent to manual hyperinflation. However, when hyperinflation is performed with the ventilator, there is greater reproducibility, maintenance of positive end-expiratory pressure (PEEP), as well as a better parameter adjustment to optimize the peak expiratory flow/peak inspiratory flow ratio, ensuring an acceleration of expiratory flow.

One of the most used forms of ventilator hyperinflation is the volume assist/control mode, using a 150% increase in tidal volume, which is supplied at a flow rate below 40 L/min, generating less swirling during air entrance and with a pressure limited to 40 $cmH_2O$ [4].

In patients with respiratory muscle weakness associated with clinical stability and an inability to breathe through spontaneous ventilation, inspiratory muscle training (IMT) is indicated, as it helps to accelerate ventilator weaning, especially for patients with prolonged weaning. For this, it is necessary to use a device that imposes a load on the inspiratory muscles, and the most used devices are those that generate linear resistance via a spring-loaded system. They are simple devices that can be attached directly to the orotracheal tube or tracheostomy tube or even through a mouthpiece for patients with functional airways (Fig. 2.1). One of the ways to perform IMT is through strength training in one shift and resistance training in another shift. First, strength training is performed with a load of 30–40% of maximal inspiratory pressure (MIP), with six to ten repetitions, performed in three to four series [7]. Subsequently, after returning to the MV, the patient will perform the resistance training with a daily progressive increase in the time on spontaneous ventilation. At

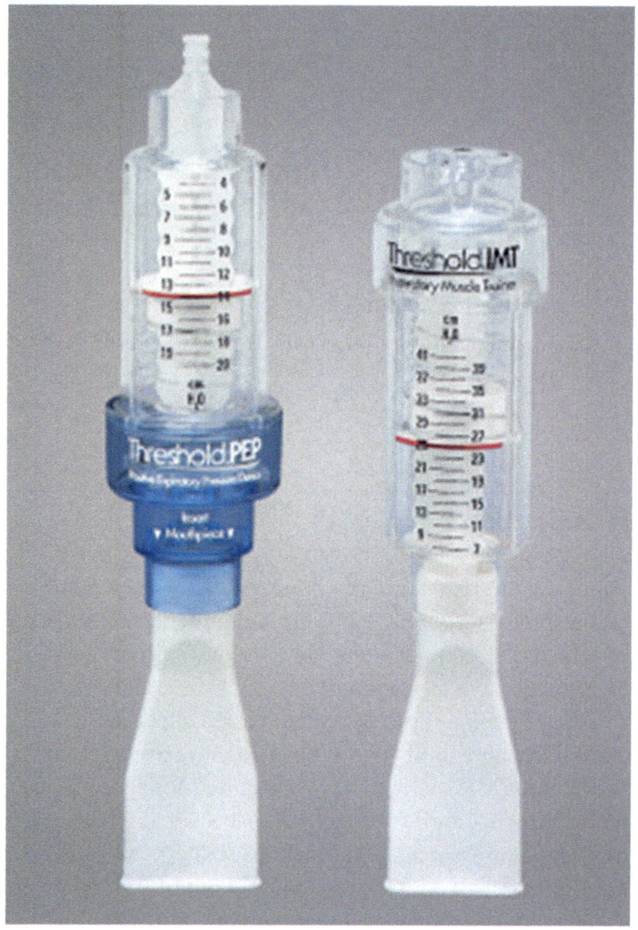


**Fig. 2.1** Threshold devices

the first moment of this intervention, the time on spontaneous ventilation should be measured, which will be called the "test window." If the patient is able to remain more than 12 h in spontaneous ventilation and, after this period, needs to be reconnected to the MV, the next day, MV should be disconnected again to assess if the patient developed a greater tolerance to spontaneous ventilation. If the first test window results in disconnection failure before the first 12 h, indicated by increased ventilation, hemodynamic changes, and/or oxygenation drop, the patient should enter a program of daily spontaneous ventilation progression, respecting the trials of 1, 2, 4, 6, 9, and 12 h. On the day after the test window, the patient should start a second trial below the duration the patient tolerated on their first and progress through subsequent times in the following days. In case of failure to maintain spontaneous ventilation for the proposed time, the time should be regressed to the nearest lower trial [7] (Fig. 2.2).

Although studies on IMT include the general population, they also include patients with TBI. Individuals in the group that received inspiratory muscle training had an increase in MIP and a higher rate of successful weaning in relation to the control group [8].

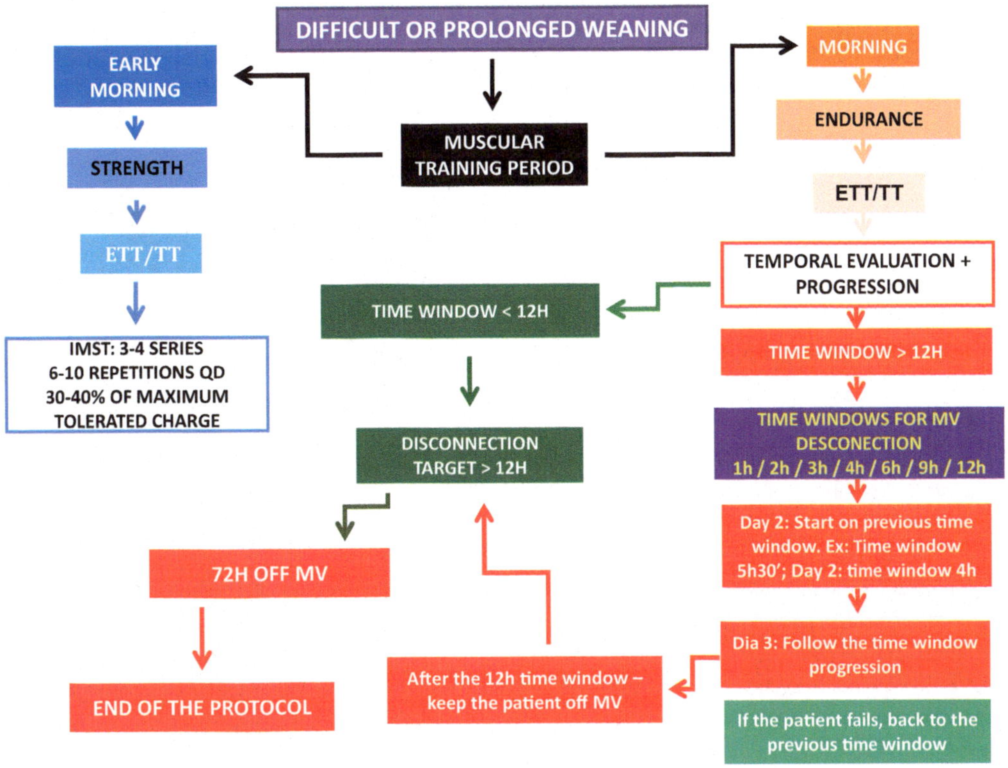


**Fig. 2.2** Respiratory muscle training protocol. ETT: endotrachel tube, TT: tracheostomy tube, IMST: inspiratory muscle strengh training, MV: mechanical ventilation

Proper management of MV in the acute phase of TBI can have a marked impact on clinical outcomes and rehabilitation.

One of the major concerns in the ventilatory management of patients with TBI is PEEP titration. Increased PEEP may lead to a higher intracranial pressure (ICP) by increasing the intrathoracic pressure, associated with the reduction of the cerebral perfusion pressure (CPP), mediated by the reduction of venous return and the consequent reduction in cardiac output. However, in recruitable patients, i.e., patients who present an increase in tidal volume after the increase in PEEP, there is in fact a decrease in ICP and an increase in CPP, mediated mainly by the reduction of $PaCO_2$ [9, 10].

Another much-discussed topic on the ventilatory management of TBI patients is the $PaCO_2$. Hypercapnia leads to increased cerebral blood flow and the consequent unwanted increase in ICP. On the other hand, hyperventilation (which means maintaining $PaCO_2$ below 35 mmHg) is a routinely used strategy to control ICP, as hypocapnia leads to reduced cerebral blood flow and consequent reduction of ICP. Conversely, the reduction of the cerebral blood flow can intensify ischemia, and the vasoconstrictor effects of $PaCO_2$ have a temporary character, being able to generate a rebound vasodilation and consequent worsening of cerebral edema if maintained for long periods [11]. Thus, we should always promote eucapnia in TBI patients receiving MV. In addition, hyperventilation should be used only temporarily, in emergencies, when an immediate ICP reduction is necessary, until safer measures of intracranial hypertension are instituted.

Patients with moderate or severe TBI have an incidence rate of approximately 25% of acute respiratory distress syndrome (ARDS). However, TBI patients were summarily excluded from the main randomized clinical trials (RCTs) that evaluated strategies for the treatment of ARDS [12]. In the main RCTs that evaluated a strategy of protective ventilation in patients with ARDS, patients, on average, remained in the normocapnia range, even using the concept of permissive hypercapnia during MV [13–15]. Thus, we should not deprive TBI patients of protective MV strategies, since these are associated with lower mortality and better rehabilitation rates.

Early mobilization of patients should also be performed to preserve movement capacity in ventilated and non-ventilated patients, taking into consideration medical criteria, stability, and functional prognosis. A cohort study conducted in an ICU with trauma patients identified that a low level of mobility at the time of hospital discharge was associated with higher 1-year mortality after discharge [16]. The study also reported that patients who had improved mobility before discharge had a higher survival rate 1 year after discharge. Procedures that can be employed in critically ill patients are functional electrostimulation in the quadriceps, mobilization of members (passive, assisted, active, or resisted), transfer training in bed, trunk balance training, orthostatic training (including orthostatic table when indicated and available), and assisted walking [17, 18]. Although they are motor interventions, these procedures can positively influence respiratory function.

## Interventions for Patients on Spontaneous Ventilation

Some procedures applied to patients on spontaneous ventilation follow the same principles as those applied to MV patients, such as manual hyperinflation for removal of secretion in patients with tracheostomy [19] (Fig. 2.3). The literature describes that manual hyperinflation can be used by slow insufflation and with an inspiratory pause to enhance and accelerate expiratory flow, consequently causing the displacement of secretions, and may be also associated with chest compression, as in patients on MV. An experimental study demonstrated that in a respiratory system model with low compliance of the respiratory system, the ideal inspiratory pause time for the displacement of secretions was 2 s, whereas for a system with normal compliance, the ideal pause time was 3 s [20].

Ideally, the individual should be able to accelerate the expiratory flow through coughing; however, as many patients are unable to cough effectively, this technique is indicated for some patients only.

Patients with low or no coughing ability may benefit from the use of mechanically assisted cough, which noninvasively provides effective removal of secretions, reducing the need for aspiration. The technique comprises the use of an apparatus, the cough assist. The cough machine is a flow generator that is connected to the patient through an interface, such as a face mask, in patients with functional airways, or directly into the tracheostomy tube (Figs. 2.4, 2.5 and 2.6). The procedure begins with the insufflation phase, using positive pressure, followed by a rapid depressurization of the respiratory system, using negative pressure, which can generate Δ pressures above 100 $cmH_2O$, promoting a sudden acceleration of the expiratory flow and thus simulating a cough, favoring the removal of secretions [21]. The use of the cough machine is a very effective intervention for individuals with a cough peak flow (CPF) <160 L/min [21]. This technique presents benefits, as the displacement of secretion to proximal airways, reaching often the nose and mouth, facilitating its removal. A limiting factor is that not every hospital has access to this very effective procedure. A study conducted with critical patients under intensive care showed that the use of this equipment in patients under a high risk of extubation failure promoted the improvement of clinical outcomes, including the increase in success rates during the use of noninvasive ventilation (NIV) after extubation [22].

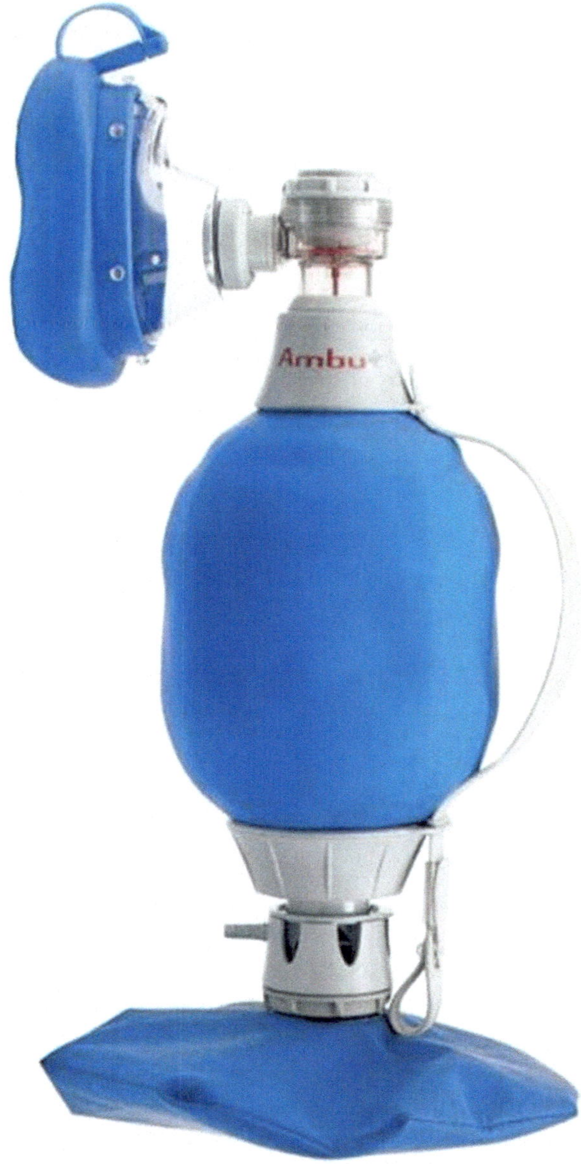

**Fig. 2.3** Bag-valve-mask for manual hyperinflation

In patients who remained on MV for more than 7 days and had a successful ventilator weaning (>48 h out of MV), a randomized clinical trial demonstrated the improvement of inspiratory muscle strength and life quality in the group that received this intervention. However, there was no difference in hospital mortality rates between the groups. IMT was employed using the Threshold IMT equipment. The Threshold PEP with nozzle inversion, which allows for the use of a higher training load (Fig. 2.7), is one of the other options available. Initially, a load of 50% of MIP can be

Fig. 2.4 Cough assist devices. NIV denotes noninvasive machanical ventilation

| | | | |
|---|---|---|---|
| 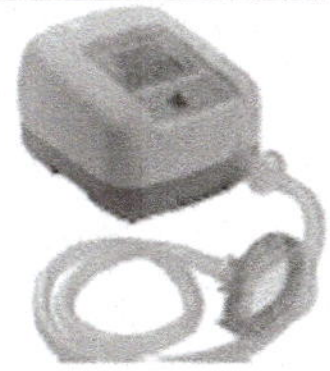 | COMFORT COUGH<br>Seoil Pacific Corporation<br><br>Korea | Positive Pressure<br>+5 to +60 $cmH_2O$<br><br>Negative Pressure<br>-5 to -60 $cmH_2O$ | Modes<br><br>Manual<br>Automatic |
| 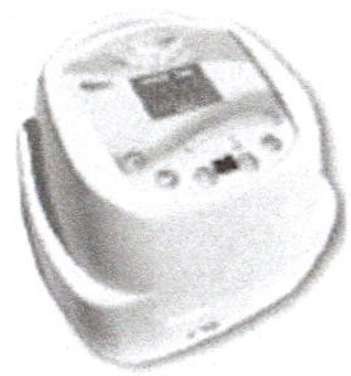 | PEGASO COUGH<br>Dima Italia<br><br>Italy | Positive Pressure<br>0 to +70 $cmH_2O$<br><br>Negative Pressure<br>-0 to -70 $cmH_2O$ | Modes<br><br>Manual<br>Automatic<br>Autoajusted<br>Percussion |
| 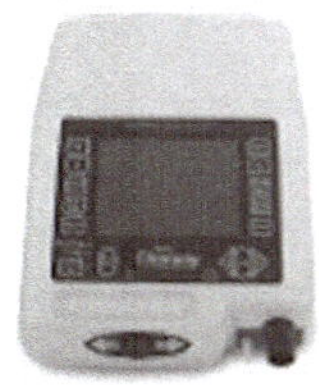 | NIPPY CLEARWAY<br>B&D Electromedical<br><br>United Kingdom | Positive Pressure<br>0 to +60 $cmH_2O$<br><br>Negative Pressure<br>0 to -60 $cmH_2O$ | Modes<br><br>Manual<br>Automatic<br>NIV |
| 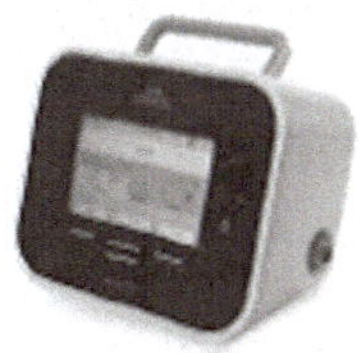 | COUGHASSIST E70<br>Philips<br><br>Netherlands | Positive Pressure<br>0 to +70 $cmH_2O$<br><br>Negative Pressure<br>0 to -70 $cmH_2O$ | Modes<br><br>Manual<br>Automatic<br>Autoajusted |

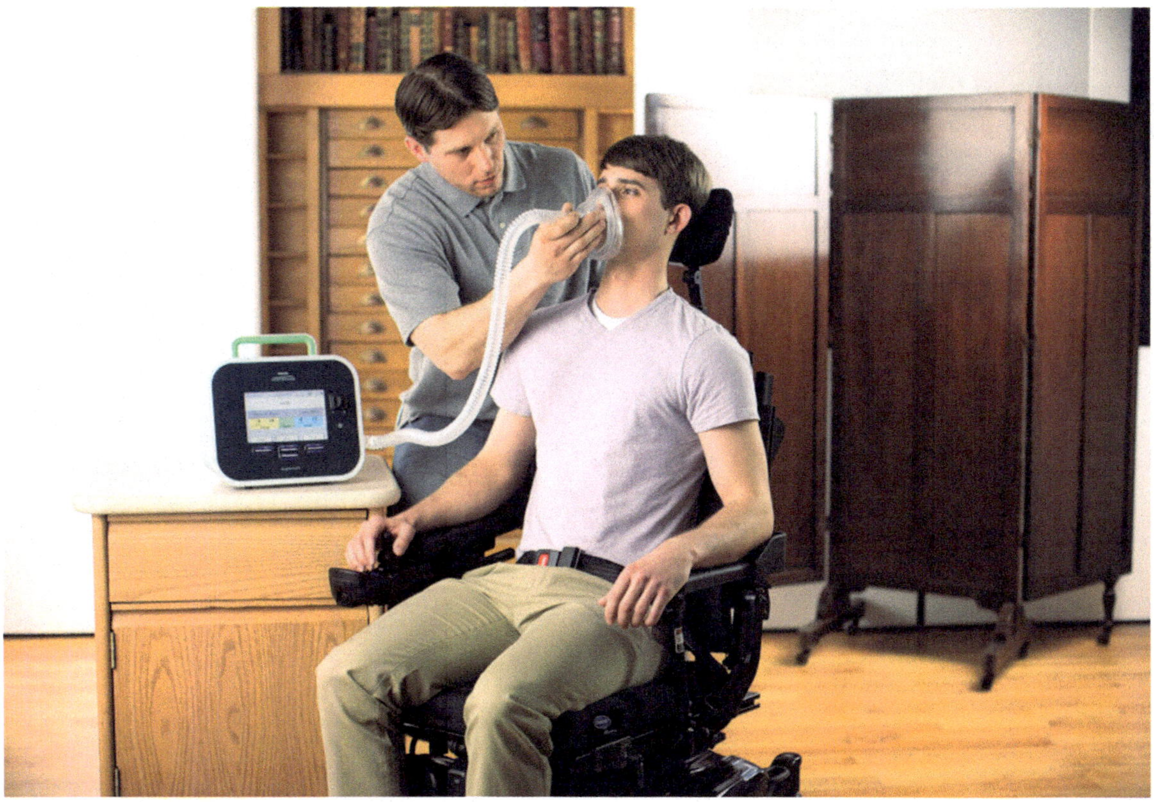

Fig. 2.5 Mechanically assisted cough with facial mask

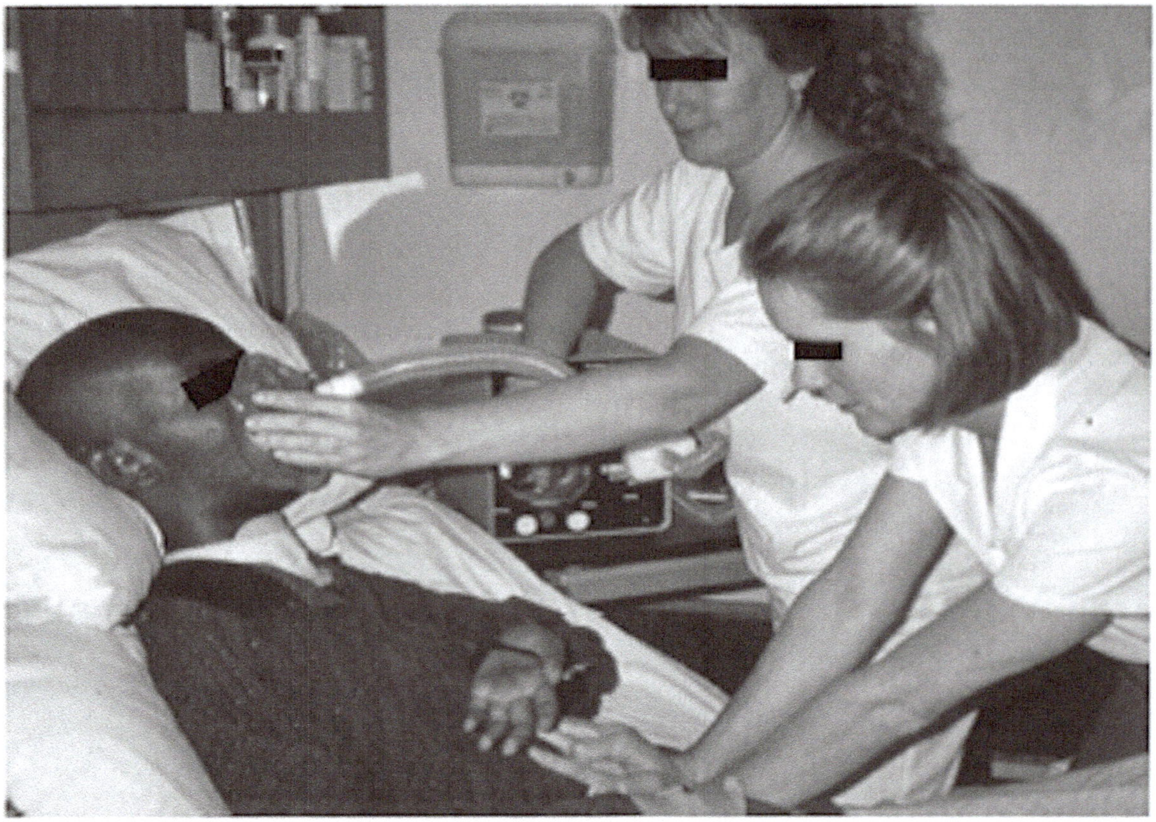

**Fig. 2.6** Mechanically assisted cough with facial mask associated with manually assisted cough

**Fig. 2.7** Inspiratory muscle training device

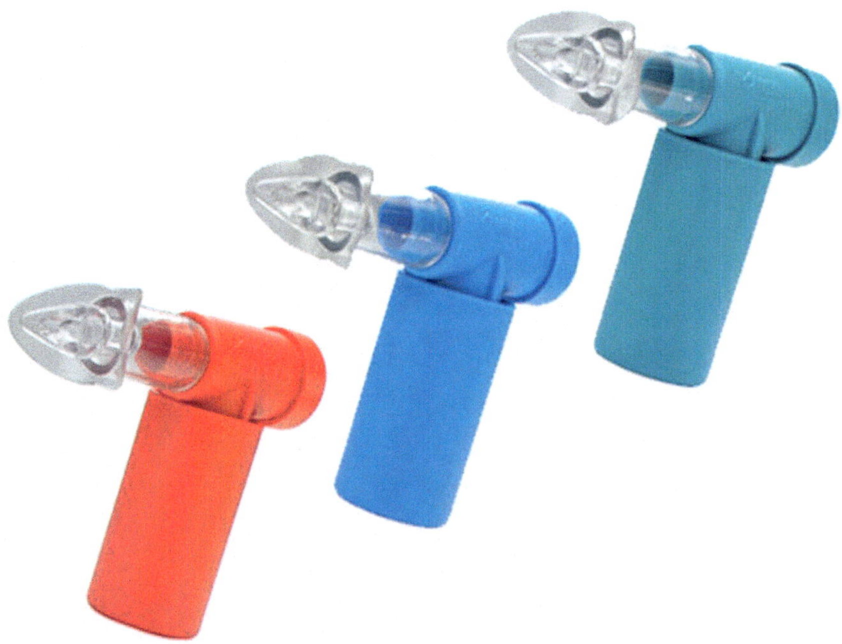

used, and, in the study, the technique was performed once a day, five times a week, for 2 weeks [23].

The goal of these techniques is to maintain a patent airway, facilitating secretion removal and improving ventilatory function, as well as strengthening the inspiratory muscles. These efforts are employed in order to keep the patient breathing spontaneously and to guarantee a greater cardiorespiratory reserve, favoring total rehabilitation of the individual.

## Final Considerations

Interventions for respiratory rehabilitation may have a positive impact on the outcomes of hospitalized TBI patients under intensive care. However, it is essential that these techniques be applied in the right moments. The main interventions are secretion removal therapies, respiratory muscle training, and early mobilization.

## References


1. Boles JM, Bion J, Connors A, Herridge M, Marsh B, Melot C, Pearl R, Silverman H, Stanchina M, Vieillard-Baron A, Welte T. Weaning from mechanical ventilation. Eur Respir J. 2007;29:1033–56.
2. McCredie VA, Alali AS, Scales DC, Adhikari NK, Rubenfeld GD, Cuthbertson BH, Nathens AB. Effect of early versus late tracheostomy or prolonged intubation in critically ill patients with acute brain injury: a systematic review and meta-analysis. Neurocrit Care. 2017;26:14–25.
3. Berney S, Denehy L. A comparison of the effects of manual and ventilator hyperinflation on static lung compliance and sputum production in intubated and ventilated intensive care patients. Physiother Res Int. 2002;7:100–8.
4. Dennis D, Jacob W, Budgeon C. Ventilator versus manual hyperinflation in clearing sputum in ventilated intensive care unit patients. Anaesth Intensive Care. 2012;40:142–9.
5. Lemes DA, Zin WA, Guimaraes FS. Hyperinflation using pressure support ventilation improves secretion clearance and respiratory mechanics in ventilated patients with pulmonary infection: a randomised crossover trial. Aust J Physiother. 2009;55:249–54.
6. Berti JS, Tonon E, Ronchi CF, Berti HW, Stefano LM, Gut AL, Padovani CR, Ferreira AL. Manual hyperinflation combined with expiratory rib cage compression for reduction of length of ICU stay in critically ill patients on mechanical ventilation. J Bras Pneumol. 2012;38:477–86.
7. Martin AD, Smith BK, Davenport PD, Harman E, Gonzalez-Rothi RJ, Baz M, Layon AJ, Banner MJ, Caruso LJ, Deoghare H, Huang TT, Gabrielli A. Inspiratory muscle strength training improves weaning outcome in failure to wean patients: a randomized trial. Crit Care. 2011;15:R84.
8. Elkins M, Dentice R. Inspiratory muscle training facilitates weaning from mechanical ventilation among patients in the intensive care unit: a systematic review. J Physiother. 2015;61:125–34.
9. Mascia L, Grasso S, Fiore T, Bruno F, Berardino M, Ducati A. Cerebro-pulmonary interactions during the application of low levels of positive end-expiratory pressure. Intensive Care Med. 2005;31:373–9.
10. Saback LM, Almeida ML, Andrade W. Traumatic brain injury and acute respiratory distress syndrome: how to ventilate? Evaluation of clinical practice. Rev Bras Ter Intensiva. 2007;19:44–52.
11. Muizelaar JP, Marmarou A, Ward JD, Kontos HA, Choi SC, Becker DP, Gruemer H, Young HF. Adverse effects of prolonged hyperventilation in patients with severe head injury: a randomized clinical trial. J Neurosurg. 1991;75:731–9.
12. Bakowitz M, Bruns B, McCunn M. Acute lung injury and the acute respiratory distress syndrome in the injured patient. Scand J Trauma Resusc Emerg Med. 2012;20:54.
13. Acute Respiratory Distress Syndrome N, Brower RG, Matthay MA, Morris A, Schoenfeld D, Thompson BT, Wheeler A. Ventilation with lower tidal volumes as compared with traditional tidal volumes for acute lung injury and the acute respiratory distress syndrome. N Engl J Med. 2000;342:1301–8.
14. Brower RG, Lanken PN, MacIntyre N, Matthay MA, Morris A, Ancukiewicz M, Schoenfeld D, Thompson BT, National Heart L, Blood Institute ACTN. Higher versus lower positive end-expiratory pressures in patients with the acute respiratory distress syndrome. N Engl J Med. 2004;351:327–36.
15. Meade MO, Cook DJ, Guyatt GH, Slutsky AS, Arabi YM, Cooper DJ, Davies AR, Hand LE, Zhou Q, Thabane L, Austin P, Lapinsky S, Baxter A, Russell J, Skrobik Y, Ronco JJ, Stewart TE, Lung Open Ventilation Study I. Ventilation strategy using low tidal volumes, recruitment maneuvers, and high positive end-expiratory pressure for acute lung injury and acute respiratory distress syndrome: a randomized controlled trial. JAMA. 2008;299:637–45.
16. Peetz AB, Brat GA, Rydingsward J, Askari R, Olufajo OA, Elias KM, Mogensen KM, Lesage JL, Horkan CM, Salim A, Christopher KB. Functional status, age, and long-term survival after trauma. Surgery. 2016;160:762–70.
17. Kayambu G, Boots R, Paratz J. Physical therapy for the critically ill in the ICU: a systematic review and meta-analysis. Crit Care Med. 2013;41:1543–54.
18. Schweickert WD, Pohlman MC, Pohlman AS, Nigos C, Pawlik AJ, Esbrook CL, Spears L, Miller M, Franczyk M, Deprizio D, Schmidt GA, Bowman A, Barr R, McCallister KE, Hall JB, Kress JP. Early physical and occupational therapy in mechanically ventilated, critically ill patients: a randomised controlled trial. Lancet. 2009;373:1874–82.
19. Paulus F, Binnekade JM, Vroom MB, Schultz MJ. Benefits and risks of manual hyperinflation in intubated and mechanically ventilated intensive care unit patients: a systematic review. Crit Care. 2012;16:R145.
20. Bennett BG, Thomas P, Ntoumenopoulos G. Effect of inspiratory time and lung compliance on flow bias generated during manual hyperinflation: a bench study. Respir Care. 2015;60:1449–58.
21. Homnick DN. Mechanical insufflation-exsufflation for airway mucus clearance. Respir Care. 2007;52:1296–305; discussion 1306-1297.
22. Goncalves MR, Honrado T, Winck JC, Paiva JA. Effects of mechanical insufflation-exsufflation in preventing respiratory failure after extubation: a randomized controlled trial. Crit Care. 2012;16:R48.
23. Bissett BM, Leditschke IA, Neeman T, Boots R, Paratz J. Inspiratory muscle training to enhance recovery from mechanical ventilation: a randomised trial. Thorax. 2016;71:812–9.

# Posttraumatic Hydrocephalus: Relevance, Mechanisms, Treatment, and Outcome

3

Fernando Campos Gomes Pinto and Matheus Fernandes de Oliveira

## Introduction

Traumatic brain injury (TBI) is the leading cause of death in children and young adults ranging from 15 to 30 years of age in the United States [1, 2]. TBI occurs at an alarming frequency of once every 23 s, resulting in 1.7 million incidences annually, including approximately 52,000 deaths [1–4].

In Brazil, although available data are limited and probably underestimated, trauma is also a major cause of death in people from 5 to 40 years old and carries an impacting posttraumatic morbidity, like impaired cognitive and motor functions [1–4].

In cases with mild TBI, most of the patients are able to return progressively to normal function. However, in moderate to severe TBI, several patients may suffer consequences, needing specialized support and rehabilitation. In some dramatic cases, patients are not able to return to basic social life, enlarging health costs and social losses [1–4].

Posttraumatic hydrocephalus (PTH) is one of the most typical consequences after different grades of TBI, and it may occur in up to 30% of TBI patients in some time along clinical recovery. In this brief chapter, we try to analyze with current evidence the causes, mechanisms, and proposed treatment and outcomes for PTH [1–4].

## Concept

Posttraumatic hydrocephalus (PTH) is the commonest neurosurgical complication in the rehabilitation setting in patients with severe TBI. Incidence varies widely from 0.7% to 29%, reflective of variable definitions of the condition (Fig. 3.1). If imaging criteria of ventriculomegaly are used, the reported incidence is higher, ranging between 30% and 86% [1–4].

F. C. G. Pinto · M. F. de Oliveira (✉)
Division of Functional Neurosurgery of the Institute of Psychiatry, Clinics Hospital, University of São Paulo, São Paulo, Brazil

PTH has been recognized since Dandy's report in 1914. Classically, it can be classified as an acquired hydrocephalus, which can be acute, subacute, or chronic. Additionally, it can be normotensive or hypertensive and communicant or obstructive, depending on the underlying pathogenesis [1–4].

## Pathogenesis

Cerebrospinal fluid (CSF) production occurs in choroid plexus and ependymal cells, and, after circulating along cranial and spinal subarachnoid spaces, it is absorbed in subarachnoid capillaries (arachnoid granulations) following a pressure gradient, with venous blood being the final route for CSF circulation and clearance [1–4]. Additional evidence has pointed to the potential role of CSF absorption and circulation through lymphatic vessels along venous sinuses, especially superior sagittal sinus [5]. The balance of this detailed system is dynamic and depends on the adequate function of the whole system.

After TBI, due to effects of mechanical forces involved in trauma, several dysfunctions may be disclosed in hydrodynamic balance. Several pathogenesis theories involve:

1. *Dramatic decrease in ependymal cilia number and function*. Ependymal cells lining ventricular system contain cilia which allow for CSF flow and, thus, waste and nutrient exchange. After TBI-induced injury, CSF flow is usually diminished with impairment of CSF clearance. Injury-induced ventricular system pathology usually resolves completely by 30 days after injury as ependymal cell ciliogenesis restores cilia density to uninjured levels. However, severe or repeated TBI may impair irreversibly ciliary function, contributing to hydrocephalus genesis and consequent disturbances [6].
2. *Matrix metalloproteinases (MMPs)* are a family of zinc-binding proteolytic enzymes that normally remodel the extracellular matrix (ECM). MMP-2 and MMP-9


R. Anghinah et al. (eds.), *Topics in Cognitive Rehabilitation in the TBI Post-Hospital Phase*,
https://doi.org/10.1007/978-3-319-95376-2_3

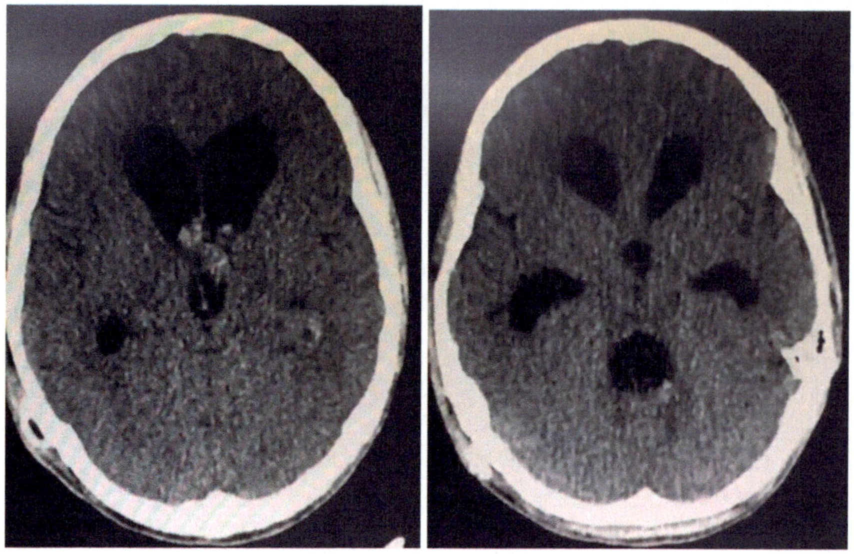

**Fig. 3.1** Example of skull CT with posttraumatic hydrocephalus

specifically degrade type IV collagen, laminin, and fibronectin, which are the major components of the basal lamina around the cerebral blood. Several trauma studies have disclosed the role of MMPs in cascades after trauma. Similarly, the role of aquaporins (family of proteins involved in transport of water) is also remarked in posttraumatic states. Their level is probably related to severity of trauma, and it is being increasingly considered a marker of acute trauma impact and outcomes [7].

3. *Direct trauma and apoptosis***.** Direct traumatic forces (acceleration and disacceleration) are responsible for primary brain lesions, including fiber rupture seen in diffuse axonal lesion and hematomas and contusions [8–12].

   Following primary effects of trauma, there is probably a complex metabolic cascade involving programmed cell death (apoptosis), neuronal remodeling, and deposition of minerals, like calcium [8, 9].

4. *Blood products*. One frequently cited theory to explain hydrocephalus after TBI involves obliteration of the arachnoid villi by microthrombi with subsequent inflammation and fibrosis causing CSF outflow obstruction [8, 11–13].

Several neuronal and glia cell changes are described, like unreactive oligodendrocytes and neurons, reactive oligodendrocytes and neurons, anoxic-ischemic oligodendrocytes and neurons, hypertrophic phagocytic oligodendrocytes, and apoptotic oligodendrocytes and neurons [14–16].

Involved cells may exhibit enlargement of endoplasmic reticulum, Golgi complex, and enlargement and disassembly of nuclear envelope. They appear in contact with degenerated myelinated axons. Hypertrophic phagocytic oligodendrocytes engulf degenerated myelinated axons exerting myelinolytic effects. A continuum oncotic and apoptotic cell death type leading to necrosis is observed [14–16].

Some products of neuronal death and loss, like deposition of proteins tau, phospho-tau, and beta-amyloid, can also be observed in posttraumatic states, similarly to what is found in Alzheimer's disease (AD)[14–18].

MRI has shown a preponderance of hemorrhagic lesions compared to ischemic lesions during the acute phase after TBI. A study found that 56% of TBI patients had at least one intracranial bleed and another showed that patients with greater initial total hemorrhagic contusion volume had more severe chronic brain atrophy. Iron released from hemoglobin contributes to brain edema, brain atrophy, and neurological deficits [8].

## Pathology

In an acute phase, main factors involved with ventricular enlargement after TBI are ventricular and subarachnoid clots, occluding natural paths for CSF clearance. In subacute to chronic phase, several degrees of neuronal loss, vessel rupture, blood, iron, and other mineral depositions can be observed [9].

## Risk Factors

Risk factors for PTH are as follows: age, duration of coma, decompressive craniectomy, and subarachnoid hemorrhage (SAH). PTH is usually correlated with the degree of hypoperfusion in the temporal lobes. Craniectomy size is also related to the chance of developing PTH. Continuous lumbar drainage of cerebrospinal fluid can greatly reduce posttraumatic hydrocephalus [14–17].

## Clinical Manifestations

CSF within the ventricular system functions as a mean of nonsynaptic volume transmission, providing a route of communication for signals mediating sleep, circadian rhythms, seasonal reproduction, and sexual behavior. Additionally, CSF has protective and immunological functions, and the imbalance in hydrodynamics may cause a myriad of symptoms [10, 16–20].

Posttraumatic hydrocephalus is typically recognized in the rehabilitation setting or during neurosurgical follow-up. Several different clinical syndromes exist, all of which fall into two general categories: patients either plateau in a trajectory of previous clinical improvement or clinically deteriorate. The clinical syndromes include (1) obtundation, (2) psychomotor retardation, (3) memory impairment, (4) gait impairment, (5) incontinence, (6) behavioral disturbances, and (7) emotional disturbances [10, 16–20].

Symptoms of hydrocephalus are not infrequently masked by the degree of brain injury sustained, making diagnosis difficult when the patient is too severely injured to display hydrocephalic symptoms or has atypical symptoms [10, 16–20].

Clinical manifestations depend especially on the time of appearance and form of onset, if acute/subacute or chronic. As a general rule, acute hydrocephalus produce pronounced symptoms as headache, vomitus, papilledema, and impaired consciousness, leading patient to coma and death. Chronic hydrocephalus, on other hand, might produce spasticity, progressive neurological deficits and dementia, urinary incontinence, and gait changes in elderly [10, 16–20].

### NPH

NPH can be divided into two categories: idiopathic and secondary. The secondary NPH occurs in the context of neurological events such as subarachnoid hemorrhage (SAH), intraventricular hemorrhage caused by trauma or aneurysm rupture, and meningitis. In contrast, idiopathic NPH usually occurs between the sixth and eighth decades of life and does not have its pathophysiological mechanisms completely understood [20].

NPH may develop especially in elderly patients after TBI, being characterized by enlarged ventricles, normal pressure of CSF and a typical clinical setting of gait apraxia, urinary incontinence, and cognitive deficits (Fig. 3.2). Posttraumatic NPH is not easily distinguished from other causes of NPH, Alzheimer's disease, and vascular dementia, and treatment should be performed to allow rehabilitation [20].

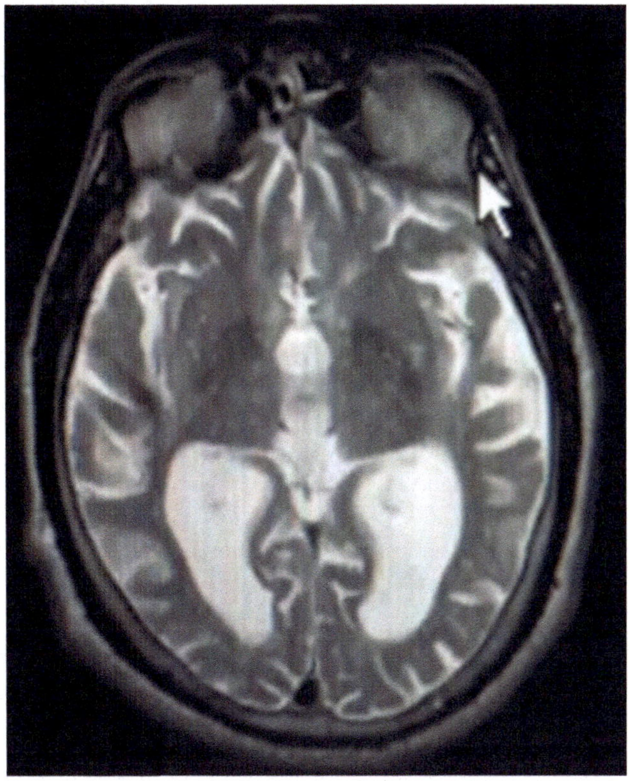

**Fig. 3.2** Normal pressure hydrocephalus following TBI

### Neuropsychological

Up to 81% of patients with PTH may present with disorders of higher integrative functions of the brain; of these, 73% get easily fatigued [4, 21, 22]. There are also frequent disorders of attention, slowing down of those processes relating to abstract thought, power of apprehension, and recent memory. Amnestic disturbances may also occur, being more common in mild to moderate trauma, while higher integrative functions prevail after severe TBI [4].

Some kind of neuropsychological improvement may be seen in 70% of PTH cases after surgery (ventriculoperitoneal shunt) of the cases. The probability of worsening despite of treatment is higher among patients with chronic installation (after 6 months of the trauma) [4].

## Differential Diagnosis and Evaluation

Selection of patients for surgery can be defined principally on a clinical basis. Ventricular enlargement is a common finding in the postacute phase of TBI. The controversy is to distinguish brain atrophy-related ventriculomegaly from active, symptomatic ventricular dilation. Typically PTH develops within 3 months from TBI, whereas ventriculomegaly because of cortical atrophy evolves over 6 or more months. Further, cortical atrophy appears to correlate with cerebral hypoxia and anoxia and diffuse axonal injury, whereas PTH is more clearly related to CSF blockage over the convexities [1–10].

Maintained lumbar puncture pressures higher than 20 cm $H_2O$ are suggestive of PTH. On imaging, ventriculomegaly is a typical finding but not always a good predictor of therapeutic response to interventions. Ventricular dilation in the absence of prominent sulci and gyri is most suggestive of PTH. Nevertheless, secondary NPH following trauma may share ventricular enlargement and have wider sulci and gyri [1–10].

Measurements of CSF dynamics may help formulate the diagnosis as might assessment of cerebral aqueduct flow void on MRI. SPECT scanning showing temporal lobe hypoperfusion may also be a useful indicator of patients that will respond to surgery [1–10].

## Treatment

Once diagnosed PTH, treatment with shunt must be considered, once hydrocephalus is a reversible condition with impact in symptoms and rehabilitation programs. Although repeated lumbar puncture with CSF removal may decrease indications for definitive surgery, in most cases, a ventriculoperitoneal shunt (VPS) is the most applied technique. If an obstructive hydrocephalus is present, neuroendoscopic approach with third ventriculostomy (ETV) may also be tried; however, the rate of converting ETV to VPS may reach 30%. Factors involved in higher risk of conversion are need for craniotomy within 48 h of admission, history of culture-positive CSF, and length of stay [1–10].

Ventriculoperitoneal shunt is one of the most applied neurosurgical procedures worldwide, and the gold standard for treating PTH is the shunt with a programmable valve, which theoretically allows for adequate and case-to-case adjustment of drainage pressure, thus reaching better functional outcomes and avoiding complications like overdrainage, subdural effusions, and additional surgery. Nevertheless, literature lacks comparative studies to answer questions about efficacy and complications of fixed pressure valves, programmable valves, and flow-regulated valves. Current evidence is based mainly in several series and personal experience [1–10, 20–23].

Improvements after surgical treatment are seen in approximately 70% of patients; however, such result varies according to patient profiles (Fig. 3.3). After treatment of PTH, there may be impact in consciousness, motor function, spasticity, and epileptic activity. If patients were submitted to decompressive craniectomy, a cranioplasty is also important before final hydrocephalus treatment. It is widely known that after cranioplasty, there is a clear improvement in CSF flow, demonstrated by functional studies. Additionally, younger patients and those with less severe hydrocephalus before shunt placement may expect a better outcome after shunt placement [1–10, 20–23].

A proportion of patients who had PTH and remained in severe conscious disturbance would benefit from shunt implantation, and the improvement may turn up late after this procedure [1–9].

Additional caution must be carried in patients undergoing VPS and still with intraventricular clots. In such cases, acute system failure may result in coma and death. External ventricular shunt should be applied in cases with acute bleeding and ongoing infection.

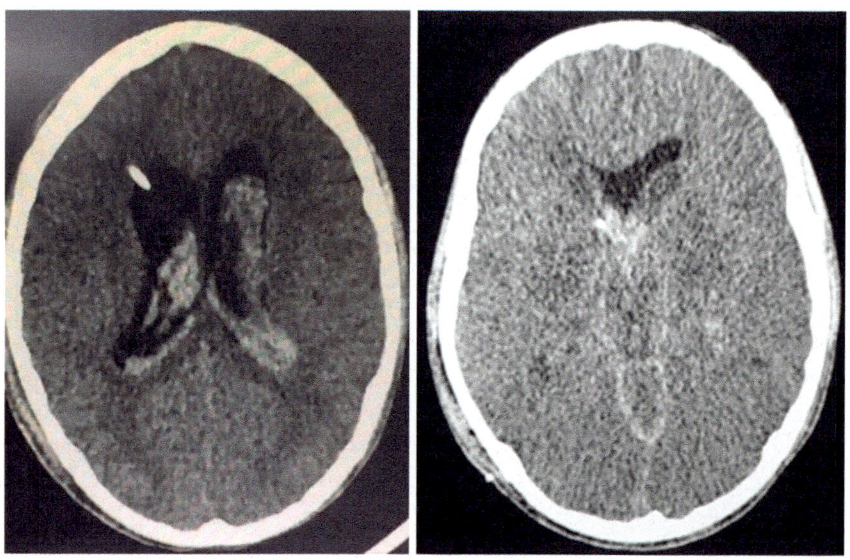

**Fig. 3.3** Ventriculoperitoneal shunt in PTH

## Rehabilitation

Most cases of PTH emerge during rehabilitation. Therefore, attention toward this complication should be present also beyond the acute stage after TBI, particularly among older patients and patients with severe disordered consciousness [25–27].

In the setting of posttraumatic patients, those with PTH are usually older, with more severe brain injury and longer acute treatment. At discharge, they have more disability, longer rehabilitation stays, and unfavorable outcome [3, 4, 19].

Those patients generally require a multidisciplinary team approach, with speech and language therapist, physical therapy, occupational therapy, nutritional support, and neuropsychological support. Rehabilitation avoids complication occurrence and allows for maximal motor and cognitive improvement. The role of hydrocephalus surgical treatment is well known, and functional techniques of brain stimulation are being matter of upcoming studies [3, 4, 19].

## Outcome

Although a high number of patients suffer from TBI and PTH, there are scarce data on the follow-up. Many patients may die due to acute hemodynamic, pulmonary, and systemic conditions while hospitalized, especially secondary to systemic and brain infections [3, 4, 19].

Among patients who survive acute phase, develop PTH, and treat it, up to 70% may have clear motor, cognitive, seizure, or consciousness benefits after shunt implantation, with widely varied final outcomes. The best predictive parameters for outcome after shunt implantation are preoperative status and patients in a better clinical condition (GOS 3 or better). Patient's age and injury did not seem to influence the outcome. Thus, outcome of posttraumatic hydrocephalus is ameliorated if proper treatment is employed [3, 4, 19].

## Specific Conditions

### Traumatic Hygroma and Hydrocephalus

Traumatic subdural hygromas (TSH) are often early lesions and can be detected after trauma, usually as small symmetrical subdural effusions (Fig. 3.4). The underlying mechanism involved includes acute hemorrhagic foci impairing CSF flow and arachnoid membrane tearing, both in different and varying degrees. They may happen as fast as 24 h after trauma and persist for months [24–27].

Most authors divide them in normotensive hygromas (no evidence of mass effect) and hypertensive hygromas (evidence of mass effect). An accompanying subarachnoid hemorrhage (SAH) may be seen in 90% of patients. Delayed hydrocephalus may occur in hygromas with remarked CSF flow imbalance, reaching until 50% of patients. Interhemispheric hygroma is predictive of PTH [24–27].

Treatment is decided based in a clinical and complementary approach. Patients with clear mass effect and those with impaired hemodynamic functions although no mass effect in neuroimage may be candidates for surgery. In the majority of cases, neurological follow-up and conservative treatment are enough [24–27].

Treatment is usually performed with trephination and drainage of hypertensive collection. In case of recurrence, repeated lumbar punctures or even a subdural subgaleal or subdural ventricular shunt can be tried [24–27].

### Decompressive Craniectomy and Hydrocephalus

Decompressive craniectomy (DC) is a neurosurgical procedure to reduce elevated intracranial pressure after severe traumatic brain injury (TBI) (Fig. 3.5). There is increasing evidence to support such procedure, impacting in brain hemodynamics, perfusion, and outcome. However, it is an emer-

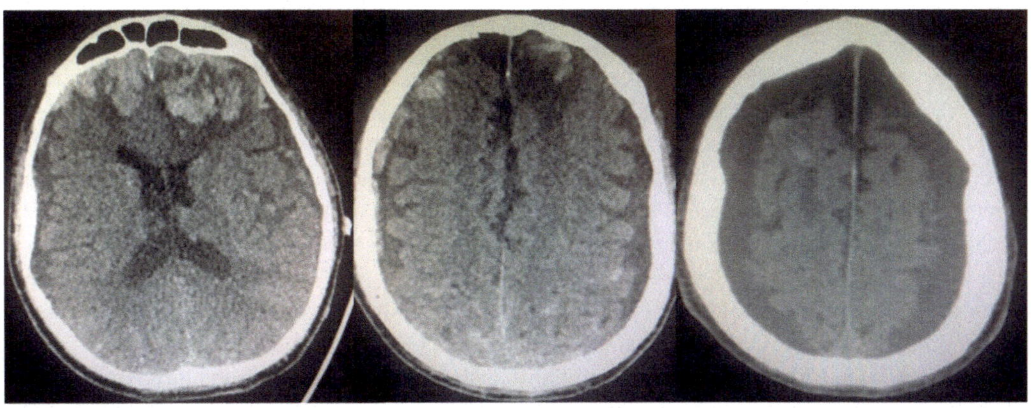

**Fig. 3.4** Posttraumatic hygroma developing after TBI

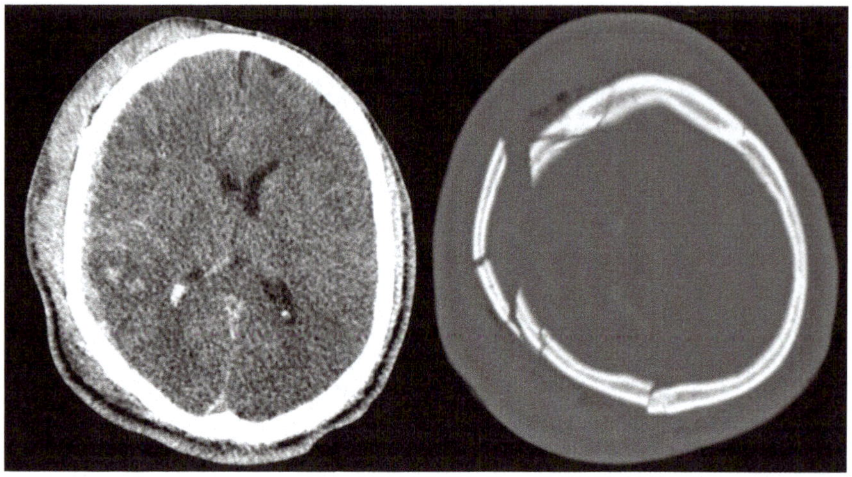

**Fig. 3.5** Severe TBI with bone and brain tissue extensive damage, needing decompressive craniectomy

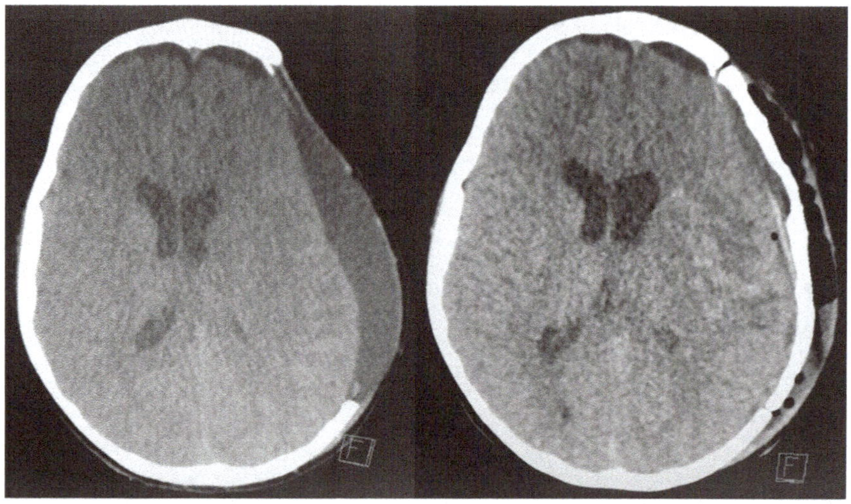

**Fig. 3.6** Bone flap repositioning after acute phase of TBI. After cranioplasty, there was a decrease in subdural effusion, suggesting improvement in hydrodynamics

gency procedure, and, after acute phase, several complications can happen. The most frequent complications after TBI and DC are formation of hygroma, aseptic bone resorption of the reimplanted bone flap, posttraumatic hydrocephalus, secondary infection or dysfunction of ventriculoperitoneal shunt or cranioplasty, and epilepsy. Because of these complications, 75% of patients may require further surgery in addition to cranioplasty [25–37].

Underlying mechanisms for late complications of DC are CSF malabsorption or obstruction of CSF flow. Some authors believe that DC play a "flattening" role in the normally dicrotic CSF pulse wave. Arachnoid granulation function is dependent on the pressure difference between the subarachnoid space and draining venous supply; so, it is possible that disruption of pulsatile intracranial pressure dynamics secondary to opening the cranial defect results in decreased CSF outflow and absorption, thus leading to hydrocephalus. SAH or IVH after TBI may promote the development of hydrocephalus after DC. Blood products may block CSF circulation or absorption via an obstructive mechanism, due to a disturbance in CSF absorption at the arachnoid granulation site. CSF absorption decreases and accumulation increases, resulting in development of chronic hydrocephalus. Thus, the initial benefit in hemodynamic parameters can be soon changed by worsening of hydrodynamic parameters [25–37].

Therefore, repositioning bone flap either with autologous bone or synthetic bone is fundamental in rehabilitation and restoring hydrodynamic function (Fig. 3.6). Such procedure is usually technically simple and should be considered as soon as acute phase of TBI has passed and clinical conditions allow for cranioplasty. When PTH is present, cranioplasty and VPS may be needed As a general rule, if there are no clear signs or symptoms of elevated intracranial pressure, a first step surgery with only cranioplasty should be tried, reserving VPS for those cases with clear signs and symptoms of intracranial pressure and persisting hydrocephalus after bone repositioning. This rationale lies on the potential improvement of PTH just due to repositioning of the bone, avoiding additional surgery (VPS) and its complications [25–37].

## References


1. Pinto FC, Oliveira MF, Prist R, Silva MR, Silva LF, Capone Neto A. Effect of volume replacement during combined experimental hemorrhagic shock and traumatic brain injury in prostanoids, brain pathology and pupil status. Arq Neuropsiquiatr. 2015;73(6):499–505.
2. Pinto FC, Capone-Neto A, Prist R, E Silva MR, Poli-de-Figueiredo LF. Volume replacement with lactated Ringer's or 3% hypertonic saline solution during combined experimental hemorrhagic shock and traumatic brain injury. J Trauma. 2006;60(4):758–63; discussion 763-4.
3. Kammersgaard LP, Linnemann M, Tibæk M. Hydrocephalus following severe traumatic brain injury in adults. Incidence, timing, and clinical predictors during rehabilitation. NeuroRehabilitation. 2013;33(3):473–80.
4. Mazzini L, Campini R, Angelino E, Rognone F, Pastore I, Oliveri G. Posttraumatic hydrocephalus: a clinical, neuroradiologic, and neuropsychologic assessment of long-term outcome. Arch Phys Med Rehabil. 2003;84(11):1637–41.
5. Louveau A, Smirnov I, Keyes TJ, Eccles JD, Rouhani SJ, Peske JD, Derecki NC, Castle D, Mandell JW, Lee KS, Harris TH, Kipnis J. Structural and functional features of central nervous system lymphatic vessels. Nature. 2015;523(7560):337–41.
6. Xiong G, Elkind JA, Kundu S, Smith CJ, Antunes MB, Tamashiro E, Kofonow JM, Mitala CM, Cole J, Stein SC, Grady MS, Einhorn E, Cohen NA, Cohen AS. Traumatic brain injury-induced ependymal ciliary loss decreases cerebral spinal fluid flow. J Neurotrauma. 2014;31(16):1396–404.
7. Liu CL, Chen CC, Lee HC, Cho DY. Matrix metalloproteinase-9 in the ventricular cerebrospinal fluid correlated with the prognosis of traumatic brain injury. Turk Neurosurg. 2014;24(3):363–8.
8. Chen Q, Tang J, Tan L, Guo J, Tao Y, Li L, Chen Y, Liu X, Zhang JH, Chen Z, Feng H. Intracerebral hematoma contributes to hydrocephalus after intraventricular hemorrhage via aggravating Iron accumulation. Stroke. 2015;46(10):2902–8.
9. Castejón OJ. Ultrastructural pathology of oligodendroglial cells in traumatic and hydrocephalic human brain edema: a review. Ultrastruct Pathol. 2015;39(6):359–68.
10. Godbolt AK, Stenberg M, Jakobsson J, Sorjonen K, Krakau K, Stålnacke BM, Nygren DeBoussard C. Subacute complications during recovery from severe traumatic brain injury: frequency and associations with outcome. BMJ Open. 2015;5(4):e007208.
11. Zhao J, Chen Z, Xi G, Keep RF, Hua Y. Deferoxamine attenuates acute hydrocephalus after traumatic brain injury in rats. Transl Stroke Res. 2014;5(5):586–94.
12. Strahle J, Garton HJ, Maher CO, Muraszko KM, Keep RF, Xi G. Mechanisms of hydrocephalus after neonatal and adult intraventricular hemorrhage. Transl Stroke Res. 2012;3(Suppl 1):25–38.
13. Bauer DF, McGwin G Jr, Melton SM, George RL, Markert JM. Risk factors for conversion to permanent ventricular shunt in patients receiving therapeutic ventriculostomy for traumatic brain injury. Neurosurgery. 2011;68(1):85–8.
14. Wen L, Wan S, Zhan RY, Li G, Gong JB, Liu WG, Yang XF. Shunt implantation in a special sub-group of post-traumatic hydrocephalus--patients have normal intracranial pressure without clinical representations of hydrocephalus. Brain Inj. 2009;23(1):61–4.
15. Licata C, Cristofori L, Gambin R, Vivenza C, Turazzi S. Posttraumatic hydrocephalus. J Neurosurg Sci. 2001;45(3):141–9.
16. Xin H, Yun S, Jun X, Liang W, Ye-Lin C, Xiao-Feng Y. Long-term outcomes after shunt implantation in patients with posttraumatic hydrocephalus and severe conscious disturbance. J Craniofac Surg. 2014;25(4):1280–3.
17. Tribl G, Oder W. Outcome after shunt implantation in severe head injury with post-traumatic hydrocephalus. Brain Inj. 2000;14(4):345–54.
18. Brandner S, Thaler C, Lelental N, Buchfelder M, Kleindienst A, Maler JM, Kornhuber J, Lewczuk P. Ventricular and lumbar cerebrospinal fluid concentrations of Alzheimer's disease biomarkers in patients with normal pressure hydrocephalus and posttraumatic hydrocephalus. J Alzheimers Dis. 2014;41(4):1057–62.
19. Linnemann M, Tibæk M, Kammersgaard LP. Hydrocephalus during rehabilitation following severe TBI. Relation to recovery, outcome, and length of stay. NeuroRehabilitation. 2014;35(4):755–61.
20. Oliveira MF, Reis RC, Trindade EM, Pinto FC. Evidences in the treatment of idiopathic normal pressure hydrocephalus. Rev Assoc Med Bras. 2015;61(3):258–62.
21. Oliveira MF, Saad F, Reis RC, Rotta JM, Pinto FC. Programmable valve represents an efficient and safe tool in the treatment of idiopathic normal-pressure hydrocephalus patients. Arq Neuropsiquiatr. 2013;71(4):229–36.
22. Pereira RM, Suguimoto MT, Oliveira MF, Tornai JB, Amaral RA, Teixeira MJ, Pinto FC. Performance of the fixed pressure valve with antisiphon device SPHERA® in the treatment of normal pressure hydrocephalus and prevention of overdrainage. Arq Neuropsiquiatr. 2015;74:55.
23. Pinto FC, Saad F, Oliveira MF, Pereira RM, Miranda FL, Tornai JB, Lopes MI, Ribas ES, Valinetti EA, Teixeira MJ. Role of endoscopic third ventriculostomy and ventriculoperitoneal shunt in idiopathic normal pressure hydrocephalus: preliminary results of a randomized clinical trial. Neurosurgery. 2013;72(5):845–53; discussion 853-4.
24. Zanini MA, de Lima Resende LA, de Souza Faleiros AT, Gabarra RC. Traumatic subdural hygromas: proposed pathogenesis based classification. J Trauma. 2008;64(3):705–13.
25. Kaen A, Jimenez-Roldan L, Alday R, Gomez PA, Lagares A, Alén JF, Lobato RD. Interhemispheric hygroma after decompressive craniectomy: does it predict posttraumatic hydrocephalus? J Neurosurg. 2010;113(6):1287–93.
26. Choi I, Park HK, Chang JC, Cho SJ, Choi SK, Byun BJ. Clinical factors for the development of posttraumatic hydrocephalus after decompressive craniectomy. J Korean Neurosurg Soc. 2008;43(5):227–31.
27. Jiao QF, Liu Z, Li S, Zhou LX, Li SZ, Tian W, You C. Influencing factors for posttraumatic hydrocephalus in patients suffering from severe traumatic brain injuries. Chin J Traumatol. 2007;10(3):159–62.
28. Oh CH, Park CO, Hyun DK, Park HC, Yoon SH. Comparative study of outcomes between shunting after cranioplasty and in cranioplasty after shunting in large concave flaccid cranial defect with hydrocephalus. J Korean Neurosurg Soc. 2008;44(4):211–6.
29. Pechmann A, Anastasopoulos C, Korinthenberg R, van Velthoven-Wurster V, Kirschner J. Decompressive craniectomy after severe traumatic brain injury in children: complications and outcome. Neuropediatrics. 2015;46(1):5–12.
30. Fotakopoulos G, Tsianaka E, Siasios G, Vagkopoulos K, Fountas K. Posttraumatic hydrocephalus after decompressive craniectomy in 126 patients with severe traumatic brain injury. J Neurol Surg A Cent Eur Neurosurg. 2015;77(2):88–92.
31. Pachatouridis D, Alexiou GA, Zigouris A, Michos E, Drosos D, Fotakopoulos G, Voulgaris S. Management of hydrocephalus after decompressive craniectomy. Turk Neurosurg. 2014;24(6):855–8.
32. Ding J, Guo Y, Tian H. The influence of decompressive craniectomy on the development of hydrocephalus: a review. Arq Neuropsiquiatr. 2014;72(9):715–20.
33. Jeon SW, Choi JH, Jang TW, Moon SM, Hwang HS, Jeong JH. Risk factors associated with subdural hygroma after decompressive craniectomy in patients with traumatic brain injury : a comparative study. J Korean Neurosurg Soc. 2011;49(6):355–8.

34. Coelho F, Oliveira AM, Paiva WS, Freire FR, Calado VT, Amorim RL, Neville IS, de Andrade AF, Bor-Seng-Shu E, Anghinah R, Teixeira MJ. Comprehensive cognitive and cerebral hemodynamic evaluation after cranioplasty. Neuropsychiatr Dis Treat. 2014;10:695–701.
35. Bor-Seng-Shu E, Paiva WS, Figueiredo EG, Fujimoto Y, de Andrade AF, Fonoff ET, Teixeira MJ. Posttraumatic refractory intracranial hypertension and brain herniation syndrome: cerebral hemodynamic assessment before decompressive craniectomy. Biomed Res Int. 2013;2013:750809.
36. Bor-Seng-Shu E, Figueiredo EG, Fonoff ET, Fujimoto Y, Panerai RB, Teixeira MJ. Decompressive craniectomy and head injury: brain morphometry, ICP, cerebral hemodynamics, cerebral microvascular reactivity, and neurochemistry. Neurosurg Rev. 2013;36(3):361–70.
37. Bor-Seng-Shu E, Figueiredo EG, Amorim RL, Teixeira MJ, Valbuza JS, de Oliveira MM, Panerai RB. Decompressive craniectomy: a meta-analysis of influences on intracranial pressure and cerebral perfusion pressure in the treatment of traumatic brain injury. J Neurosurg. 2012;117(3):589–96.

# Challenges and Complications of Immobility

**4**

Christina May Moran de Brito, Linamara Rizzo Battistella, and Maria Lúcia Costacurta Guarita

The conception, among many others, that the human being was created to work [1] is one of the oldest and most debated principles that guide humanity. However, without addressing the merit of the anthropological discussion of this concept, what is increasingly proved by science is that the body was made to function. Vital function is intrinsically associated with the production of energy, and an organ that is not stimulated degenerates, atrophies, and may even irreversibly lose its function [2].

Indicated as a "medical treatment" since the nineteenth century [3], most of the scientific community ignored the deleterious effects of bed rest until the mid-1950s [4]. Bed rest, in principle harmless, was seen as something that allowed body restoration by reducing metabolic demand [5], and so it was of the utmost importance for one's recovery. Thus, prescriptions recommended excessive bed resting periods or even contained incorrect indications [6]. Vestiges of this conduct exist to this day, not because of the persistence of the bed rest culture in the popular scope but because of its persistence also in the medical environment [7].

Many studies published in subsequent years analyzed the effects of immobilization from the organic and functional points of view and its impact on the quality of life of bedridden patients [8].

A meta-analysis consisting of 39 randomized studies about the effect of bed rest on 15 different diseases and after 24 medical procedures showed that immobilization was not beneficial; on the contrary, it could be harmful [6].

The advancement of aerospace science and the development of studies submitting normal individuals to experimental models of forced bed rest ("elevated limb," "casted limb," and "bed rest and microgravity") provided better physiological understanding of immobilization [9].

In addition to the most evident complications, such as deformities, joint pain, loss of muscle mass, deep vein thrombosis, and atelectasis [10], injuries to the cardiovascular [11], endocrine [12], immune [13], gastrointestinal [14], excretory [15], vestibular [16], cognitive [17], and psychological [18] systems have also been reported.

With the growing survival of individuals in critical conditions [19], this fact became even more evident. This occurred because scientific and technological knowledge increased the number of so-called intensive care unit survivors, which resulted in a threefold increase in the number of patients referred to rehabilitation centers to treat hospital-acquired disabilities [20].

Roughly, 60–70% of individuals who are released from intensive care units present some degree of motor disability [21], and 50–70% have some type of neurocognitive impairment, both acquired during hospital stay [22].

According to the World Health Organization [23], quality of life is directly related to the degree of independence and physical, psychological, social, and spiritual statuses of individuals. Hence, as bed rest can have a negative impact on most of these domains, many studies have correlated immobilization with worse quality of life in hospitalized patients submitted to prolonged bed rest [24–26].

Given above, medical services around the world have been working on the development and implementation of early intervention protocols aiming at fast mobilization of bedridden patients in detriment of harmful bed rest [27–29].

Until now, early mobilization provided by an effective multidisciplinary approach has proven a positive, viable, and low-risk strategy [10, 30].

C. M. M. de Brito (✉)
Rehabilitation Department, Institute of Cancer of São Paulo, Clinics Hospital – School of Medicine – University of São Paulo, São Paulo, Brazil

L. R. Battistella
Legal Medicine, Medical Ethics, Social and Occupational Medicine and Physical and Rehabilitation Medicine Institute, Clinics Hospital – School of Medicine – University of São Paulo, São Paulo, Brazil

M. L. C. Guarita
Institute of Cancer of São Paulo – Rehabilitation Department, São Paulo, São Paulo, Brazil


R. Anghinah et al. (eds.), *Topics in Cognitive Rehabilitation in the TBI Post-Hospital Phase*, https://doi.org/10.1007/978-3-319-95376-2_4

Older patients or patients with chronic diseases or disabilities are especially more susceptible to the adverse effects of immobilization [31].

However, studies in the literature correlating immobilization in patients with traumatic brain injury are scarce. The few studies on the topic reported that bed rest did not provide a positive, but possibly a negative, contribution to the recovery of these patients [32–34].

Thus, debating and further studying this topic are of the utmost importance, not only because of the long hospital stays that these individuals experience but also because of the harm caused by the incorrect management of orthosis and the disabling nature of this type of injury. The earlier an injured nervous system is stimulated, the better the prognosis [35].

The objective of this chapter is to review the negative effects of bed rest on many systems, correlating them to the peculiarities of patients with traumatic brain injury. The available interventional strategies in the rehabilitation scope for early, effective, and safe mobilization will also be approached.

## Musculoskeletal, Nervous, and Integumentary Systems

The integumentary, nervous, and musculoskeletal systems have an intrinsic relationship with one's degree of functionality and independence.

Given the neuromuscular impairment inherent to traumatic brain injury, patients who suffer this type of injury are more susceptible to the deleterious effects of immobilization of these systems as a result of many factors, which will be discussed.

The main musculoskeletal and neurological complications related to immobilization cited in the literature, regarding these systems, are muscle atrophy, fatigue, changes in bone density, heterotopic ossification, contracture deformities, peripheral and central nervous system involvement, behavioral and cognitive changes, pressure ulcers, and pain.

### Muscle Atrophy and Fatigue

A person in complete bed rest loses from 1% to 3% of their muscle strength per day of immobilization [36]. In 4 weeks, immobilized individuals are estimated to lose 69% of their net muscle weight [37], the loss being more significant between the second and tenth day of bed rest due to edema and tissue fatty replacement [8, 31, 38].

The lower limbs of a healthy individual in complete bed rest are more affected than the upper limbs [39], and among muscles, the most affected are those composed predominantly of type II fibers and related to movement instead of joint stabilization, such as the rectus femoris muscle compared with the vastus intermedius muscle [8], and especially antigravitational movement.

The mechanism responsible for muscle atrophy and weakness involves a complex group of interrelated processes [10]. Lack of use and inflammation seems to be the main factors related to the deterioration of the muscular system, promoting mass loss, reduction of the number of contraction fibers, and reduction of contraction strength, especially of type II fibers [40].

Muscle immobilization seems to change the balance between muscle protein synthesis and lysis, affecting the former more intensely [41]. Low protein synthesis would stem from 4E-BP-1 mRNA inhibition of protein synthesis initiation factors. Excessive protein lysis would be triggered by three distinct pathways: the calcium-dependent protease calpain, lysosomal cathepsins, and the ubiquitin-proteasome system [10].

Meanwhile, the inflammatory pathway would be triggered in later phases of prolonged bed rest by increasing pro-inflammatory cytokines (IL-1 beta, IL-2, and interferon gamma) [42] and producing reactive oxygen species (ROS), which promotes a negative protein balance [43]. This same pathway includes the relationship between the extra cytokines and higher insulin resistance, since hyperglycemia has been demonstrably associated with higher neuromuscular involvement. Simultaneously, low oxidative enzyme capacity, which decreases the contraction of type II fibers, associated with low vascular flow in the immobilized muscles and changes in the size of the plaque of terminal acetylcholine receptors, induces low fatigue resistance.

The majority of patients with traumatic brain injury in the first stages of recovery have low protein intake, which, when associated with the motor and cognitive impairments caused by the trauma, further increase the abovementioned muscle degradation. On the other hand, studies of spastic patients have found an increase in the muscle mass of the most spastic limbs compared with those with mild or without spasticity [44].

### Changes in Bone Density

Numerous are the factors that affect bone quality, such as age and genetic factors, pharmaceuticals, and diseases, among others. Nevertheless, one of the main factors associated with inactivity that reduce bone mineral density is the absence or decreased level of gravity-induced mechanic compression and traction stimuli and/or muscle contraction stimuli [45].

Animals submitted to different gravities present changes in the trabecular and cortical bone structures, mineralization pathways, collagen metabolism, and calcium excretion [46].

These losses begin quickly, occurring a few weeks after immobilization. They are self-limited and reach a peak after

20–30 weeks. In more severe cases, they are partly irreversible, even years after resuming mobility [47]. The immobilization of forearms and wrists in males and females for almost 5 weeks resulted in significant bone loss, which was not recovered after 5 weeks of hand remobilization and therapy [48]. Individuals submitted to microgravity had bone deficiency in the calcaneus bone as long as 5 years after exposure [49].

In the first months of immobilization, bone mineral loss is mainly attributed to higher bone resorption [50]. Although the pathophysiology has not been well established, osteoblasts in vitro in microgravity environments responded differently to systemic hormones and growth factor [51].

Given that the fluid movement inside bone gap junctions and canaliculi provides a significant collaboration to the preservation of the skeletal matrix, studies in vivo have found that bone movements change the pressure of this liquid in the skeletal cells, which in turn stimulate the release of signaling molecules that mediate bone remodeling [52, 53].

Another bone remodeling mechanism, also impaired by the lack of mechanic bone stressors and increasingly accepted by the scientific community, is promoted by the sympathetic nervous system, which stimulates remodeling via beta-adrenergic receptors. This pathway could also be influenced by lesions in the central nervous system, which, in turn, would cause metabolic, neurovascular, and molecular disorders, generating the so-called neurogenic osteoporosis.

Hence, one can speculate that individuals with traumatic brain injury are more susceptible to bone involvement because they have more than one causal trigger of bone mass reduction stimuli.

Age and injury location aside, this fact could also be reinforced by bone density changes, which indicate the different bone qualities of a healthy and a compromised limb of patients with stroke or spinal cord injury [54, 55].

Additionally, in the initial critical stage of traumatic brain injury, patients often present nutritional changes, severe weight loss, inflammatory processes and hormonal changes secondary to thyroid and gonadal disorders, and changes related to the growth hormone and insulin-like growth factor 1 [56]. All these factors may have a negative impact on bone integrity, along with immobilization and nervous system injury.

Although many studies have found a negative correlation between spasticity and bone mineral density, some studies have reported a positive correlation between high spasticity and worse bone mass quality [57, 58].

## Heterotopic Ossification

Still on bone involvement, heterotopic ossification [HO] could not be omitted. This disease develops in situations of immobilization and is usually associated with central nervous system lesions [59].

HO is defined as the presence of bone tissue in places where bone normally does not exist. This abnormality stems from a metaplastic process with bone neoformation in soft tissues, usually adjacent to large joints (hip, elbows, knees, and shoulders) [60]. Its etiology is still unknown, but many factors responsible for osteoblastic activation through bone-forming proteins have been studied, such as the stimulus caused by the central neurological lesion itself [61].

Potential HO-related complications are limited joint amplitude with functional impairment, pain, nerve compression, and worsening of spasticity [62].

## Contracture Deformities

As mentioned earlier, significant changes in the muscle tissues of previously healthy limbs occur after some weeks of immobilization. These, in addition to changes of the other structures that involve the joints, such as ligaments, capsules, disks, and menisci, may cause structural and disabling deformities.

Experimental animal studies have found roughly a 12.5° loss of amplitude of joint movement after 2 weeks of immobilization, which may increase to 51.4° after 32 weeks of bed rest [63].

The pathophysiology of this joint phenomenon has not been well defined, but replacement of type III collagen fibers by type I collagen fibers after 1 week of immobilization of a healthy joint has been described, with reduction of total elasticity [64]. Yet, low production of collagen fibrils in the ligaments reduces their long-term resistance and increases osteoclastic activity in the ligament-bone interface [65].

An inflamed joint deserves special attention given that short-term immobilization is indicated to reduce the concentration of type I interleukin and increase proteoglycans, necessary for cartilage protection. However, the presence of inflammation and pain increases the risk of long-term contracture deformities, so the former cannot be excessive [31].

Given the traumatic nature of the lesion, patients with traumatic brain injury may have three factors that promote the development of contracture deformities in addition to immobilization: motor changes, spasticity, and/or other joint inflammation processes stemming directly from the polytrauma, such as fractures, ligament lesions, etc.

Since paresis or paralysis in traumatic brain injury patients in the initial stages of the trauma can even progress to complete functional recovery, segmental immobilization, with the introduction and maintenance of orthosis, should be done carefully and under supervision.

## Pressure Ulcers

In addition to the collagen changes mentioned earlier, which increases contracture deformities, another frequent and disabling change in patients that remain immobilized for prolonged periods is pressure ulcers.

A 3-month study of 530 patients hospitalized for clinical or surgical reasons found that 11.3% of these patients had pressure ulcers, and immobilization was the main risk factor for pressure ulcer development [66].

Likewise, a study proposing an early mobilization program over a period of 12 months in 3233 intensive care unit patients found a 3% reduction in the incidence of pressure ulcers [67].

In addition to motricity changes stemming from the central nervous system lesion, traumatic brain injury patients may also present other risk factors for skin lesions, such as sensory changes, nutritional deficiencies, metabolic changes, spasticity, neurotrophic changes, and long intensive care unit stays. The strategies proposed to lower the incidence of pressure wounds in patients with traumatic central nervous system lesions include not only early mobilization, with assistive position change when active movement is impaired, and assistive devices that reduce friction and shear, but also rigorous surveillance and, if necessary, correction of plasma hemoglobin level and introduction of oral feeding, as soon as possible, and skin hydration [68].

## Neuronal Involvement and Cognitive and Behavioral Changes

Neuroplasticity occurs in adulthood in response to natural cell maturation associated with neuronal use or lack of use [69]. As the field of diagnostic tests involving functional analyses of the various levels of the nervous system advances, more pieces of evidence of the negative impacts of immobilization on this system are frequently being discovered.

The changes seen in bedridden patients or patients in microgravity environments for prolonged periods include sensory disorders, altered vestibular reflex responses, lack of coordination, balance changes, reaction speed, attention, planning, memory, spatial-temporal orientation, body perception, level of anxiety, depression, and insomnia [9, 16, 17, 64, 70, 71].

The pathophysiology of these changes has not been well defined, but some studies have suggested a correlation between stimulus to the vagal tone and growth of white and gray masses in the prefrontal cortex after observing the higher brain volume of individuals submitted to frequent aerobic exercises [17]. Regarding the peripheral nervous system, animal nerve diameter changes proportionally to immobilization duration [72].

Two entities often mentioned in the current literature, which have immobilization and sensory deprivation as their greatest risk factors, must also be cited: delirium and post-intensive care syndrome. The latter is proof that the sequelae of immobilization may continue after the patient is released from the hospital and may even become permanent.

In addition to the damages to central nervous system and motor system secondary to trauma, traumatic brain injury patients may also develop post-traumatic stress disorder, further aggravating the cognitive-behavioral domain [73].

Strategies must be addressed toward the provision of information to promote better orientation of the patient, and stimulus must be done during the day, in respect to the physiological sleep-wake cycle.

## Pain

Pain may be related to immobilization in many domains, but little is known about its pathophysiology. It may result from involvement of the nociceptive, neuropathic, and mixed pathways.

Patients exposed to stress or excessive sensory deprivation present low tolerance to painful stimuli because of neuroplasticity changes [74, 75]. Likewise, changes in integumentary and muscle tissues (atrophy, contracture deformities, skin lesions) may trigger constant unpleasant stimuli, which generate even greater suffering in underweight, restrained, and/or functionally dependent patients, who often have impaired communication skills.

Traumatic brain injury patients are no exception, and to make matters worse, they may have various inflammatory processes due to the etiology of the disease and to nervous system lesions that may evolve to sensory changes (allodynia/ dysesthesia) and/or presence of pain of central nervous system origin.

About 51.5% of traumatic brain injury patients will develop significant chronic pain after the accident, including patients with mild lesions. This pain does not appear to be associated with a history of depression or the development of post-traumatic stress disorder [76].

Analgesic measures must watch out for sedative effects and may include physical modalities.

## Cardiovascular and Pulmonary Systems

The cardiovascular and pulmonary systems are two other systems that may suffer significantly with immobilization. The first one suffers from the rapid adaptation of the blood vessels and the cardiac pump to the decubitus position, and the slow and often risky recovery of their function as orthostatism is regained. The second one suffers because of adaptations to the lower oxygen demand during bed rest, adaptations associated with numerous complications, such as pneumonia and atelectasis.

## Cardiovascular Adaptation

When a healthy person stands up from a lying position, the heart rate increases by 32%, 62%, and 89% after 3 days, 1 week, and 6 weeks, respectively, of complete bed rest. Systolic volume may reduce by 15% after 2 weeks of bed rest [77]. After 20 days of bed rest, VO2 max can decrease by roughly 27% [78]. Three weeks of immobilization may decrease cardiac performance by 25% [79]. In addition to the physiological cardiovascular adaptations to the horizontal position, time will promote further pathological changes to the structures responsible for the adaptive cardiac response to postural changes, impairing cardiovascular function recovery as patients exposed to immobilization stand up [9].

## Deep Vein Thrombosis

Another known complication of immobilization is deep vein thrombosis, promoted mainly by venous blood stagnation and increased blood coagulability [80]. Stagnation may lead to an increase of thrombin, which promotes platelet aggregation and thrombosis [81]. If left untreated, venous thrombosis may evolve to potentially fatal pulmonary embolism. In traumatic brain injury patients, the presence of lower-limb paralysis and the trauma itself may increase the risk of developing this complication [82].

Trauma patients with prolonged bed rest, frequently combined with segmental paralysis that might result from brain injury, are at high risk for deep vein thrombosis and demand mechanical and pharmacological interventions for its prevention.

## Postural Hypotension

As mentioned earlier, in addition to cardiovascular changes, immobilization also causes changes to the sympathetic-adrenergic system [83]. Hence, the response to baroreceptor stimulation in individuals not exposed to bed rest is different in individuals exposed to approximately 3 weeks of bed rest [84]. This process may take from 20 to 72 days to recover once mobilization is resumed [31]. Increased beta-adrenergic activity caused by immobilization may be responsible for this intolerance [85], associated with the more recent finding of intolerance associated with changes in the vestibulosympathetic reflex [16].

Progressive early mobilization strategies, care of fluid balance and systemic hydration, and surveillance toward the possible adverse effects of the medication in use must be applied.

## Atelectasis and Pneumonia

Immobilization causes changes in the respiratory system, namely, changes in pulmonary blood flow, tissue structure, and ciliary movement, and decreased diaphragmatic excursion, with repercussions on functional residual capacity and effectiveness of coughing [86, 87]. In turn, these changes increase the risk of atelectasis and risk of airway infection.

Traumatic brain injury patients are four times more susceptible to Pneumonia than the general population [88]. Among other reasons, this higher susceptibility occurs as a result of dysphagia and the frequent use of invasive mechanical ventilation [89].

Hence, preventive measures to the deleterious effects of immobilization on the respiratory system are critical in this type of patient to reduce their morbidity and mortality rates. Respiratory exercises, with or without the use of support and assistive devices, must be part of the rehabilitation interventions, as adequate positioning and early mobilization.

## Endocrine and Metabolic Disorders

The greatest and best known changes in the endocrine system associated with immobilization are increased peripheral insulin resistance, which is related to higher morbidity [90]; high parathormone associated with low growth hormone, which changes bone density [91]; and high adrenocorticotrophic hormone, possibly triggered by the stress experienced by critical care patients [31].

With respect to metabolic changes, potassium-, sodium-, nitrogen-, magnesium-, and calcium-related disorders have been associated with immobilization. Immobilization rarely causes severe electrolyte imbalance, but it is important to bear in mind patients with renal failure [31] and the association between high serum potassium, sodium, and calcium and low cerebral blood flow in traumatic brain injury patients [92].

## Digestive and Excretory Systems

Immobilization repercussions on absorptive functions are commonly found in these two systems, such as atrophy of the intestinal mucosa and glands; intestinal motility disorder, which causes constipation and reflux; and sphincter dysfunction, which generates urinary stasis with the formation of calculi and higher incidence of infections [31].

Traumatic brain injury patients already have a high incidence of gastrointestinal tract changes due to the nature of the lesion. These changes can be related to deglutition disorders, fecal incontinence, and intestinal constipation [93]. The excretory system may also be affected, resulting in urinary incontinence, which may affect up to 62% of these patients during the acute phase [94].

Given the negative repercussion of these problems on the patient's social and clinical domains, and the high susceptibility of traumatic brain injury patients to these problems, the implementation of early mobilization strategies is vital to avoid the deleterious effects of immobilization. They include pharmacological and non-pharmacological interventions, which include dietetic measures, adequate positioning, abdominal maneuvers, and the use of the gastrocolic reflex, apart from the early mobilization strategies.

## Early Mobilization

The mainstay of treatment lies on early mobilization strategies, since the acute phase, and that include critical ill patients. The early rehabilitation of critically ill patients has proven a feasible and safe approach that may promote improved physical function, greater independence in activities of daily living [ADL], and an accelerated process of the return to premorbidity activities, with reduced symptoms of fatigue and dyspnea [24, 28, 95–99]. In addition to those benefits, early rehabilitation has also been associated with other relevant clinical outcomes, including preventing the incidence of ICU-acquired muscle weakness and reducing the time of weaning from mechanical ventilation [MV], the length of hospital stay, and costs [27, 100–104].

Bedridden and comatose patients unable to cooperate with the therapy should receive passive mobilization and multisensory stimulation. Stimulation and activities must be applied in an organized, planned, and isolated manner during daytime. Family and caregivers should be involved. Passive mobilization should include progressive passive orthostatic training with the monitoring of vital signs. Orthostatic training contributes to sensory stimulation toward arousal, cardiovascular response, and the prevention of orthostatic hypotension [104], total lung capacity [105], gastrointestinal regulation and the prevention of contracture deformities and also to the alleviation of the pressure of some skin areas. As the patient improves collaboration and mobility, the use of active exercises and neuromuscular stimulation may be introduced. Contracture deformity prevention might demand the introduction of orthosis, and pharmacologic interventions might be needed if spasticity is present.

Regarding bone loss prevention, pharmacologic interventions must be added to mobilization strategies especially in the presence of paralysis to minimize bone reabsorption. Vitamin D must also be maintained or replaced, and minimum calcium intake must be provided [54, 58].

## References


1. The Holy Bible. The new American Bible. Genesis. 1970;2:15.
2. Bortz WM. The disuse syndrome. West J Med. 1984;141(5):691–4.
3. Stiles A. The rest cure, 1873–1925. In: Felluga DF, editor. BRANCH: Britain, representation and nineteenth-century history; 2012. p. 1–11.
4. Needham DM. Mobilizing patients in the intensive care unit: improving neuromuscular weakness and physical function. JAMA. 2008;300(14):1685–90.
5. Pavy-Le Traon A, Heer M, Narici MV, Rittweger J, Vernikos J. From space to earth: advances in human physiology from 20 years of bed rest studies (1986-2006). Eur J Appl Physiol. 2007;101:143–94.
6. Allen C, Glasziou P, Del Mar C. Bed rest: a potentially harmful treatment needing more careful evaluation. Lancet. 1999;354(9186):1229–33.
7. Corcoran PJ. Use it or lose it--the hazards of bed rest and inactivity. West J Med. 1991;154(5):536–8.
8. Parry SM, El-Ansary D, Cartwright MS, Sarwal A, Berney S, Koopman R, et al. Ultrasonography in the intensive care setting can be used to detect changes in the quality and quantity of muscle and is related to muscle strength and function. J Crit Care. 2015;30(5):1151.e9–1151.e14.
9. Liu Q, Zhou R, Zhao X, Oei TPS. Effects of prolonged head-down bed rest on working memory. Neuropsychiatr Dis Treat. 2015;11:835–42.
10. Truong AD, Fan E, Brower RG, Needham DM. Bench-to-bedside review: mobilizing patients in the intensive care unit--from pathophysiology to clinical trials. Crit Care. 2009;13(4):216.
11. Bringard A, Pogliaghi S, Adami A, De Roia G, Lador F, Lucini D, et al. Cardiovascular determinants of maximal oxygen consumption in upright and supine posture at the end of prolonged bed rest in humans. Respir Physiol Neurobiol. 2010;172(1–2):53–62.
12. Belavy DL, Seibel MJ, Roth HJ, Armbrecht G, Rittweger J, Felsenberg D. The effects of bed rest and counter measure exercise on the endocrine system in male adults - evidence for immobilization induced reduction in SHBG levels. J Endocrinol Investig. 2011;35(1):54–62.
13. Hoff P, Belavy DL, Huscher D, Lang A, Hahne M, Kuhlmey AK, et al. Effects of 60-day bed rest with and without exercise on cellular and humoral immunological parameters. Cell Mol Immunol. 2015;12(4):483–92.
14. Iovino P, Chiarioni G, Bilancio G, Cirillo M, Mekjavic IB, Pisot R, et al. New onset of constipation during long-term physical inactivity: a proof-of-concept study on the immobility-induced bowel changes. PLoS One. 2013;8(8):e72608.
15. Okada A, Ohshima H, Itoh Y, Yasui T, Tozawa K, Kohri K. Risk of renal stone formation induced by long-term bed rest could be decreased by premedication with bisphosphonate and increased by resistive exercise. Int J Urol. 2008;15(7):630–5.
16. Dyckman DJ, Sauder CL, Ray CA. Effects of short-term and prolonged bed rest on the vestibulosympathetic reflex. Am J Physiol Heart Circ Physiol. 2012;302:H368–74.
17. Lipnicki DM, Gunga HC, Belavý DL, Felsenberg D. Bed rest and cognition: effects on executive functioning and reaction time. Aviat Space Environ Med. 2009;80(12):1018–24.
18. Ishizaki Y, Fukuoka H, Katsura T, Nishimura Y, Kiriyama M, Higurashi M, et al. Psychological effects of bed rest in young healthy subjects. Acta Physiol Scand Suppl. 1994;616:83–7.

19. Needham DM, Davidson J, Cohen H, Hopkins RO, Weinert C, Wunsch H, et al. Improving long-term outcomes after discharge from intensive care unit: report from a stakeholders' conference. Crit Care Med. 2012;40(2):502–9.
20. Wischmeyer PE, San-Millan I. Winning the war against ICU-acquired weakness: new innovations in nutrition and exercise physiology. Crit Care. 2015;19(Suppl 3):S6.
21. Latronico N, Bolton CF. Critical illness polyneuropathy and myopathy: a major cause of muscle weakness and paralysis. Lancet Neurol. 2011;10:931–41.
22. Girard TD, Jackson JC, Pandharipande PP, Pun BT, Thompson JL, Shintani AK, et al. Delirium as a predictor of long-term cognitive impairment in survivors of critical illness. Crit Care Med. 2010;38(7):1513–20.
23. Division of Mental Health and Prevention of Substance Abuse WHO. WHOQOL: measuring quality of life (Internet). Geneva: World Health Organization; 1997. Available from: http://apps.who.int/iris/bitstream/10665/63482/1/WHO_MSA_MNH_PSF_97.4.pdf.
24. Adler J, Malone D. Early mobilization in the intensive care unit: a systematic review. Cardiopulm Phys Ther J. 2012;23(1):5–13.
25. Gorecki C, Brown JM, Nelson EA, Briggs M, Schoonhoven L, Dealey C, et al. Impact of pressure ulcers on quality of life in older patients: a systematic review. J Am Geriatr Soc. 2009;57(7):1175–83.
26. Parker A, Sricharoenchai T, Needham DM. Early rehabilitation in the intensive care unit: preventing physical and mental health impairments. Curr Phys Med Rehabil Rep. 2013;1(4):307–14.
27. Murakami FM, Yamaguti WP, Onoue MA, Mendes JM, Pedrosa RS, Maida ALV, et al. Functional evolution of critically ill patients undergoing an early rehabilitation protocol. Rev Bras Ter Intensiva. 2015;27(2):161–9.
28. Gosselink J, Bott J, Johnson M, Dean E, Nava S, Norrenberg M, Schonhofer B, Stiller K, van de Leur H, Vincent JLRB. Physiotherapy for adult patients with critical illness: recommendations of the European Respiratory Society and European Society of Intensive Care Medicine Task Force on Physiotherapy for Critically Ill Patients. Intensive Care Med. 2008;34(7):1188–99.
29. Stiller K. Safety issues that should be considered when mobilizing critically ill patients. Crit Care Clin. 2007;23:35–53.
30. Clark DE, Lowman JD, Griffin RL, Matthews HM, Reiff DA. Effectiveness of an early mobilization protocol in a trauma and burns intensive care unit: a retrospective cohort study. Phys Ther. 2012;93(2):186–96.
31. Halar EM, Bell KR. Imobilidade. In: DeLisa JA, Gans BM, editors. Tratado de Medicina de Reabilitação. 3rd ed. São Paulo: Editora Manole Ltda; 2002. p. 1067–89.
32. de Kruijk JR, Leffers P, Meerhoff S, Rutten J, Twijnstra A. Effectiveness of bed rest after mild traumatic brain injury: a randomised trial of no versus six days of bed rest. J Neurol Neurosurg Psychiatry. 2002;73(2):167–72.
33. Singer BJ, Jegasothy GM, Singer KP, Allison GT, Dunne JW. Incidence of ankle contracture after moderate to severe acquired brain injury. Arch Phys Med Rehabil. 2004;85(9):1465–9.
34. Carlile M, Nicewander D, Yablon SA, Brown A, Brunner R, Burke D, et al. Prophylaxis for venous thromboembolism during rehabilitation for traumatic brain injury: a multicenter observational study. J Trauma. 2010;68(4):916–23.
35. Grüner ML, Terhaag D. Multimodal early onset stimulation (MEOS) in rehabilitation after brain injury. Brain Inj. 2000;14(6):585–94.
36. Nicks DK, Beneke WM, Key RM, Timson BF. Muscle fibre size and number following immobilisation atrophy. J Anat. 1989;163:1–5.
37. Haggmark T, Eriksson E, Jansson E. Muscle fiber type changes in human skeletal muscle after injuries and immobilization. Orthopedics. 1986;9(0147-7447 (Print)):181–5.
38. Puthucheary ZA, Phadke R, Rawal J, McPhail MJW, Sidhu PS, Rowlerson A, et al. Qualitative ultrasound in acute critical illness muscle wasting. Crit Care Med. 2015;43(8):1603–11.
39. LeBlanc D, Schneider VS, Evans HJ, Pientok C, Rowe R, Spector E. Regional changes in muscle mass following 17 weeks of bed rest. J Appl Physiol. 1992;73:2172–8.
40. Stevenson EJ, Giresi PG, Koncarevic A, Kandarian SC. Global analysis of gene expression patterns during disuse atrophy in rat skeletal muscle. J Physiol. 2003;551(Pt 1):33–48.
41. Ashmore CR, Summers PJ. Stretch-induced growth in chicken wing muscles: myofibrillar proliferation. Am J Phys. 1981;241(3):C93–7.
42. Schmitt DA, Schwarzenberg M, Tkaczuk J, Hebrard S, Brandenberger G, Mauco G, et al. Head-down tilt bed rest and immune responses. Pflügers Arch Eur J Physiol. 2000;441(2–3 Suppl):R79–84.
43. Pawlak W, Kedziora J, Zolynski K, Kedziora-Kornatowska K, Blaszczyk J, Witkowski P. Free radicals generation by granulocytes from men during bed rest. J Gravit Physiol. 1998;5(1):P131–2.
44. Lofvenmark I, Werhagen L, Norrbrink C. Spasticity and bone density after a spinal cord injury. J Rehabil Med. 2009;41(13):1080–4.
45. Giannotti S, Bottai V, Dell'osso G, De Paola G, Bugelli G, Pini E, et al. Disuse osteoporosis of the upper limb: assessment of thirty patients. Clin Cases Miner Bone Metab (Internet). 2013 (cited 2016 Apr 30);10(2):129–32. Available from: http://www.ncbi.nlm.nih.gov/pubmed/24133531.
46. Zerath E. Effects of microgravity on bone and calcium homeostasis. Adv Space Res Off J Comm Space Res (COSPAR). 1998;21:1049–58.
47. Steinberg FU. The immobilized patient. Boston: Springer US; 1980. p. 34–43.
48. Houde JP, Schulz LA, Morgan WJ, Breen T, Warhold L, Crane GK, et al. Bone mineral density changes in the forearm after immobilization. Clin Orthop Relat Res. 1995;(317):199–205.
49. Tilton FE, Degioanni JJ, Schneider VS. Long-term follow-up of Skylab bone demineralization. Aviat Space Environ Med. 1980;51(11):1209–13.
50. Gross TS, Rubin CT. Uniformity of resorptive bone loss induced by disuse. J Orthop Res. 1995;13(5):708–14.
51. Carmeliet G, Nys G, Bouillon R. Microgravity reduces the differentiation of human osteoblastic MG-63 cells. J Bone Miner Res. 1997;12(5):786–94.
52. Mullender MG, Dijcks SJ, Bacabac RG, Semeins CM, Van Loon J, Klein-Nulend J. Release of nitric oxide, but not prostaglandin E2, by bone cells depends on fluid flow frequency. J Orthop Res. 2006;24(6):1170–7.
53. Knothe Tate ML, Steck R, Forwood MR, Niederer P. In vivo demonstration of load-induced fluid flow in the rat tibia and its potential implications for processes associated with functional adaptation. J Exp Biol. 2000;203(Pt 18):2737–45.
54. Brito CMM, Battistella LR, Sakamoto H, Saito ET. Densidade Mineral Óssea após Lesão Medular. Acta Fisiátrica. 2002;9:127–33.
55. Sato Y, Kuno H, Kaji M, Ohshima Y, Asoh T, Oizumi K. Increased bone resorption during the first year after stroke. Stroke. 1998;29(7):1373–7.
56. Daci E, Van Cromphaut S, Bouillon R. Mechanisms influencing bone metabolism in chronic illness. Horm Res. 2002;58:44–51.
57. Pang MYC, Ashe MC, Eng JJ. Muscle weakness, spasticity and disuse contribute to demineralization and geometric changes in the radius following chronic stroke. Osteoporos Int. 2007;18(9):1243–52.

58. De Brito CMM, Garcia ACF, Takayama L, Fregni F, Battistella LR, Pereira RMR. Bone loss in chronic hemiplegia: a longitudinal cohort study. J Clin Densitom. 2013;16(2):160–7.
59. Hudson SJ, Brett SJ. Heterotopic ossification – a long-term consequence of prolonged immobility. Crit Care (Internet). 2006 (cited 2016 Apr 30);10(6):174. Available from: http://www.ncbi.nlm.nih.gov/pubmed/17129365.
60. Hartmann APB, Ximenes AR, Hartmann LG, Fernandes AR, Natour J, D'Ippolito G. Diagnóstico por imagem na avaliação da ossificação heterotópica. Rev Bras Reumatol. Sociedade Brasileira de Reumatologia. 2004;44(4):291–3.
61. Argyropoulou MI, Kostandi E, Kosta P, Zikou AK, Kastani D, Galiatsou E, et al. Heterotopic ossification of the knee joint in intensive care unit patients: early diagnosis with magnetic resonance imaging. Crit Care (Internet). 2006 (cited 2016 Apr 30);10(5):R152. Available from: http://www.ncbi.nlm.nih.gov/pubmed/17074077.
62. Vanden Bossche L, Vanderstraeten G. Heterotopic ossification: a review. (Review) (80 refs). J Rehabil Med. 2005;37(Sweden PT - Journal Article PT - Review LG - English DC - 20050725):129–36.
63. Trudel G, Uhthoff HK. Contractures secondary to immobility: is the restriction articular or muscular? An experimental longitudinal study in the rat knee. Arch Phys Med Rehabil. 2000;81(1):6–13.
64. Oliveira RCC, Haddad MSCM, Koyama RCC. Síndrome da imobilização In: Greve JMGG, Amatuzzi MM, editors. Medicina de reabilitação aplicada à ortopedia e traumatologia. 1st ed. São Paulo: Rocca; 1999. p. 381–98.
65. Newton PO, Woo SL, Kitabayashi LR, Lyon RM, Anderson DR, Akeson WH. Ultrastructural changes in knee ligaments following immobilization. Matrix. 1990;10(5):314–9.
66. Lindgren M, Unosson M, Fredrikson M, Ek AC. Immobility - a major risk factor for development of pressure ulcers among adult hospitalized patients: a prospective study. Scand J Caring Sci. 2004;18(1):57–64.
67. Azuh O, Gammon H, Burmeister C, Frega D, Nerenz D, DiGiovine B, et al. Benefits of early active mobility in the medical intensive care unit - a pilot study. Am J Med. 2016;129:866.
68. Dhandapani M, Dhandapani S, Agarwal M, Mahapatra AK. Pressure ulcer in patients with severe traumatic brain injury: significant factors and association with neurological outcome. J Clin Nurs. 2014;23(7–8):1114–9.
69. Lundbye-Jensen J, Nielsen JB. Immobilization induces changes in presynaptic control of group Ia afferents in healthy humans. J Physiol. 2008;586(17):4121–35.
70. Dupui P, Montoya R, Costes-Salon MC, Séverac A, Güell A. Balance and gait analysis after 30 days –6 degrees bed rest: influence of lower-body negative-pressure sessions. Aviat Space Environ Med. 1992;63(11):1004–10.
71. De la Torre G. Cognitive neuroscience in space. Life. 2014;4(3):281–94.
72. Malathi S, Batmanabane M. Effects of varying periods of immobilization of a limb on the morphology of a peripheral nerve. Acta Morphol Neerl Scand. 1983;21:185–98.
73. Bryant R. Post-traumatic stress disorder vs traumatic brain injury. Dialogues Clin Neurosci. 2011;13(3):251–62.
74. Dufton LM, Konik B, Colletti R, Stanger C, Boyer M, Morrow S, et al. Effects of stress on pain threshold and tolerance in children with recurrent abdominal pain. Pain. 2008;136(1–2):38–43.
75. Petrie A, Collins W, Solomon P. The tolerance for pain and for sensory deprivation. Am J Psychol. 1960;73(1):80.
76. Nampiaparampil DE. Prevalence of chronic pain after traumatic brain injury: a systematic review. JAMA. 2008;300(6):711–9.
77. Taylor HL, Henschel A. Effects of bed rest on cardiovascular function and work performance. J Appl Physiol. 1949;2(5):223–39.
78. Chobanian AV, Lille RD, Tercyak A, Blevins P. The metabolic and hemodynamic effects of prolonged bed rest in normal subjects. Circulation. 1974;49(3):551–9.
79. Demida BF, Machinskiĭ GV. Use of rehabilitation measures for restoration of human physical work capacity after the prolonged limitation of motor activity. Kosm Biol Aviakosm Med. 1979;13(1):74–5.
80. Gibbs NM. Venous thrombosis of the lower limbs with particular reference to bed-rest. Br J Surg. 1957;45(191):209–36.
81. Okoye GC, Evans JH, Beattie J, Lowe GD, Lorimer AR, Forbes CD. Response of femoral venous oxygen tension to graduated pressure stockings--possible relationship to deep vein thrombosis. Thromb Haemost. 1984;51(1):103–4.
82. Reiff DA, Haricharan RN, Bullington NM, Griffin RL, McGwin G, Rue LW. Traumatic brain injury is associated with the development of deep vein thrombosis independent of pharmacological prophylaxis. J Trauma. 2009;66(5):1436–40.
83. Melada GA, Goldman RH, Luetscher JA, Zager PG. Hemodynamics, renal function, plasma renin, and aldosterone in man after 5 to 14 days of bedrest. Aviat Space Environ Med. 1975;46(8):1049–55.
84. Lamb LE, Stevens PM, Johnson RL. Hypokinesia secondary to chair rest from 4 to 10 days. Aerosp Med (Internet). 1965 (cited 2016 Apr 30);36:755–63. Available from: http://www.ncbi.nlm.nih.gov/pubmed/14334709.
85. Pequignot JM, Guell A, Gauquelin G, Jarsaillon E, Annat G, Bes A, et al. Epinephrine, norepinephrine, and dopamine during a 4-day head-down bed rest. J Appl Physiol. 1985;58(1):157–63.
86. Schulz H, Hillebrecht A, Karemaker JM, ten Harkel AD, Beck L, Baisch F, et al. Cardiopulmonary function during 10 days of head-down tilt bedrest. Acta Physiol Scand Suppl. 1992;604:23–32.
87. Svanberg L. Influence of posture on the lung volumes, ventilation and circulation in normals; a spirometric-bronchospirometric investigation. Scand J Clin Lab Invest. 1957;9(Suppl 25):1–195.
88. Harrison-Felix CL, Whiteneck GG, Jha A, DeVivo MJ, Hammond FM, Hart DM. Mortality over four decades after traumatic brain injury rehabilitation: a retrospective cohort study. Arch Phys Med Rehabil. 2009;90(9):1506–13.
89. Katzan IL, Cebul RD, Husak SH, Dawson NV, Baker DW. The effect of pneumonia on mortality among patients hospitalized for acute stroke. Neurology. 2003;60(4):620–5.
90. Jeschke MG, Klein D, Herndon DN. Insulin treatment improves the systemic inflammatory reaction to severe trauma. Ann Surg. 2004;239(4):553–60.
91. Bloomfield SA. Changes in musculoskeletal structure and function with prolonged bed rest. Med Sci Sports Exerc. 1997;29(2):197–206.
92. Weber JT. Altered calcium signaling following traumatic brain injury. Front Pharmacol. 2012;3:60.
93. Lim YH, Kim DH, Lee MY, Joo MC. Bowel dysfunction and colon transit time in brain-injured patients. Ann Rehabil Med. 2012;36(3):371–8.
94. Chua K, Chuo A, Kong KH. Urinary incontinence after traumatic brain injury: incidence, outcomes and correlates. Brain Inj. 2003;17(6):469–78.
95. Schweickert WD, Pohlman MC, Pohlman AS, Nigos C, Pawlik A, Esbrook CL, et al. Early physical and occupational therapy in mechanically ventilated, critically ill patients: a randomised controlled trial. Lancet. 2009;373(9678):1874–82.
96. Feliciano V, Albuquerque CG, Andrade FM, Dantas CM, Lopez A, Ramos FF, et al. A influência da mobilização precoce no tempo de internamento em unidade de terapia intensiva. ASSOBRAFIR Ciênc. 2012;3(2):31–42.
97. Dantas CM, Silva PF, Siqueira FH, Pinto RM, Matias S, Maciel C, et al. Influence of early mobilization on respiratory and peripheral

muscle strength in critically ill patients. Rev Bras Ter Intensiva. 2012;24(2):173–8.
98. Soares TR, Avena KM, Olivieri FM, Feijó LF, Mendes KM, Souza Filho SA, et al. Retirada do leito após a descontinuação da ventilação mecânica: há repercussão na mortalidade e no tempo de permanência na unidade de terapia intensiva? Rev Bras Ter Intensiva. 2010;22(1):27–32.
99. Pires-Neto RC, Pereira AL, Parente C, Sant'anna GN, Esposito DD, Kimura A, et al. Characterization of the use of a cycle ergometer to assist in the physical therapy treatment of critically ill patients. Rev Bras Ter Intensiva. 2013;25(1):39–43.
100. Morris PE, Goad A, Thompson C, Taylor K, Harry B, Passmore L, et al. Early intensive care unit mobility therapy in the treatment of acute respiratory failure. Crit Care Med. 2008;36(8):2238–43.
101. Pinheiro AR, Christofoletti G. Motor physical therapy in hospitalized patients in an intensive care unit: a systematic review. Rev Bras Ter Intensiva. 2012;24(2):188–96.
102. McWilliams D, Weblin J, Atkins G, Bion J, Williams J, Elliott C, et al. Enhancing rehabilitation of mechanically ventilated patients in the intensive care unit: a quality improvement project. J Crit Care. 2015;30(1):13–8.
103. Lord RK, Mayhew CR, Korupolu R, Mantheiy EC, Friedman MA, Palmer JB, et al. ICU early physical rehabilitation programs: financial modeling of cost savings. Crit Care Med. 2013;41(3):717–24.
104. Sibinelli M, Maioral DC, Falcão ALE, Kosour C, Dragosavac D, Lima NMFV. Efeito imediato do ortostatismo em pacientes internados na unidade de terapia intensiva de adultos. Rev Bras Ter Intensiva. 2012;24(1):64–71.
105. Smelt WL, de Lange JJ, Booij LH. Cardiorespiratory effects of the sitting position in neurosurgery. Acta Anaesthesiol Belg. 1988;39(4):223–31.

# Motor Rehabilitation Program and Robotics

# 5

Rebeca Boltes Cecatto and Linamara Rizzo Battistella

## Introduction

The Brain Injury Association of America (BIAA) defines TBI as brain injury, neither degenerative nor congenital, caused by external physical force. TBI is normally caused by a dynamic impact to the head, resulted from localized shock or from sudden movements produced by shock in other parts of the body. This can result in a combination of compression, expansion, acceleration, deceleration, and rotation of the brain inside the cranium. The complex pathophysiology of TBI includes secondary pathologic processes in the brain as inflammation, ischemia, edema, oxidative stress, apoptosis, excitotoxicity, mitochondrial dysfunction, and many chronic secondary changes [1]. In general the lesion site after TBI may be more diffuse than after stroke and the common region of lesions differ among TBI patients. So TBI lesion can produce altered or diminished state of conscience and disabilities on cognitive, behavioral, emotional, or physical performance. There are also several common neurobehavioral complications after TBI [2]. Moreover behavioral symptoms such as depression and anxiety can overlap with cognitive and motor symptoms. Apathy, fatigue, and attention also modify the clinical pattern of motor, cognitive, and mood clinical complications [3–5]. TBI involves a gradual reactivation of brain function as compensatory and associative circuits. The entire recovery process is in itself dynamic and can be significantly altered by external events, stimulation, and training. But while cognitive dysfunction after TBI is the most common claim cited by caregivers, the extent of injury to the motor system and to motor-related cognitive circuits often overlaps. So rehabilitation includes all four function domains: physical, mental, affective, and social [6].

There are multiple therapeutic strategies that are currently employed for improved neurologic disabilities of TBI patients. Despite continued progress and efforts in occupational, physical, and cognitive rehabilitation, there are many significant unmet clinical needs for more specific and effective therapies [6]. Thus, functional use combined with stimulation may improve late outcome in TBI. Recent advances in our understanding of neural circuitry have support innovative neuromodulation approaches to enhance the functional recovery in patients with acquired brain disorders. A large area of rehabilitation has translated the concept of activity-induced recovery. This emerging approach to motor restoration is now multimodal. It engages the traditional multidisciplinary rehabilitation team with highly structured activity-based therapies, pharmacology, brain stimulation, and robotics [7–17]. Similarly, there is continued support for intensity as a key factor in activity-based therapies and skilled and nonskilled interventions. Aerobic training appears to have multiple benefits: increasing the capacity of gait improvement and endurance for activities of daily living and promoting cognition and mood [18].

Because external stimulation involves constant exchange between outputs from the brain and inputs to brain activation, these approaches may enhance neural circuitry over time, strengthening endogenous plasticity. Thus, in addition to treating specific clinical symptoms of TBI, an early target stimulation of function as robotic therapy may enhance connectivity since brain functional recovery depends in part of activity-dependent mechanisms. In this way numerous rehabilitation robotic devices have been developed since the late 1990s [19, 20].

R. B. Cecatto (✉)
Rehabilitation Department, Institute of Cancer of São Paulo, Clinics Hospital – School of Medicine – University of São Paulo, São Paulo, Brazil
e-mail: boltes@einstein.br

L. R. Battistella
Legal Medicine, Medical Ethics, Social and Occupational Medicine and Physical and Rehabilitation Medicine Institute, Clinics Hospital – School of Medicine – University of São Paulo, São Paulo, Brazil


R. Anghinah et al. (eds.), *Topics in Cognitive Rehabilitation in the TBI Post-Hospital Phase*,
https://doi.org/10.1007/978-3-319-95376-2_5

## Robotic Therapy

Robotic rehabilitation technology can be classified as "service," "assistive," or "therapeutic." Service-based devices are compensatory for patients who cannot provide sufficient voluntary movement to perform a task. Therapeutic devices provide task-specific training. Assistive devices provide variable amounts and types of assistance to help the patient complete a task [20]. Rehabilitation robotic devices may also be described as end-effector type or exoskeleton type. End-effector-type devices apply mechanical forces to the distal segments of limbs, whereas exoskeleton-type devices provide direct control or support of multiple joints to enable functional movement [21, 22]. Although training robots may be clinically useful in many neurological disorders (cerebral palsy, traumatic brain injury, spinal cord injury), stroke therapy is the most studied application. The reasons for this focus on stroke include the large number of people affected; the well-documented motor, cognitive, and behavioral deficits; and the relatively focal deficits that commonly leave stroke survivors capable and motivated to participate in robotic therapy [23].

Although the optimal amount of therapeutic exercise post-TBI remains unknown, an advantage of robotic assistance is the possibility for patients to carry out a great number of movement repetitions, increasing the intensity of therapy. So it's capacity to deliver highly intense and repetitive motor practice is the most obvious benefit of robotic therapy. Robot therapy is still interesting since it improves more movement opportunities than standard therapy. Moreover rehabilitation robotic therapy should be able to respond to any grade of movement made by the patient (thus minimum pathological). This must be based on a fine control of the mechanical interaction with the patient's limb [24]: more than assisting the movement, the goal is to help the patient recover his/her sensorimotor capability. It is important to know that studies describing randomized rehabilitation strategies in TBI patients are restricted [25]. Happily, animal studies have support us to obtain reliable biomarkers for neuroplasticity that have been used to study stimulation therapies in TBI. Physical activity is increasingly being reported as producing beneficial effects on the brain [26]. Rats that are exercised in a voluntary running wheel after injury show increases in BDNF, CREB, synapsin at hippocampus [27, 28], and clinical cognitive improvements [29]. On the other hand, despite the neuroprotective effects of exercise, premature postconcussive exercise has been linked with an exacerbation of post-concussive symptomatology such as depression and cognitive deterioration [30, 31], even as animal studies have shown that forced exercise administered early following cortex injury increases the brain lesion size resulting in a behavioral impairment [32]. So effects of exercise after TBI are time-dependent, and this could explain why many studies about robotic therapy and TBI have better results at chronic patients failing to show good results in the acute phase.

Another important advantage of robots is their ability to deliver a well-defined and reproducible form of exercise therapy. Human therapists vary from person-to-person and from session-to-session in the specific activities that constitute exercise therapy. This lack of standardized therapy makes it difficult to compare different therapy techniques. In contrast, robots deliver exercise therapy based on their programming that varies only based on the patient's performance and as determined by their own pre-established parameters, and this ability to precisely control the therapy delivered enables reliable studies to compare different treatment options and optimize motor retraining. Beside this, the goal of the rehabilitation training is not only to maximize the number of repetition but to maximize the patient attention and voluntary sensorimotor and cognitive participation. Moreover, studies suggest us that monotonous exercises provide worse retention of a skill compared with exciting training. In this way again, robotic therapy seems to be a very promising therapeutic option. Many robots can incorporate virtual reality or gaming scenarios to make exercises more interesting for the patient and to maintain a high level of patient motivation. Besides, while the pioneer devices only controlled articular motion in a single plane, more recently approaches provide 3D interaction at the joint level. These characteristics offer new and interesting perspectives for rehabilitation [20, 23].

In spite of these advantages, robotic therapies have not yet proven to be more effective than dose-matched human delivered treatment. While upper-limb and lower-limb exoskeletons have been used in the clinical practice for several years now (see InMotion© and the Lokomat© by Hocoma), their clinical effects have been little studied. Moreover while robots can be programmed to provide motivating stimuli, they lack the nuanced ability of a human therapist to detect the patient's emotional state, motivation, and engagement. So robots are unable to adjust therapeutic strategies accordingly humor patient. In this way, in TBI rehabilitation, more than stroke patients, this kind of fine control is essential. We know that the main difference about stroke and TBI patients is the fact that stroke patients exhibit more motor than cognitive impairments, while TBI patients present devastating emotional, behavioral, and cognitive impairments within general more slight motor impairments. Moreover most of the literature reviews on robotic devices for rehabilitation concentrate their results in study of just motor functions and rarely cognitive or motor cognitive association impairments. Unhappily this is very disappointing; once at TBI patients, the cognition is a major therapeutic goal.

In this way a very interesting study by Debert et al. (2012) [33] shows the potential of robotic assessments as a refined model to identifying deficits in visuomotor control and position sense following TBI. For each subject with TBI, a review of the initial injury and neuroradiologic findings was conducted. Following this, each subject completed a number of standardized clinical measures (Fugl-Meyer Assessment, Purdue Pegboard, Montreal Cognitive Assessment, Rancho Los Amigos Scale), followed by two robotic tasks. A visually guided task was performed to assess visuomotor control of the limb. Robotic task performance in the subjects with TBI was compared with findings in a cohort of 170 human healthy without disabilities. Subjects with TBI demonstrated a broad range of sensory and motor deficits on robotic testing. Notably, several subjects with TBI displayed significant deficits in one or both of the robotic tasks, despite normal scores on traditional clinical motor and cognitive assessment measures.

Subbian et al. (2014) [34] present the results of robotic-assisted neurologic testing on mild TBI patients in acute period and its ability to predict post-concussion syndrome (PCS) at 3 weeks post-injury. Preliminary results show that abnormal proprioception, as measured using robotic testing, is associated with higher risk of developing PCS following mild TBI.

Kiguchi et al. (2007) [35] compared the mechanical design of selected robotic devices for upper extremity rehabilitation. Robotic interventions can offer kinetic measurements (force and torque trends) and electrograms (such as EEG and EMG) to provide further cognitive insights on the improvement of motor function. They further recommend that the assessment should focus on kinematic analysis more than in electrograms analysis, even this kind of data are currently searched.

Lapitskaya et al. (2011) [36] perform a study with 12 TBI patients, and 14 healthy controls underwent a single training session on a computer-driven gait orthosis (Lokomat®). The sensory pathways were assessed using sensory evoked potentials (SEPs). The global delta-alpha EEG power ratio (DAR) and latency of the P300 component of the event-related potentials were assessed prior to and following a training session. Baseline measurements showed impaired SEPs in the majority of patients and significantly larger DAR in patients compared to healthy controls. Robotic gait training resulted in a reduction of the DAR in healthy subjects but not in patients. No changes were observed in P300 latencies after training in either patients or healthy controls. The study showed that robotic gait training induced measurable changes in the EEG power spectrum in healthy individuals, while no changes were observed in patients with severe TBI. The absence of the EEG changes following training might be an indicator of the severity of brain dysfunction and highlight the importance of minimal cognitive participation of patients for better results.

Recent extensive clinical testing of upper- and lower-limb robot devices (which has been used in clinical practice for many years) has demonstrated its effectiveness with significant improvements in motor capacity of many neurological conditions [37–46]. However, it is controverse if it has a qualitative benefit of robotic devices over a therapist performing the same quantity of movements at TBI patients [47–49].

Several studies have been done using robotic body weight-supported treadmill training (RBWSTT). Although some of the results were encouraging, there is still uncertainty regarding the right patient selection, the right timing, and the best protocol for RBWSTT treatment following TBI. The major benefit of training with the RBWSTT is that patients can practice intensive gait training in a safe and controlled environment. This added security allows individuals to begin walking as soon as they are medically stable at an early stage of very severe motor impairment which is important not only for functional returns but also for prevention of secondary complications such as deep venous thrombosis (DVT), muscle atrophy, cardiovascular deterioration, and pneumonia. The intensity of the training can be also graded by walking speed. In addition, unlike treadmill training sessions that may be limited by therapist fatigue, training sessions on robotic devices like the Lokomat are time-unlimited. Besides the possible neuromodulator effect of robotic therapy, treadmill training following brain has significant cardiovascular and muscular effects.

Beretta et al. (2015) [50] evaluate a group of 23 patients with TBI who underwent 20 sessions of robotic-assisted gait training (RAGT) in addition to traditional manual physiotherapy (PT). All the patients were evaluated before and after the training by using the Gross Motor Function Measures (GMFM) and the Functional Assessment Questionnaire. Ambulant children were also evaluated through the 6-min walk test (6MinWT). After the training, the GMFM showed significant improvement in both dimensions "D" (standing) and "E" (walking). In ambulant patients the 6MinWT showed significant improvement after training, and robotic parameters highlighted a significant increase in cadence, velocity, and stride length. Moreover, hip kinematics on the sagittal plane revealed a statistically significant increase in range of motion (ROM) during the whole gait cycle, increased hip extension during terminal stance, and increased ROM during the swing phase. The data suggest that the combined program, RAGT+PT, induces improvements in functional activities and gaits pattern in children and adolescents with TBI.

Esquenazi et al. (2013) [51] perform a randomized prospective study with 16 participants with TBI randomly assigned to either the robotic-assisted treadmill training (RATT) or manually assisted treadmill training (MATT) group to compare the effects of RATT and MATT on walking self-selected velocity (SSV). Gait training for 45 min,

3 times a week with either RATT or MATT for a total of 18 training sessions, was performed. As results they found that between-group differences were not statistically significant for any measure. However, from pretraining to post-training, the average SSV increased by 49.8% for the RATT group ($P = 0.01$) and by 31% for MATT group ($P = 0.06$). The average maximal velocity increased by 14.9% for the RATT group ($P = 0.06$) and by 30.8% for the MATT group ($P = 0.01$). Step-length asymmetry ratio improved during SSV by 33.1% for the RATT group ($P = 0.01$) and by 9.1% for the MATT group ($P = 0.73$). The distance walked increased by 11.7% for the robotic group ($P = 0.21$) and by 19.3% for manual group ($P = 0.03$). The results of this study demonstrate greater improvement in symmetry of gait for RATT and no significant differences between RATT and MATT with regard to improvement in gait velocity and endurance, providing evidence that participants with a chronic TBI can experience improvements in gait parameters with gait training with either MATT or RATT.

In 2015 the Cochrane Library published a review performed to assess the effects of multidisciplinary rehabilitation following TBI in adults 16–65 years of age, including studies about robotic therapy [52]. As results we have that within the subgroup of predominantly mild brain injury, "strong evidence" suggested that most individuals made a good recovery when appropriate information was provided, without the need for additional specific interventions as robotic. For moderate to severe injury, "strong evidence" showed benefit from formal intervention, and "limited evidence" indicated that commencing rehabilitation early after injury results in better outcomes. For participants with moderate to severe TBI already in rehabilitation, "strong evidence" revealed that more intensive programs such as robotic treatment are associated with earlier functional gains. The context of multidisciplinary rehabilitation appears to influence outcomes. "Strong evidence" supports the use of a coordinated rehabilitation model for patients with severe brain injury, in which comprehensive cognitive rehabilitation takes place in a therapeutic environment and involves a peer group of patients with intensive motor training.

Unhappily no currently available robot can assist TBI patients with home activities of daily living (ADLs) as learning dressing tasks or with bathroom transfers. Thus robots tend to be used to supplement, rather than substitute for, conventional therapy. Systematic review and meta-analysis of the trials performed in stroke patients suggest that robotic training improves motor impairment and strength but do not improve ability to perform ADLs.

All together these results show us that there may be multiple roles for development of robotic technology in TBI, depending on the specific purpose needed and particularly symptoms to be treated. These may vary from simply detecting the presence of mild TBI to more complex moderate and severe TBI issues. Consequently, different interventions and combinations of interventions are required to meet the needs of patients with different problems. Once intensive intervention appears to lead to earlier gains, and once group-based rehabilitation in a therapeutic-enrolled environment (where patients undergo neuropsychological rehabilitation with a peer group of individuals facing similar challenges submitted to intensive motor training) represents an effective approach for TBI patients, robotic therapy could be a valuable tool in the TBI rehabilitation. Thus the most important advantage of robotic systems could be their ability to provide more intensive repetitive training than human therapists. But this should not be used in isolation, but in conjunction with other traditional therapies.

## Conclusion

Robotic therapy and neuromodulation approaches may enhance recovery from TBI, by directly enhancing axonal sprouting and other mechanisms of neural compensation, as well as modulating endogenous neural recovery plasticity and cardiovascular, metabolic, and muscular effects.

The limitations to the application of robotics is defining the more promising symptoms to be treated, how to optimize predictive function, and the better therapy parameters.

Robots provide a safe method for providing well-defined, reproducible therapeutic exercises. Advantages of robots compared with dose-matched human therapy remain exciting but still unproven. Some of the advantages of robotic devices in delivering intensive therapy have been designed. These advantages are very useful to TBI patients for which it is precious to make the motor training coupled with cognitive training. Adding measures of cardiac and metabolic responses would make these devices better to rehabilitation clinics.

However, these devices break down the rehabilitation routine service, and they are very expensive. Moreover the biggest disadvantage is they do not have the same "feel" as therapists do. While robots have high-resolution sensors that can also monitor such events, they uncommonly are programmed to do so. Integrating advanced concepts such as virtual reality and quantifying impairments such as weakness and spasticity are not in the routine.

Another future research point is to move robotic therapy into the home environment, where patients require less supervision. This approach requires devices that are easier to use and also less expensive.

The effectiveness of robotics over conventional therapy is exciting, but the best therapy strategy is still not clear. Advances in robotic therapy and research are likely to profoundly change the way we treat patients with TBI in the future and the use of various rehabilitation modalities together likely be the most promise.

## References


1. Park E, Bell JD, Baker AJ. Traumatic brain injury: can the consequences be stopped? CMAJ. 2008;178(9):1163–70.
2. Bombardier CH, Fann JR, Temkin NR, Esselman PC, Barber J, Dikmen SS. Rates of major depressive disorder and clinical outcomes following traumatic brain injury. JAMA. 2010;303(19):1938–45.
3. Hoofien D, Gilboa A, Vakil E, Donovick PJ. Traumatic brain injury (TBI) 10-20 years later: a comprehensive outcome study of psychiatric symptomatology, cognitive abilities and psychosocial functioning. Brain Inj. 2001;15(3):189–209.
4. Hoofien D, Gilboa A, Vakil E, Barak O. Unawareness of cognitive deficits and daily functioning among persons with traumatic brain injuries. J Clin Exp Neuropsychol. 2004;26(2):278–90.
5. Hoofien D, Barak O, Vakil E, Gilboa A. Symptom checklist-90 revised scores in persons with traumatic brain injury: affective reactions or neurobehavioral outcomes of the injury? Appl Neuropsychol. 2005;12(1):30–9.
6. Almeida TLT, Falkenburg L, Nascimento RZR, Reis CA, Sales VC, Pedroso TD, et al. Traumatismo cranioencefálico: reabilitação. Acta Fisiátrica. 2012;19(2):130. ISSN 0104–7795
7. Fu MJ, Knutson JS, Chae J. Stroke rehabilitation using virtual environments. Phys Med Rehabil Clin N Am. 2015;26(4):747–57.
8. Knutson JS, Fu MJ, Sheffler LR, Chae J. Neuromuscular electrical stimulation for motor restoration in hemiplegia. Phys Med Rehabil Clin N Am. 2015;26(4):729–45.
9. Caleo M. Rehabilitation and plasticity following stroke: insights from rodent models. Neuroscience. 2015;311:180–94.
10. Pin-Barre C, Laurin J. Physical exercise as a diagnostic, rehabilitation, and preventive tool: influence on neuroplasticity and motor recovery after stroke. Neural Plast. 2015;2015:608581.
11. Mrachacz-Kersting N, Jiang N, Stevenson AJ, Niazi IK, Kostic V, Pavlovic A, et al. Efficient neuroplasticity induction in chronic stroke patients by an associative brain-computer interface. J Neurophysiol. 2016;115(3):1410–21.
12. Xu Y, Hou QH, Russell SD, Bennett BC, Sellers AJ, Lin Q, et al. Neuroplasticity in post-stroke gait recovery and noninvasive brain stimulation. Neural Regen Res. 2015;10(12):2072–80.
13. Livingston-Thomas J, Nelson P, Karthikeyan S, Antonescu S, Jeffers MS, Marzolini S, et al. Exercise and environmental enrichment as enablers of task-specific neuroplasticity and stroke recovery. Neurotherapeutics. 2016;13(2):395–402.
14. Kantak SS, Zahedi N, McGrath RL. Task-dependent bimanual coordination after stroke: relationship with sensorimotor impairments. Arch Phys Med Rehabil. 2016;97(5):798–806.
15. Dobkin BH. Collaborative models for translational neuroscience and rehabilitation research. Neurorehabil Neural Repair. 2009a;23(7):633–40.
16. Dobkin BH. Motor rehabilitation after stroke, traumatic brain, and spinal cord injury: common denominators within recent clinical trials. Curr Opin Neurol. 2009b;22(6):563–9.
17. Cheeran B, Cohen L, Dobkin B, Ford G, Greenwood R, Howard D, et al. The future of restorative neurosciences in stroke: driving the translational research pipeline from basic science to rehabilitation of people after stroke. Neurorehabil Neural Repair. 2009;23(2):97–107.
18. Breceda EY, Dromerick AW. Motor rehabilitation in stroke and traumatic brain injury: stimulating and intense. Curr Opin Neurol. 2013;26(6):595–601.
19. Brewer BR, McDowell SK, Worthen-Chaudhari LC. Poststroke upper extremity rehabilitation: a review of robotic systems and clinical results. Top Stroke Rehabil. 2007;14(6):22–44.
20. Maciejasz P, Eschweiler J, Gerlach-Hahn K, Jansen-Troy A, Leonhardt S. A survey on robotic devices for upper limb rehabilitation. J Neuroeng Rehabil. 2014;11:3.
21. Jarrassé N, Proietti T, Crocher V, Robertson J, Sahbani A, Morel G, et al. Robotic exoskeletons: a perspective for the rehabilitation of arm coordination in stroke patients. Front Hum Neurosci. 2014;8:947.
22. Chang WH, Kim YH. Robot-assisted therapy in stroke rehabilitation. J Stroke. 2013;15(3):174–81.
23. Poli P, Morone G, Rosati G, Masiero S. Robotic technologies and rehabilitation: new tools for stroke patients' therapy. Biomed Res Int. 2013;2013:153872.
24. Maclean N, Pound P. A critical review of the concept of patient motivation in the literature on physical rehabilitation. Soc Sci Med. 2000;50(4):495–506.
25. Rimmer JH, Chen MD, McCubbin JA, Drum C, Peterson J. Exercise intervention research on persons with disabilities: what we know and where we need to go. Am J Phys Med Rehabil. 2010;89(3):249–63.
26. van Praag H, Kempermann G, Gage F. Running increases cell proliferation and neurogenesis in the adult mouse dentate gyrus. Nat Neurosci. 1999;2(3):266–70.
27. Griesbach GS, Gomez-Pinilla F, Hovda DA. The upregulation of plasticity-related proteins following TBI is disrupted with acute voluntary exercise. Brain Res. 2004a;1016(2):154–62.
28. Griesbach GS, Hovda DA, Molteni R, Wu A, Gomez-Pinilla F. Voluntary exercise following traumatic brain injury: brain-derived neurotrophic factor upregulation and recovery of function. Neuroscience. 2004b;125(1):129–39.
29. Piao CS, Stoica BA, Wu J, Sabirzhanov B, Zhao Z, Cabatbat R, et al. Late exercise reduces neuroinflammation and cognitive dysfunction after traumatic brain injury. Neurobiol Dis. 2013;54:252–63.
30. Guskiewicz KM, Goldman SB. A changing landscape: traumatic brain injury in military combat and civilian athletics. FASEB J. 2013;27(11):4327–9.
31. Guskiewicz KM. When treating sport concussion, check the boxes, but also go the extra mile. J Athl Train. 2013;48(4):441.
32. Humm J, Kozlowski D, James D, Gotts J, Schallert T. Use-dependent exacerbation of brain damage occurs during an early post-lesion vulnerable period. Brain Res. 1998;783(2):286–92.
33. Debert CT, Herter TM, Scott SH, Dukelow S. Robotic assessment of sensorimotor deficits after traumatic brain injury. J Neurol Phys Ther. 2012;36(2):58–67.
34. Subbian V, Meunier JM, Korfhagen JJ, Ratcliff JJ, Shaw GJ, Beyette FR. Quantitative assessment of post-concussion syndrome following mild traumatic brain injury using robotic technology. Conf Proc IEEE Eng Med Biol Soc. 2014;2014:5353–6.
35. Kiguchi K, Imada Y, Liyanage M. EMG-based neuro-fuzzy control of a 4DOF upper-limb power-assist exoskeleton. Conf Proc IEEE Eng Med Biol Soc. 2007;2007:3040–3.
36. Lapitskaya N, Nielsen JF, Fuglsang-Frederiksen A. Robotic gait training in patients with impaired consciousness due to severe traumatic brain injury. Brain Inj. 2011;25(11):1070–9.
37. Krebs HI, Ferraro M, Buerger SP, Newbery MJ, Makiyama A, Sandmann M, et al. Rehabilitation robotics: pilot trial of a spatial extension for MIT-Manus. J Neuroeng Rehabil. 2004;1(1):5.
38. Krebs HI, Volpe BT, Williams D, Celestino J, Charles SK, Lynch D, et al. Robot-aided neurorehabilitation: a robot for wrist rehabilitation. IEEE Trans Neural Syst Rehabil Eng. 2007;15(3):327–35.
39. Krebs HI, Volpe B, Hogan N. A working model of stroke recovery from rehabilitation robotics practitioners. J Neuroeng Rehabil. 2009;6:6.
40. Krebs HI, Volpe BT. Rehabilitation robotics. Handb Clin Neurol. 2013;110:283–94.
41. Krebs HI, Krams M, Agrafiotis DK, DiBernardo A, Chavez JC, Littman GS, et al. Robotic measurement of arm movements after stroke establishes biomarkers of motor recovery. Stroke. 2014;45(1):200–4.
42. Krebs HI, Volpe BT. Robotics: a rehabilitation modality. Curr Phys Med Rehabil Rep. 2015;3(4):243–147.

43. Lo AC, Guarino P, Krebs HI, Volpe BT, Bever CT, Duncan PW, et al. Multicenter randomized trial of robot-assisted rehabilitation for chronic stroke: methods and entry characteristics for VA ROBOTICS. Neurorehabil Neural Repair. 2009;23(8):775–83.
44. Volpe BT, Ferraro M, Lynch D, Christos P, Krol J, Trudell C, et al. Robotics and other devices in the treatment of patients recovering from stroke. Curr Atheroscler Rep. 2004;6(4):314–9.
45. Volpe BT, Ferraro M, Lynch D, Christos P, Krol J, Trudell C, et al. Robotics and other devices in the treatment of patients recovering from stroke. Curr Neurol Neurosci Rep. 2005;5(6):465–70.
46. Schwartz I, Meiner Z. Robotic-assisted gait training in neurological patients: who may benefit? Ann Biomed Eng. 2015;43(5):1260–9.
47. Lo AC, Guarino PD, Richards LG, Haselkorn JK, Wittenberg GF, Federman DG, et al. Robot-assisted therapy for long-term upper-limb impairment after stroke. N Engl J Med. 2010;362(19):1772–83.
48. Volpe BT, Lynch D, Rykman-Berland A, Ferraro M, Galgano M, Hogan N, et al. Intensive sensorimotor arm training mediated by therapist or robot improves hemiparesis in patients with chronic stroke. Neurorehabil Neural Repair. 2008;22(3):305–10.
49. Volpe BT, Huerta PT, Zipse JL, Rykman A, Edwards D, Dipietro L, et al. Robotic devices as therapeutic and diagnostic tools for stroke recovery. Arch Neurol. 2009;66(9):1086–90.
50. Beretta E, Romei M, Molteni E, Avantaggiato P, Strazzer S. Combined robotic-aided gait training and physical therapy improve functional abilities and hip kinematics during gait in children and adolescents with acquired brain injury. Brain Inj. 2015;29(7–8):955–62.
51. Esquenazi A, Lee S, Packel AT, Braitman L. A randomized comparative study of manually assisted versus robotic-assisted body weight supported treadmill training in persons with a traumatic brain injury. PM R. 2013;5(4):280–90.
52. Turner-Stokes L, Pick A, Nair A, Disler PB, Wade DT. Multidisciplinary rehabilitation for acquired brain injury in adults of working age. Cochrane Database Syst Rev. 2015;12:CD004170.

# Extrapyramidal Syndromes After Traumatic Brain Injury

6

Egberto Reis Barbosa, Sara Carvalho Barbosa Casagrande, and Christian Henrique de Andrade Freitas

Traumatic brain injury (TBI) may account for a range of neurologic syndromes. Generally, the resulting symptoms depend on the trauma location and severity. In severe trauma with structural brain abnormalities, the occurrence of movement disorders is well recognized, mainly hyperkinesias such as tremor, dystonia, and parkinsonism. The presence of clinical-neuroanatomic correlations and the timing between TBI and symptom onset are essential for the diagnosis. The purpose of this chapter is to provide an overview of the movement disorders associated with head trauma, their usual characteristics and pathophysiology, as well as the appropriate management of these disorders.

## Tremor

Tremor is an involuntary and rhythmic muscle contraction leading to trembling or shaking movement in one or more parts of the body. It is the most common posttraumatic movement disorder. Different types of tremor can emerge after a TBI such as resting, postural, kinect, intention, and Holmes tremor. The mean time between the TBI and the symptom onset ranges from 1 to 3 weeks [1]. Usually, direct lesions on cerebellar input/output or thalamic pathways or midbrain connections are the main reasons for trauma-induced tremor. Those brain areas are part of or play a role on the dentate-rubro-thalamic tract [2]. Another important etiology is the diffuse axonal injury (DAI), which typically results from shearing forces from rotational accelerations/deceleration, which have a predilection for axons at the gray-white matter junction. Thus, multiple brain areas are damaged at the same time, disturbing the motor neurons input and output and promoting different movement disorders such as tremor. It is classic associated with high-energy close head trauma [3]. However, Biary and colleagues published seven cases of mild to moderate TBI followed by postural and kinect tremor after days to weeks of latency. At that time, CT scan and MRI scan were without abnormalities, and the cause of posttraumatic tremor remained unknown. Therefore, small lesions or biochemical changes were hypothesized as possible causes [3–6] reported damage of the dentate-rubro-thalamic tract by mild TBI in two patients. After a latency of 1–2 weeks, those patients developed a resting and intention tremor.

Two retrospective studies (Table 6.1) analyzed the association between severity of TBI and tremor. A larger number of patients were evaluated. The collected data showed that either mild or severe head trauma could cause a disabling tremor. The onset latency of tremor was just a little higher in severe head injury. That is explained by the diffuse brain damage and longer coma time which cause a delay in motor recovery and consequently a delay in tremor onset [6–8].

Holmes tremor is described as a rest and intention tremor with irregular amplitude and slow frequency and is also known as rubral or mesencephalic tremor. However, such terms are not used anymore because typical Holmes tremor has been described in other brain area lesions, and guided injury of red nucleus lesions fails to cause such tremor. It is a very disabling condition. According to a recent review, head trauma was the second main cause of Holmes tremor [9]. Despite the poor or minimal results in posttraumatic tremor, a few possibilities of oral medications can be used such as levodopa, propranolol, and clonazepam [1, 10]. In some cases, thalamic or zona incerta stereotactic lesional surgery seems to be an effective treatment option [9–11]. Deep brain stimulation (DBS) is an emerging therapy with encouraging results for post-TBI tremor. The main targets are ventral intermediate nucleus of thalamus and globus pallidus internus [12].

E. R. Barbosa (✉) · S. C. B. Casagrande · C. H. de Andrade Freitas
Movement Disorders Unit, Department of Neurology, Clinics Hospital – School of Medicine – University of São Paulo, São Paulo, Brazil
e-mail: egbertob@8415.com.br



R. Anghinah et al. (eds.), *Topics in Cognitive Rehabilitation in the TBI Post-Hospital Phase*,
https://doi.org/10.1007/978-3-319-95376-2_6

**Table 6.1** Data from two studies analyzing the relationship between severity of TBI and tremor onset

| Author | Severity TBI | Number of patients | Tremor (%) | Types of tremor | Latency |
|---|---|---|---|---|---|
| Krauss, et al. (Neurology [6, 7]) | Severe head injury (GCS < 9) | 221 | 42 (19%) | Postural/kinect /intention | LF: 2 weeks to 6 months<br>HF: Days to few weeks |
| Krauss, et al. (Movement Disorders [8]) | Mild or moderate head injury (GCS > 8) | 158 | 15 (9.5%) | Postural/ intention | HF only<br>Hours to few days |

*GCS* Glasgow Coma Scale, *LF* low frequency, *HF* high frequency

## Dystonia

Dystonia is defined as a movement disorder characterized by sustained or intermittent muscle contractions causing abnormal, often repetitive, movements, postures, or both [12]. Other involuntary movements like tremor or myoclonia can be associated. Krauss et al. [8] studied the occurrence of post-TBI movement disorders in 398 survivors (with Glasgow Coma Scale of eight or less) of severe head injury, and 4.1% of them had dystonia. It may be difficult to distinguish dystonia from superimposed spasticity, and this can compromise the treatment. The onset of dystonia can be variable, from minutes to years after trauma [13, 14]. Usually the progression is slow and tends to stabilized. The diagnostic criteria of posttraumatic dystonia require a temporal and anatomic relationship between the movement and the injury. The subtypes are focal, segmental, and generalized hemidystonia. Hemidystonia is the most common presentation of post-TBI dystonia [13, 16–18].

Hemidystonia is one of the most common manifestations of secondary dystonia associated with brain structural lesions. Perinatal injury, closed-head injury, encephalitis, and thalamotomy have been reported to cause hemidystonia [19]. Krauss et al. published a series of nine patients with posttraumatic dystonia, seven of eight patients with pure hemidystonia had lesions involving the contralateral caudate or putamen, and one patient with hemidystonia plus torticollis had a contralateral mesencephalic lesion [13]. Dystonia due to head injury accounts for 7–9% of all cases of symptomatic hemidystonia [15]. Posttraumatic hemidystonia frequently is associated with ipsilateral hemiparesis [14]. The mean latency between injury and the onset of dystonia is 20 months [13]. It is possible that the delay of onset of dystonia after static brain lesions is associated with the age at trauma. Young patients (less than 7 years old) with hemidystonia secondary to brain lesions had a longer latency between the lesion and the manifestation of dystonia compared to adults [20]. Manifestations of posttraumatic dystonia such as cervical dystonia, segmental axial dystonia, and spasmodic dysphonia are rare [13, 21, 22]. Lesions in the striatum, particularly in the putamen, thalamus, pontomesencephalic region, and rarely in caudate nucleus and globus pallidus can cause dystonia [23, 24]. It is very common in posttraumatic dystonia the presence of focal cerebral lesions. Dystonia secondary to pallidal lesions are unusual [25, 26]. The mechanisms involved are not understood.

Oral medication like anticholinergic drugs can be tried; however, in posttraumatic dystonia, the response is usually minimal. For post-TBI torticollis and other focal dystonias, botulinum toxin (BTx) injections are indicated [27, 28]. In case of refractory symptoms in post-TBI hemidystonia or generalized and disabling dystonia, functional stereotactic surgery is a treatment option [13]. DBS or ablative lesions can be indicated. Usually the targets include the ventrolateral thalamus, the subthalamic nucleus, and the globus pallidus internus [29]. There are some studies comparing thalamic targets versus pallidal surgery. The response to surgery for dystonia is variable and dependent on cause. Patients with secondary dystonia presented less improvement compared with primary dystonia [29–32]. The effect can be earlier, and a few reports demonstrated long-term efficacy of DBS [33–35]. Selected patients with posttraumatic hemidystonia, including following penetrating head injury, represent one group of secondary dystonias that might benefit from DBS surgery [36]. In patients with generalized dystonia associated with spasticity or hemiballism, an intrathecal baclofen via an implanted pump may provide improvement of the symptoms [37–39]. In dystonia secondary to subdural hematoma, including in a report of Pisa syndrome (tonic flexion of trunk), the outcome is favorable after drainage of the hematoma [40–42].

## Parkinson Disease

Parkinson disease (PD) is the second most common neurodegenerative disease around the world. According to the Movement Disorder Society, the core feature of this disease includes bradykinesia plus rest tremor or rigidity [43].

The discussion regarding PD and traumatic brain injury (TBI) has been going on for a long time. The first one that hypothesized a relationship between TBI and PD was James Parkinson, in his *An Essay on the Shaking Palsy* in 1817. Since then, much research has been done on that topic [1].

An important epidemiologic study suggested that several environmental factors, including TBI, may increase the risk of PD [44]. Crane and colleagues analyzed the late effects of TBI with loss of consciousness through clinical signs and autopsy and its association with neurodegenerative process. After collecting data from three prospective cohort studies, an increased risk for Lewy body accumulation and PD was found [45]. A recent retrospective cohort study was performed among the emergency departments from California hospitals. A total of 165,799 patients were enrolled in the study, including 52,393 (32%) with TBI. Comparing to a trauma to the rest of the body, TBI in later life has increased 44% the risk of PD over a follow-up period of just 5 to 7 years [46, 47]. Interesting data was found in a survey performed by Taylor and colleagues [48]. After excluding TBI that occurred less than 10 years prior to the diagnosis of PD, the results suggested that head injury in early life increases the risk of PD [51]. A large systematic review and meta-analysis about head trauma and risk of PD concluded that severe TBI, describe as head trauma followed by cerebral concussion, should be considered an environmental risk factor for PD [49].

TBI can promote lesions on multiple sites of the dopaminergic pathways and secondary lesions due to release of oxidative cytokines, glutamate excitotoxicity, inflammatory damage, and the toxicity of metabolites that can be disseminated by the circulatory system, triggering the neurodegenerative process and accumulation of Lewy bodies [45, 50]. Experimental essays demonstrated that mice exposed to TBI show a significant accumulation of α-synuclein in microglia compared to astrocytes. Besides there is significant decrease of tyrosine hydroxylase, an enzyme required for the synthesis of dopamine in neurons. Those results suggest that PD-related molecular events can be triggered upon TBI [51]. Based on these data, the association between TBI and PD seems to be clear. However, a systematic review published by the International Collaboration on Mild Traumatic Brain Injury Prognosis in 2014 argues that there is no strong evidence for casual association between TBI and PD due the lack of high-quality studies [52]. One year later, a Danish case-control study explored the same subject, enrolling more than 3000 patients. Its results did not support the hypothesis that head injury increases the risk for PD [53].

Therefore, the true relationships of TBI and risk of PD remain inconclusive. It is a challenging neurodegenerative disorder that requires a multidisciplinary approach. Despite all the available medication option, levodopa remains as the most effective drug in the treatment of PD. A selected group of patients may benefit from surgical treatment, which can be a stereotactic ablative procedure or an implant of DBS electrode in subthalamic nucleus or globus pallidus internal [54, 55].

## Parkinsonism

There are several cases of parkinsonism secondary to TBI described on literature. Krauss et al. studied the occurrence of posttraumatic movement disorders in 398 survivors (with Glasgow Coma Scale of 8 or less) of severe head injury. Posttraumatic movement disorders were found in 22.6% of 221 patients, and 0.9% were parkinsonism [5]. The onset of the symptoms is usually after a month of the injury. The relationship between trauma and parkinsonism in some cases is unclear, but others are related to the interruption of dopaminergic pathways connecting the midbrain, substantia nigra, basal ganglia, and frontal lobes. However, some cases of post-TBI parkinsonism had lesions in other parts of the central nervous system [56].

Parkinsonism syndrome has been observed after TBI or as part of chronic traumatic encephalopathy (CTE), which is a tauopathy neurodegenerative disease secondary to TBI. In 2013 a review publish by Wong and Hazrati [57] tried to elucidate the potential relationship between TBI and subsequent development of parkinsonism. It is important to know the difference between idiopathic PD versus parkinsonism. The first one is a synucleinopathy with specific clinical and neuropathological diagnostic criteria, and parkinsonism is a set of signs and symptoms like rigidity, tremors, and bradykinesia. While it remains unclear the association between TBI and idiopathic PD, there are many reports and studies of parkinsonism syndrome secondary to TBI [57]. In 1934 Grimberg et al. described the first cases of posttraumatic parkinsonism and proposed that the diagnosis could be made only if the patient had a trauma with a sufficient severity to produce definite damage to the brain, directly to the head, and with clear and definite connection between trauma and the disease [58]. Repetitive closed-head injury occurs in a wide variety of contact sports, including football, boxing, rugby, hockey, skiing, and soccer. Boxing is the most frequent sport associated with CTE, and disease duration is the longest in boxers [59, 60]. The pugilistic parkinsonism is a chronic encephalopathy secondary to several years of cumulative concussions and direct repeat trauma to the head, mainly in boxers athletes. The frequency has been estimated 20 to 50% of professional boxers. The clinical presentation can be variable including dementia, behavioral changes, tremor at rest, cerebellar symptoms, dysarthria, and hypophonia [61–65]. The severity correlates to how long the patient has been professionally active [66]. Positron emission tomographic studies have revealed uniform nigrostriatal involvement but relative sparing of caudate function in these patients [65]. Neuropathological studies have revealed depigmentation of the substantia nigra but an absence of Lewy bodies [67]. In amateur boxers the development of chronic encephalopathy is controversial [68, 69]. Studies suggest a genetic predisposition in patients that developed the disease [70]. In a recent research published by Jesse Mez et al. involving 202 donated brains from football players who died in 2014 or later, a high proportion (87%) had neuropathological evidence of CTE. Professional players had severe pathology. The majority of patients presented behavioral and mood symptoms, cognitive symptoms, and signs of dementia (mainly in severe CTE pathology) [71]. Except for penetrating injury, parkinsonism is a rare complication of a single head injury. Lesions of substance nigra can develop hemiparkinsonism, and weeks after a subdural hematoma, there are some case reported of secondary parkinsonism with favorable outcome after drainage [72].

The treatment of posttraumatic parkinsonism is the same as for Parkinson disease, but the response to medications is less predictable. Patients with established lesions in substantia nigra may benefit from levodopa therapy [73]. To optimize the management of post-TBI parkinsonism, it is important to recognize the disease early. Matsuda et al. described three patients in vegetative state (3–12 months) post-TBI with parkinsonism after lesions in the substantia nigra that presented a dramatic improvement of consciousness after levodopa therapy [74]. Jelling K.A et al. described 19 patients at the same condition that have some levodopa response as well [75]. Deep brain stimulation of the thalamus or subthalamic nucleus (STN) may be an option in selected medically refractory patients [76, 77].

## Other Hyperkinetic Posttraumatic Movement Disorders

### Myoclonus

Myoclonus is a hyperkinetic movement disorder consisting of brief, quick, and involuntary jerks caused by muscle contractions (positive myoclonus) or interruptions of tonic muscle activity (negative myoclonus) [78]. It is a common movement disorder that happens due to a cortical irritability. It can happen in 0.5% of posttraumatic movement disorders and normally resolve after few weeks of the trauma [79]. Only single cases of posttraumatic myoclonus have been described [79–81]. Normally, the dentate or olivary nucleus is involved. Pharmacological treatment with levetiracetam can be tried, and in selected cases, the stereotactic surgery is indicated, and the targets usually are thalamus (ventrolateral nucleus) or Forel's campotomy [82].

### Tics

Tics are repeated, intermittent, simple, or complex movements; they are usually preceded by a premonitory sensation (urge feeling) that relief after the movement. Characteristic features include predictability, suggestibility, and voluntary suppressibility [78]. Posttraumatic tics and tourettism after head trauma have been described in few reports [83, 84, 85]. The diagnosis of posttraumatic tics needs history of well-documented head trauma, negative history of tics prior to TBI, and presence of other sequelae of TBI [83]. The onset of the tics starts after weeks to years following the trauma [85]. Most of the patients with early posttraumatic tics developed the symptoms after a mild to moderate TBI and had normal brain imaging [86]. Basal ganglia lesions can happen in 9% of subjects with secondary tics, and there is one case of posttraumatic tics described by Screecher et al. with these findings on MRI [83, 86]. In one patient reported by Krauss et al. with a severe head injury, in whom the tics were accompanied by marked obsessive-compulsive behavior, diffuse subcortical white matter changes were observed [87]. However, early posttraumatic tics could be aggravation of childhood tics. Neuronal regeneration after injury often results in aberrant neuronal connections. Posttraumatic movement disorders are due to these late effects of TBI [88]. Similarly, late onset posttraumatic tics could be due to a delayed effect of TBI on neural circuits connecting the frontal cortex and basal ganglia. The pharmacological treatment can relieve the severity of tics and include alpha agonist, benzodiazepine, antipsychotics, and tetrabenazine. Deep brain stimulation and botulinum toxin have been reported to be beneficial in selected cases of tics [89, 90].

### Ballism and Chorea

Ballism is characterized by high amplitude, almost violent movements that mainly involve the proximal limb joints [78]. Chorea is an irregular, unpredictable, and involuntary random-appearing sequence of one or more involuntary movements that spread from one muscle group to another [78]. There are some reports on literature of hemiballism and chorea secondary to trauma brain injury [25, 91, 92]. Hemiballismus happens usually secondary to lesions of the subthalamic nucleus [7, 91]. Posttraumatic hemiballism is associated with severe closed-head injury. The mechanism of posttraumatic chorea is poorly understood and can be secondary of loss of normal pallidal inhibitory input. The onset may occur after weeks or several months after TBI. In contrast to vascular hemiballism, posttraumatic hemiballism seems to be more persistent with less tendency for spontaneous improvement [10, 25]. Pharmacological intervention can control significantly the symptoms [91], and patients with persistent movements can benefit from functional stereotactic surgery. Targets include globus pallidum, thalamus, or zona incerta [93, 94]. Choreic movements caused by epidural or subdural hematoma are rare and considered reversible symptom, usually with favorable prognosis after drainage of the hematoma [95–97].

## Akathisia

Akathisia (from the Greek, meaning "unable to sit still") refers to a feeling of inner, general restlessness, which is reduced or relieved by moving about [98]. There are few cases in literature describing akathisia and paroxysmal dyskinesia after TBI. The onset is described minutes to month after TBI [98–101]. In both cases the diagnosis can be difficult with several differential diagnosis including anxiety, psychomotor agitation, seizures, and confusional status. Collateral effects of medication administration should always be considered [98]. These movements can respond favorably to oral medication (benzodiazepines, beta-adrenergic blockers, bromocriptine, and anticholinergic agents) [98, 101].

## Psychogenic Movement Disorders

Psychogenic movement disorder is suggested by inconsistent and incongruent movements, with abrupt onset after trauma and spontaneous remissions [78]. It is more reported after peripheral than central injury, usually involved in minor traumatic events, and occurs probably because of psychological component associated by the trauma [102, 103].

## References


1. Koller WC, Wong GF, Lang A. Posttraumatic movement disorders: a review. Mov Disord. 1989;4:20–36.
2. Jang SH, Kwon HG. Injury of the dentato-rubro-thalamic tract in a patient with mild traumatic brain injury. Brain Inj. 2015;29(13–14):1725–8.
3. Yaguchi H, Niida H, Yaguchi M, Tachikawa H, Sekihara Y. A case of postural and kinetic tremor caused by diffuse axonal injury. Rinsho Shinkeigaku. 2003;43(1–2):41–4.
4. Biary N, Cleeves L, Findley L, Koller W. Post-traumatic tremor. Neurology. 1989;39:103–6.
5. Jang SH, Lee HD. Severe and extensive traumatic axonal injury following minor and indirect head trauma. Brain Inj. 2017;31(3):416–9.
6. Krauss JK, Tränkle R, Kopp KH. Post-traumatic movement disorders in survivors of severe head injury. Neurology. 1996;47(6):1488–92.
7. Krauss JK, Borremans JJ, Nobbe F, Mundinger F. Ballism not related to vascular disease: a report of 16 patients and review of the literature. Parkinsonism Relat Disord. 1996;2:35–45.
8. Krauss JK, Trankle R, Kopp KH. Posttraumatic movement disorders after moderate or mild head injury. Mov Disord. 1997;12(3):428–31.
9. Raina GB, Cersosimo MG, Folgar SS, Giugni JC, Calandra C, Paviolo JP, et al. Holmes tremor: clinical description, lesion localization, and treatment in a series of 29 cases. Neurology. 2016;86(10):931–8.
10. Krauss JK. Movement disorders secondary to craniocerebral trauma. Handb Clin Neurol. 2015;128:475–96.
11. Contreras Lopez WO, Azevedo AR, Cury RG, Alencar F, Neville IS, Reis PR, et al. Caudal zona Incerta/VOP radiofrequency lesioning guided by combined stereotactic MRI and microelectrode recording for posttraumatic midbrain resting kinetic tremor. World Neurosurg. 2016;86:316–20.
12. Issar NM, Hedera P, Phibbs FT, Konrad PE, Neimat JS. Treating post-traumatic tremor with deep brain stimulation: report of five cases. Parkinsonism Relat Disord. 2013;19(12):1100–5.
13. Albanese A, Bathia K, Bressman SB, et al. Phenomenology an classification of dystonia: a consensus update. Mov Disord. 28(7):863–73.
14. Krauss JK, Mohadjer M, Braus DF, Wakhloo AK, Nobbe F, Mundinger F. Dystonia following head trauma: a report of nine patients and review of the literature. Mov Disord. 1992;7:263–72.
15. Silver JK, Lux WE. Early onset dystonia following traumatic brain injury. Arch Phys Med Rehabil. 1994;75:885–8.
16. Pettigrew LC, Jankovic J. Hemidystonia: a report of 22 patients and a review of the literature. J Neurol Neurosurg Psychiatry. 1985;48:650–7.
17. Burke RE, Fahn S, Gold AP. Delayed-onset dystonia in patients with "static" encephalopathy. J Neurol Neurosurg Psychiatry. 1980;43:789–97.
18. Lee MS, Rinne JO, Ceballos-Baumann A, Thompson PD, Marsden CD. Dystonia after head trauma. Neurology. 1994;44:1374–8.
19. Mauro AJ, Fahn S, Russman B. Hemidystonia following "minor" head trauma. Trans Am Neurol Assoc. 1980;105:229–31.
20. Scott BL, Jankovic J. Delayed-onset progressive movement disorders after static brain lesions. Neurology. 1996;46:68–74.
21. Jabbari B, Paul J, Scherokman B, Van Dam B. Posttraumatic segmental axial dystonia. Mov Disord. 1992;7:78–81.
22. Lee MS, Lee SB, Kim WC. Spasmodic dysphonia associated with a left ventrolateral putaminal lesion. Neurology. 1996;47:827–8.
23. Marsden CD, Obeso JA, Zarranz JJ, Lang AE. The anatomical basis of symptomatic hemidystonia. Brain. 1985;108:463–83. PMID 4005532.
24. Loher TJ, Krauss JK. Dystonia associated with pontomesencephalic lesions. Mov Disord. 2009;24(2):157–67.
25. King RB, Fuller C, Collins GH. Delayed onset of hemidystonia and hemiballismus following head injury: a clinicopathological correlation. J Neurosurg. 2001;94:309–14.
26. Münchau A, Mathen D, Cox T, Quinn NP, Marsden CD, Bhatia KP. Unilateral lesions of the globus pallidus: report of four patients presenting with focal or segmental dystonia. J Neurol Neurosurg Psychiatry. 2000;69:494–8.
27. Lee SY, Lim JY. Atypical posttraumatic dystonia treated successfully by botulinum toxin injection. Am J Phys Med Rehabil. 2015;94(3):246–9.
28. Truong DD, Dubinsky R, Hermanowicz N, Olson WL, Silverman B, Koller WC. Posttraumatic torticollis. Arch Neurol. 1991;48(2):221–3.
29. Krauss JK. Deep brain stimulation for dystonia in adults. Overview and developments. Stereotact Funct Neurosurg. 2002;78(3–4):168–82.
30. Alkhani A, Khan F, Lang AE, Hutchison WD, Dostrovsky J. The response to pallidal surgery for dystonia is dependent on the etiology. Neurosurgery. 2000;47(504):504.
31. Teive HA, Sá DS, Grande CV, Antoniuk A, Werneck LC. Bilateral pallidotomy for generalized dystonia. Arq Neuropsiquiatr. 2001;59(2-B):353–7.
32. Yoshor D, Hamilton WJ, Ondo W, Jankovic J, Grossman RG. Comparison of thalamotomy and pallidotomy for the treatment of dystonia. Neurosurgery. 2001;48:818–26.
33. Carvalho KS, Sukul VV, Bookland MJ, Koch SA, Connolly PJ. Deep brain stimulation of the globus pallidus suppresses

posttraumatic dystonic tremor. J Clin Neurosci. 2014;21(1):153–5. PMID 23896546.
34. Kang DW, Kang JH, Lee MS, Chang JW. Posttraumatic hemidystonia treated with unilateral globus pallidus interna stimulation: long-term follow up and radiologic features. Neuromodulation. 2010;13(4):261–4. PMID 21992879.
35. Loher TJ, Hasdemir M, Burgunder JM, Krauss JK. Long-term follow-up of chronic globus pallidus internus stimulation for posttraumatic hemidystonia. J Neurosurg. 2000;92:457–60.
36. Kwon CS, Hasegawa H, Sokratous G, U-King-Im JM, Samuel M, Ashkan K. Globus pallidus internus deep brain stimulation for traumatic Hemidystonia following penetrating head injury. World Neurosurg. 2016;92:586.
37. Francisco GE. Successful treatment of posttraumatic hemiballismus with intrathecal baclofen therapy. Am J Phys Med Rehabil. 2006;85(9):779–82.
38. Meythaler JM, Guin-Renfroe S, Grabb P, Hadley MN. Long-term continuously infused intrathecal baclofen for spasticdystonic hypertonia in traumatic brain injury: 1-year experience. Arch Phys Med Rehabil. 1999;80(1):13–9.
39. Penn RD, Gianino JM, York MM. Intrathecal baclofen for motor disorders. Mov Disord. 1995;10:675–7.
40. Dressler D, Schönle PW. Bilateral limb dystonia due to chronic subdural hematoma. Eur Neurol. 1990;30:211–3.
41. Krauss JK. Subdural hematoma as a cause of contralateral dystonia. Clin Neurol Neurosurg. 1997;99:37–9.
42. Marquione P, Spallone A, Valente M. Reversible Pisa syndrome associated to subdural haematoma: case –report. BMC Neurol. 2014;14:149.
43. Postuma RB, Berg D, Stern M, Poewe W, Olanow CW, Oertel W, et al. MDS clinical diagnostic criteria for Parkinson's disease. Mov Disord. 2015;39(12):1591–601.
44. Lee PC, Bordelon Y, Bronstein J, Ritz B. Traumatic brain injury, paraquat exposure, and their relationship to Parkinson disease. Neurology. 2012;79:2061–6.
45. Crane PK, Gibbons LE, Dams-OÇonnor K, Trittschuc E, Leverenz JB, Keene CD, Sonnen J, Montine TJ, Bennett DA, Leurgans S, Schneider JA, Larson EB. Association of Traumatic Brain Injury with Late-Life Neurodegenerative Conditions and Neuropathologic Findings. JAMA Neurol. 2016;73:1062–9.
46. Chase A. Parkinson disease: traumatic brain injury increases the risk of Parkinson disease. Nat Rev Neurol. 2015;11:184.
47. Gardner RC, Burke JF, Nettiksimmons J, Goldman S, Tanner CM, Yaffe K. Traumatic brain injury in later life increases risk for Parkinson disease. Ann Neurol. 2015;77:987–95.
48. Taylor KM, Saint-Hilaire MH, Sudarsky L, Simon DK, Hersh B, Sparrow D, Hu H, Weisskopf MG. Head injury at early ages is associated with risk of Parkinson's disease. Parkinsonism Relat Disord. 2016;23:57–61.
49. Jafari S, Etminan M, Aminzadeh F, Samii A. Head injury and risk of Parkinson disease: a systematic review and meta-analysis. Mov Disord. 2013;28(9):1222–9.
50. Newell KL, Boyer P, Gomez-Tortosa E, Hobbs W, Hedley-Whyte ET, Vonsattel JP, Hyman BT. Alpha-synuclein immunoreactivity is present in axonal swellings in neuroaxonal dystrophy and acute traumatic brain injury. J Neuropathol Exp Neurol. 1999;58(2):1263–8.
51. Acosta SA, Tajiri N, de la Pena I, Bastawrous M, Sanberg PR, Kaneko Y, Borlongan CV. Alpha-synuclein as a pathological link between chronic traumatic brain injury and Parkinson's disease. J Cell Physiol. 2015;230(5):1024–32.
52. Marras C, Hincapié CA, Kristman VL, Cancelliere C, Soklaridis S, Li A, Borg J, af Geijerstam JL, Cassidy JD. Systematic review of the risk of Parkinson's disease after mild traumatic brain injury: results of the international collaboration on mild traumatic brain injury prognosis. Arch Phys Med Rehabil. 2014;95(3):238–4.
53. Kenborg L, Rugbjerg K, Lee PC, Ravnskjaer L, Christensen J, Ritz B, Lassen CF. Head injury and risk for Parkinson disease. Neurology. 2015;84(11):1098–103.
54. Fasano A, Lozano AM. Deep brain stimulation for movement disorders: 2015 and beyond. Curr Opin Neurol. 2015;28(4):423–36.
55. Lotia M, Jankovic J. New and emerging medical therapies in Parkinson's disease. Expert Opin Pharmacother. 2016;17(7):895–909.
56. Formisano R, Cicinelli P, Buzzi MG, et al. Blink reflex changes in parkinsonism following severe traumatic brain injury correlates with diffuse axonal injury. Med Sci Monit. 2009;15:CR101–6.
57. Wong JC, Hazrati L-N. Parkinson's disease, parkinsonism, and traumatic brain injury. Crit Rev Clin Lab Sci. 2013;50(4–5):103–6.
58. Grimberg L. Paralysis agitans and trauma. J Nerv Ment Dis. 1934;79:14–42.
59. McKee AC, Cantu RC, Nowinski CJ, et al. Chronic traumatic encephalopathy in athletes: progressive tauopathy following repetitive head injury. J Neuropathol Exp Neurol. 2009;68(7):709–35.
60. Bailes JE, Cantu RC. Head injury in athletes. Neurosurgery. 2001;48:26–46.
61. Friedman JH. Progressive parkinsonism in boxers. South Med J. 1989;82:543–6.
62. Mawdsley C, Ferguson FR. Neurological disease in boxers. Lancet. 1963;2:795–801. MRI. J Neurol Neurosurg Psychiatry 2003;74:1571–3.
63. Roberts AH. Brain damage in boxers. London: Pitman Medical Scientific Publishing; 1969.
64. Roberts GW, Allsop D, Bruton C. The occult aftermath of boxing. J Neurol Neurosurg Psychiatry. 1990;53:373–8.
65. Turjanski N, Lees AJ, Brooks DJ. Dopaminergic function in patients with posttraumatic parkinsonism: an 18F-dopa PET study. Neurology. 1997;49:183–9.
66. Lampert PW, Hardman JM. Morphological changes in brains of boxers. JAMA. 1984;251:2676–9.
67. Ryan AJ. Intracranial injuries resulting from boxing. Clin Sports Med. 1998;17:155–68.
68. Butler RJ, Forsythe WI, Beverly DW, Adams LM. A prospective controlled investigation of the cognitive effects of amateur boxing. J Neurol Neurosurg Psychiatry. 1993;56:1055–61.
69. Haglund Y, Eriksson E. Does amateur boxing lead to chronic brain damage? A review of some recent investigations. Am J Sports Med. 1993;21:97–109.
70. Jordan BD, Relkin NR, Ravdin LD, Jacobs AR, Bennett A, Gandy S. Apolipoprotein E _4 associated with chronic traumatic brain injury in boxing. JAMA. 1997;278:136–40.
71. Mez J, Daneshvar DH, Kiernan PT, et al. Clinicopathological evaluation of chronic traumatic encephalopathy in players of American football. JAMA. 2017;318(4):360–70. https://doi.org/10.1001/jama.2017.8334.
72. Wiest RG, Burgunder JM, Krauss JK. Chronic subdural hematomas and parkinsonian syndromes. Acta Neurochir. 1999;141:753–7.
73. Bhatt M, Desai J, Mankodi A, Elias M, Wadia N. Posttraumatic akinetic-rigid syndrome resembling Parkinson's disease: a report on three patients. Mov Disord. 2000;15:313–7.
74. Matsuda W, Matsumura A, Komatsu Y, et al. Awakenings from persistent vegetative state: report of three cases with parkinsonism and brain stem lesions on MRI. J Neurol Neurosurg Psychiatry. 2003;74(11):1571.
75. Jellinger KA. Parkinsonism and persistent vegetative state after head injury. J Neurol Neurosurg Psychiatry. 2004;75:1082.
76. Baizabal-Carvallo JF, Jankovic J. Deep brain stimulation of the subthalamic nucleus for peripherally induced parkinsonism. Neuromodulation. 2014;17(1):104–6.
77. Krauss JK, Jankovic J. Head injury and posttraumatic movement disorders. Neurosurgery. 2002;50:927–39.

78. Albanese A, Jankovic J. Hyperkinetic movement disorders : differential diagnosis and treatment, 1st ed, ISBN-10 1444333526; 2012.
79. Jankovic J. Post-traumatic movement disorders: central and peripheral mechanisms. Neurology. 1994;44:2006–14.
80. Birbamer G, Gerstenbrand F, Kofler M, Buchberger W, Felber S, Aichner F. Post-traumatic segmental myoclonus associated with bilateral olivary hypertrophy. Acta Neurol Scand. 1993;87(6):505–9.
81. Obeso JA, Narbona J. Post-traumatic tremor and myoclonic jerking. J Neurol Neurosurg Psychiatry. 1983;46(8):788.
82. Eiras J, García Cosamalón J. Post-traumatic myoclonic syndrome. Effectiveness of the thalamic lesions on the action myoclonus. Arch Neurobiol. 1980;43(1):17–28.
83. Gaul J. Posttraumatic tic disorder. Mov Disord. 1994;9:121.
84. Nishant R, Ranjan I, et al. Tics after traumatic brain injury. Brain Inj. 2011;25(6):629–33.
85. Singer C, Sanchez-Ramos J, Weiner WJ. A case of post traumatic tic disorder. Mov Disord. 1989;4:342–4.
86. Siemers E, Pascuzzi R. Post traumatic tic disorder. Mov Disord. 1990;5:183.
87. Krauss JK, Jankovic J. Tics secondary to craniocerebral trauma. Mov Disord. 1997;12:776–82.
88. Meja NI, Jankovic J. Secondary tics and tourettism. Rev Bras Psiquiatr. 2005;27:11–7.
89. Shprecher D, Kurlan R. The management of tics. Mov Disord. 2009;24:15–24.
90. Bullard DE, Nashold BS Jr. Stereotaxic thalamotomy for treatment of posttraumatic movement disorders. J Neurosurg. 1984;61:316–21.
91. Kant R, Zeiler D. Hemiballismus following closed head injury. Brain Inj. 1996;10:155–8.
92. Drake ME Jr, Jackson RD, Miller CA. Paroxysmal choreoathetosis after head injury. J Neurol Neurosurg Psychiatry. 1986;49(7):837–8.
93. Krauss JK, Mundinger F. Functional stereotactic surgery for hemiballism. J Neurosurg. 1996;85:278–86.
94. Levesque MF, Markham C, Nakasato N. MR-guided ventral intermediate thalamotomy for posttraumatic hemiballismus. Stereotact Funct Neurosurg. 1992;58:88.
95. Adler JR Jr, Winston KR. Chorea as a manifestation of epidural hematoma. J Neurosurg. 1984;60:856–7.
96. Kotagal S, Shuter E, Horenstein S. Chorea as a manifestation of bilateral subdural hematoma in an elderly man. Arch Neurol. 1981;38:195.
97. Sung YF, Ma HI, Hsu YD. Generalized chorea associated with bilateral chronic subdural hematoma. Eur Neurol. 2004;51(4):227–30. Epub 2004.
98. Fanh S, Jankovic J, Hallet M. Principles and practice of movement disorders. 2nd ed; 2011. ISBN: 978-1-4377-2369-4.
99. Desai A, Nierenberg DW, Duhaime AC. Akathisia after mild traumatic head injury. J Neurosurg Pediatr. 2010;5(5):460–4.
100. Silver BV, Yablon SA. Akathisia resulting from traumatic brain injury. Brain Inj. 1996;10:609–14.
101. Stewart JT. Akathisia following traumatic brain injury: treatment with bromocriptine. J Neurol Neurosurg Psychiatry. 1989;52:1200–1.
102. Ganos C, Edwards MJ, Bhatia KP. Posttraumatic functional movement disorders. Handb Clin Neurol. 2016;139:499–507.
103. Gupta A, Lang AE. Psychogenic movement disorders. Curr Opin Neurol. 2009;22(4):430–6.

# Post-traumatic Epilepsy

7

Arezoo Rezazadeh, Danielle M. Andrade, and Aylin Reid

## Introduction

Epilepsy is a common neurologic complication of traumatic brain injury (TBI) [1–3]. Five percent of all referrals to specialized epilepsy centers are due to confirmed post-traumatic epilepsy (PTE) [4]. Patients with PTE comprise a regular part of the care provided by epilepsy specialists, as well as general neurologists and primary care physicians throughout the world [5]. The objective of this chapter is to provide an overview of post-traumatic seizures and epilepsy by reviewing the definition, epidemiology, and risk factors of epileptic events in TBI. Subsequently, we will discuss the pathophysiology of PTE particularly through animal studies. Finally, the clinical aspects of PTE will be discussed, and we provide a summary of the clinical approach to epileptic events associated with TBI, including diagnostic and therapeutic measures.

A. Rezazadeh (✉)
Division of Neurology, Department of Medicine, University of Toronto, Toronto, ON, Canada

Krembil Neuroscience Collaborative Program, Toronto Western Hospital, University Health Network, Toronto, ON, Canada

Krembil Neurosciences Epilepsy Genetics Program, Toronto Western Hospital, University of Toronto, Toronto, ON, Canada
e-mail: arezoo.rezazadeh@one-mail.on.ca

D. M. Andrade
Division of Neurology, Department of Medicine, University of Toronto, Toronto, ON, Canada

Krembil Neuroscience Collaborative Program, Toronto Western Hospital, University Health Network, Toronto, ON, Canada

Krembil Neurosciences Epilepsy Genetics Program, Toronto Western Hospital, University of Toronto, Toronto, ON, Canada

Krembil Research Institute, University Health Network, Toronto, ON, Canada
e-mail: danielle.andrade@uhn.ca

A. Reid
Division of Neurology, Department of Medicine, University of Toronto, Toronto, ON, Canada

Krembil Neuroscience Collaborative Program, Toronto Western Hospital, University Health Network, Toronto, ON, Canada

Krembil Research Institute, University Health Network, Toronto, ON, Canada
e-mail: aylin.reid@uhn.ca

## Definition

An epileptic seizure is defined as "a transient occurrence of signs and/or symptoms due to abnormal excessive or synchronous neuronal activity in the brain" [6]. According to the latest definition proposed by the task force of the International League Against Epilepsy (ILAE), epilepsy is "a disease of the brain defined by any of the following conditions: (1) At least two unprovoked (or reflex) seizures occurring >24 h apart; (2) one unprovoked (or reflex) seizure and a probability of further seizures similar to the general recurrence risk (at least 60%) after two unprovoked seizures, occurring over the next 10 years; (3) diagnosis of an epilepsy syndrome" [6].

The epileptic events occurring following TBI are classified in one of these categories: [1, 7] immediate post-traumatic seizures (PTSs) occur less than 24 h after TBI, while early PTSs occur within the first week post-injury. Both immediate and early seizures after TBI are considered provoked seizures. They do not meet the definition of epilepsy since they are not necessarily mediated by the pathogenic mechanisms that predispose the patient to manifest spontaneous seizures [6]. Late recurring seizures, or PTE, are unprovoked seizures occurring more than 1 week after TBI.


R. Anghinah et al. (eds.), *Topics in Cognitive Rehabilitation in the TBI Post-Hospital Phase*,
https://doi.org/10.1007/978-3-319-95376-2_7

## Epidemiology

### Post-traumatic Seizures

The incidence of immediate seizures is reported to be 1–4% and of early seizures is 4–25% in civilian head injuries [2, 8, 9]. The occurrence of early PTSs depends in part on TBI severity [2, 8]. There are several classification systems for TBI severity. A widely used system is that of Annegers and colleagues (Table 7.1) [1]. Recently, a newer classification, the Mayo Classification System for TBI Severity, has been designed to distinguish between different severities of TBI correlated with the general outcome of the patients after injury (Table 7.2) [10]. Age also plays an important role in the development of PTSs, as children seem to be more likely to develop PTSs compared to adults [1]. In children PTSs are more common than later development of PTE (97% vs 3%) [11]. In addition, other important risk factors have been implicated in the development of PTS, listed in Table 7.3.

Subclinical seizures are seizures which show electrophysiological changes with electroencephalogram (EEG) recordings but display no overt behavioral changes [12]. Subclinical seizures, including nonconvulsive status epilepticus (NCSE), are relatively common after severe TBI in the intensive care unit (ICU) setting [13, 14]. Thirty-three percent of adult TBI patients requiring ICU were reported to have seizures as detected by continuous EEG monitoring [15]. In a pediatric study, the reported incidence of seizures was as high as 42.5%, of whom 7% only had subclinical seizures [14]. Intracranial EEG with electrodes implanted after TBI was able to detect electrographic seizures in 71% of patients that were not apparent on scalp EEG [16], suggesting seizure rates may be even higher than reported. Detection of subclinical seizures is crucial as reports have shown early nonconvulsive PTSs are associated with increased intracranial pressure, metabolic derangements, and long-term hippocampal atrophy [17, 18].

The occurrence of status epilepticus (SE) at onset is high, estimated to be 6.39% in an adult population, comprising 28.57% of the patients with moderate to severe TBI who developed clinical and subclinical PTS [13]. SE rates are even higher in the pediatric population compared to adults. In one study, an average of 18.4% of children with acute TBI developed SE in a pediatric ICU, ranging between 12.5% and 31.3%, depending on the severity of TBI [14]. Seventy

**Table 7.1** Annegers' classification of severity of traumatic brain injury

| Severity | Description |
|---|---|
| Mild TBI | Loss of consciousness for less than 30 min and no skull fracture |
| Moderate TBI | Loss of consciousness 30 min to 24 h, with or without skull fracture |
| Severe TBI | Loss of consciousness greater than 24 h, with brain contusion, intracranial hematoma, or skull fracture |

*TBI* traumatic brain injury
Data taken from [1]

**Table 7.2** Mayo classification system for traumatic brain injury severity

| A | B | C |
|---|---|---|
| Moderate to severe (definite) | Mild (probable) | Symptomatic (possible) |
| Meets one or more of the following criteria:<br>1. Death due to this TBI<br>2. Loss of consciousness of 30 min or more<br>3. Post-traumatic anterograde amnesia of 24 h or more<br>4. Worst Glasgow Coma Scale full score in first 24 h 13 (unless invalidated upon review, e.g., attributable to intoxication, sedation, systemic shock)<br>5. One or more of the following present:<br>Intracerebral hematoma<br>Subdural hematoma<br>Epidural hematoma<br>Cerebral contusion<br>Hemorrhagic contusion<br>Penetrating TBI (dura penetrated)<br>Subarachnoid hemorrhage<br>Brain stem injury | If none of Criteria A apply,<br>If one or more of the following criteria apply:<br>1. Loss of consciousness of momentary to less than 30 min 2. Post-traumatic anterograde amnesia of momentary to less than 24 h 3. Depressed, basilar, or linear skull fracture (dura intact) | If none of Criteria A or B apply,<br>If one or more of the following symptoms are present:<br>Blurred vision<br>Confusion (mental state changes)<br>Dazed<br>Dizziness<br>Focal neurologic symptoms<br>Headache<br>Nausea |

Malec et al. [10]

**Table 7.3** Risk factors of post-traumatic seizures and post-traumatic epilepsy

| Post-traumatic seizures | Post-traumatic epilepsy |
|---|---|
| Acute subdural hematoma | Acute subdural hematoma |
| Acute intracerebral hematoma | Prolonged post-traumatic amnesia (>24 h) |
| Younger age | Age older than 65 years |
| Injury severity | Injury severity |
| Chronic alcoholism | Midline shift >5 mm |
| Multiple contusions | Multiple contusions |
| Depressed skull fractures | Depressed skull fractures |
| Neurosurgical procedures | Male gender |
| | Development of an EEG focus 1 month after TBI |
| | Frontal or temporal lesions on acute computed tomography |
| | Cortical MRI hyperintense areas |
| | Comorbid conditions |
| | Depression |

*EEG* electroencephalography, *MRI* magnetic resonance imaging, *TBI* traumatic brain injury

percent of these children showed subclinical SE [14]. Younger age, abusive head trauma, and intracranial hemorrhage were the risk factors of developing SE in this study.

## Post-traumatic Epilepsy

PTE accounts for 5–6% of all epilepsies [19]. The frequency rate of PTE varies in different studies between 1.9% and 53% [1, 2, 8, 9, 20, 21], depending on injury severity and mechanism. Patients with TBI have increased risk of developing epilepsy compared to the general population, and the relative risks of developing epilepsy after mild, moderate, and severe TBI are 1.5, 2.9, and 17, respectively [2]. Furthermore, the mechanism of injury in penetrating head trauma and closed-head injuries is different, and the former is more likely associated with PTE (50% in penetrating injuries versus up to 23.6% for the closed-head injuries) [2, 3, 9]. The bone and iron-containing metal fragments in the wounds of war survivors are potentially more epileptogenic than lead fragments from bullets. Hence, civilian injuries with bone fragments alone do not significantly increase the risk for PTE [9, 21, 22]. Furthermore, the duration of epilepsy, seizure frequency, and response to antiepileptic drug (AED) therapy is correlated with severity of TBI [2, 23]. In 27% of patients with penetrating war injuries, epilepsy persisted up to 15-year post-injury as compared with the risk in the general population [9]. Whether early PTS is a risk factor for PTE is a matter of controversy. While some studies found that PTSs were not an independent risk factor for PTE [2], other studies have demonstrated the presence of early PTSs as a precursor [21, 24], or even the most consistently significant risk factor for PTE in adults [7, 24], but this is certainly not true for children [7].

**Family History/Genetic Associations** Hereditary predisposition to PTE and related genetic polymorphisms has been long debated [25–27]. Although some studies have linked certain genes to PTE, many of them need to be duplicated.

While Schaumann and colleagues showed that family history of epilepsy could precipitate individuals into early PTSs and PTE [28], others found that family history of epilepsy increases the risk of PTE in children [29, 30] but not in older patients [9, 31].

Genetic association studies propose that there might be a genetic element to the development of PTE. A study showed that TBI patients with an apolipoprotein Eε4 (APOEε4) allele, a gene encoding a cholesterol transporter into neurons, experienced a higher risk of PTS [32]. In a review made by Cotter and colleagues, the most promising candidates were the pro-inflammatory gene Interleukin-1beta (IL-1b) SNP (rs1143634) and A1 adenosine receptor (A1AR) SNP (rs10920573) by which the individuals with heterozygous genotype seemed to be at higher risk for developing PTE. However, other genes such as glutamic acid decarboxylase 1 (GAD1) and methylenetetrahydrofolate reductase (MTHFR) C677T have been associated with early PTSs [33].

More recently, a genetic variation in solute carrier family 1 member 1 (SLC1A1), a gene encoding the neuronal glutamate transporters, was associated with reduced time to first seizure and increased seizure risk up to 3-year post-injury. When individuals were homozygous (GG) for the SLC1A1 SNP rs10974620 minor allele, the risk of seizure over this period increased significantly. Likewise, in individuals who were homozygous (TT) for the SLC1A1 SNP rs7858819 minor allele, the risk of PTE was higher when follow-up began on day 2 post-injury [34].

Mechanistic target of rapamycin (mTOR) complex 1 (mTORC1) is a protein involved in the regulation of cell proliferation and cell metabolism that widely has been associated with tumors including tuberous sclerosis. In a review recently published by Myers and colleagues, mTORC1 activation was considered as a contributing factor causing mossy fiber sprouting and neurogenesis, predisposing the patients to develop epilepsy after TBI although the significance of it has not been confirmed yet [35].

## Pathophysiology

Human studies and animal models have attempted to discover the pathophysiological mechanisms for PTE, and various mechanisms have been proposed. A number of animal models have been employed at different developmental stages and with injuries of varying severity and location. One of the most well-studied models is fluid percussion injury (FPI), a model of closed-head TBI [36]. In this model, injury is delivered through a craniotomy by rapid fluid injection. The fluid pulse first strikes the intact dura and then moves into the epidural space [37]. Craniotomies can be applied to the midline to produce more diffuse injuries or laterally to produce mixed focal and diffuse injury [37]. Early electrophysiological changes [38] as well as PTE have been described [36, 39, 40]. Controlled cortical impact (CCI) injury is another widely used experimental model of closed-head injury that was recently identified as a model of injury-induced epilepsy [41]. This model often utilizes an electronically controlled pneumatic impactor to apply a focal contusion injury to the brain surface through a craniotomy [42].

Experimental models have described potential biological changes after TBI in three distinct temporal phases. The first phase ranges from a few seconds to minutes [43], consisting of immediate release of excitatory neurotransmitters including glutamate, followed by ion channel activation and calcium influx [44]. Hyperexcitation results in energy depletion and cell death [44]. One of the underlying ionic changes identified early after the injury is potassium accumulation that is caused by failure of the ionic ATP pump [45] leading to altered resting membrane potential and neuronal excitability, with a loss of inhibitory postsynaptic potentials [46]. In addition, an increase in extracellular potassium converts spikers to a burster state in the CA3 region of the hippocampus [47]. Also, hyperexcitability in the CA1 subregion of the hippocampus has been reported by in vitro studies [48, 49].

Secondary injury is characterized by altered local cerebral blood flow regulation, breakdown in the blood brain barrier (BBB), and initiation of inflammatory and neuronal death, occurring within hours to days after TBI. During the inflammatory response, cytokines are released [50] which inhibit the uptake of glutamate by astrocytes [51] and modulate excitatory neurotransmission in the brain through glutamate receptors [52, 53]. For instance, IL-1β modulates neuronal hyperexcitability through $Ca^{2+}$, glutamatergic, and GABAergic pathways [54]. Glial glutamate transporter protein (GLT) which regulates the extracellular glutamate level also decreases after TBI, particularly in the neocortical and hippocampal regions leading to increased level of glutamate and hyperexcitability [55, 56]. Patients with PTE are more likely to show BBB disruption compared to non-epileptic patients after TBI, and slow waves are identified in EEG in 70% of cases [57].Tomkins and colleagues also showed that the size of lesion with BBB disruption was significantly larger in PTE patients [57].

The third phase is the latent period between the injury and the first successive seizure and is when epileptogenesis takes places [58]. It is characterized by morphological changes including mossy fiber sprouting, dendritic modifications, interneuron loss, rewiring of synaptic circuits, glial cell activation, ectopic cell proliferation, and gliosis [41, 59–62]. During this phase, excitability is increased both in CA1 [63] and dentate gyrus [64]. Loss of GABAergic interneurons decreases the inhibition on pyramidal cells [65–67]. Moreover, not only mossy fiber sprouting and loss of inhibition but also the increased connections on the dentate granule cells together enhance the excitability of hippocampus [47, 68–72]. This could also explain how injury at the neocortex progresses to mesial temporal seizures at a later time. Some groups have shown that seizures are originally neocortical at onset, but over time, the mesial temporal region transforms to an epileptogenic zone [73]. In fact, in approximately 61% of patients with PTE, seizures emanate from the temporal lobe [74], and magnetic resonance imaging (MRI) has shown that about 35% of these patients have mesial temporal lobe sclerosis (MTS). It is unclear, however, if MTS could be a secondary phenomenon [74]. Furthermore, prolonged seizures at the acute post-TBI phase have been implicated in hippocampal atrophy at the later phase of injury [18]. It is, however, worth mentioning that it is not uncommon that TBI results in multifocal pathology [74]. In conclusion, neuronal loss, chronic neuroinflammation, and network reorganization in the overlaying cortical regions are implicated in epileptogenesis.

## Clinical or Natural History

Forty-seven percent of late PTSs recur after 1 month, while an 86% recurrence rate is observed within 2 years after injury [75]. In general, the relative risk of developing PTE after severe TBI remains significantly high even after 10 years both in adults [2] and in children [30], whereas patients with mild TBI exhibit a normalization of the risk after the first 5 years [2]. Christensen and colleagues believe that the absolute risk of PTE decreases significantly, and the yearly absolute risk remains below 1% for all types of brain injury including severe TBI by 5 years of follow-up [76]. One study showed that the mean latency to seizure was 3.5 years [77], ranging from 2.1 years for MTS to 5.1 years for all lesional neocortical cases. Age may be a determining factor in the latency period of seizures after trauma. There was a latency period of about 3 years in the patients who were over 15 years at time of injury versus a 13-year latency period in those who were 2 years or younger at the time of injury [78].

Seizure onset location can be very variable after TBI. In a study of 60 patients with moderate to severe TBI and PTE, 52% developed generalized seizures, 34% had focal seizures, and 15% showed focal seizures with secondary generalization; however, this was based on seizure semiology and not electrophysiology [75]. By contrast, in a 10-year retrospective study based on EEG recordings from the epilepsy monitoring unit, 93% had localization-related epilepsy arising most commonly from temporal or frontal lobes [77], and 4.8% displayed generalized epilepsy. Of temporal lobe epilepsy cases, just under half had MTS, and about one-third were nonlesional. In humans, owing to the shape of the skull, the frontal and temporal cortices are susceptible to contusion, accounting for the greater prevalence of post-traumatic contusion [79–81]. Likewise, in most animal studies, frontal neocortical or limbic epilepsy are more common than parietal/occipital seizures regardless of FPI location [82]. The other explanation for the predilection of the frontal lobe to epileptogenesis, although not well established, could be higher intrinsic susceptibility to tissue damage or the known tendency of prefrontal neurons to burst discharges and hypersynchronization [82]. In experimental models, frontal neocortical foci develop within 1 month following FPI, while it takes several months for limbic regions to transform to an epileptogenic zone [73]. Whether frontal neocortical seizures are capable to kindle the hippocampus through propagation [73] is a proposed explanation. Direct hippocampal injury could also cause limbic epileptogenesis although more slowly [82]. In two studies, 24% to 35% of patients had mesial TLE (MTLE), while neocortical foci were identified in 12–48% of patients [74, 83]. TBI can induce MTLE in children younger than 5 years, while neocortical epilepsy tends to occur later in life [74]. However, recently, Gupta and colleagues reported that 83% of patients with MTS following TBI had their injury after the age of 5 years. Englander and colleagues believe that although TBI has a propensity toward frontal and temporal lobes, parietal lobe involvement may also reduce the overall seizure threshold [21].

The remission rates of seizures vary between 25% and 40% once PTE is diagnosed (and treated), and up to half of patients with PTE show prolonged periods of seizure freedom [84].This is slightly lower than remission rates in other epilepsy populations [85]. Patients with high frequencies of seizures during the first year following injury are less likely to achieve remission [86].

## Investigations

Following a seizure associated with acute head injury, investigation should involve assessment of the biochemical parameters, such as hyponatremia, along with exploring for possible intracranial hemorrhage. Hyponatremia induced by head trauma may lower the seizure threshold [86]. Acute brain edema, perioperative events including cerebral interventions or stress from general anesthesia, and metabolic disturbances account for a high proportion of seizures which develop during the first month after brain injury [21]. In patients developing PTS after moderate to severe TBI, CT scan should be performed urgently. If the seizures occur after initial imaging, a repeat CT is indicated.

Patients with PTE should be approached similarly to patients with a first non-traumatic epileptic seizure. All patients with epilepsy should be asked specifically about head trauma, since patients do not usually volunteer certain incidences of head trauma such as sports-related concussions [87]. In addition, psychogenic non-epileptic seizures (PNES) are common after TBI [88, 89] and are frequently mistaken for epileptic seizures [90]. They should be ruled out with appropriate investigations, including video-EEG monitoring if necessary.

Magnetic resonance imaging (MRI) is the most sensitive means in identifying the extent and severity of brain injury and is the recommended neuroimaging modality in patients with PTE. Conventional MRI sequences, including T1-weighted, T2-weighted, gradient echo, and diffusion-weighted imaging, may discover parenchymal hemorrhages, extra-axial blood products (hemosiderin deposits), early ischemia, edema, and gliosis [91]. While the epileptogenic role of hemosiderin deposits has been established [20], precocious formation of a gliotic scar around a hemosiderin deposit reduces the risk of PTE [92]. Advanced MRI modalities including diffusion tensor imaging (DTI) and functional MRI (fMRI) identify early and late changes that might correlate with epileptogenic foci [93]. Susceptibility-weighted imaging and DTI are more sensitive to microhemorrhages and white matter injury, respectively [94].

The EEG findings in TBI are usually nonspecific, and the presence of epileptiform activity does not predict the development of PTE [95] or disability outcome [96]. As described earlier, continuous EEG monitoring is worthwhile to rule out subclinical seizures, particularly NCSE in the ICU setting. The scalp EEG is negative in more than 20% of patients with PTE during the first 3 months after TBI [95]. However, it remains useful for localization of the epileptogenic zone as well as measurements of the extent of damage and in predicting relapse before AED is withdrawn [97]. Intracranial recordings also have demonstrated interictal spikes and fast ripples early during the epileptogenic process in patients with established PTE, representing a more sensitive method than routine scalp recordings in identifying the epileptic activity in these patients [16].

## Management

The decision to initiate pharmacotherapy depends on the temporal relationship between the inciting brain injury and onset of seizures. In immediate seizures which occur immediately following head trauma, antiepileptic therapy is not indicated. Indeed, the pathophysiological mechanism of immediate seizures might be related to transient functional decerebration with loss of cortical inhibition and is characterized by initial tonic phase within 2 s of impact, followed by a clonic or myoclonic phase, which may last for several minutes. Immediate seizures do not lead to development of PTE [98].

In contrast, since early seizures increase cerebral perfusion pressure and intracranial pressure, seizure prophylaxis is the recommended therapy during the first 7 days of moderate to severe TBI based on the latest guideline (2016) of the Brain Trauma Foundation. Phenytoin treatment significantly reduces the incidence of early PTSs (3.6–14.2%) [99]. While phenytoin has been widely used to prevent early PTS, levetiracetam recently has gained attention for seizure prophylaxis in TBI [100]. However, a high-quality, head-to-head randomized clinical trial (RCT) between phenytoin and levetiracetam is lacking. Levetiracetam has demonstrated comparable efficacy to phenytoin in non-controlled studies [101–103] and is associated with fewer adverse effects, monitoring considerations [104], and better long-term outcomes [103]. An observational study on severe TBI revealed that epileptiform EEG abnormalities are more likely to persist in patients treated with levetiracetam compared to phenytoin [105]. Compared to placebo, carbamazepine has been documented to be effective in the prevention of early PTSs only in one true RCT [106]. Although similar results have been reported for valproate [107], this drug has lesser capacity to prevent early PTSs compared with phenytoin.

Compared to the established efficacy of early PTS, there is no evidence for pharmacological prophylaxis of the development of PTE [86, 99, 108]. Nevertheless, patients with early PTS, dural-penetrating injuries, multiple contusions, and/or SDH requiring evacuation may benefit from antiepileptic therapy beyond the first week post-injury [21, 107, 109, 110]. Principles of AED selection in PTE are identical to other patients with epilepsy, and no specific AED has been recommended for PTE [111, 112]. Neuropsychological consideration is required to be taken prior to starting AEDs [22]. Inappropriate treatment with AEDs may impair neurorehabilitation after TBI [113], and patients with post-TBI PNES could benefit from antidepressants, such as selective serotonin reuptake inhibitors and/or cognitive–behavioral therapy [114] rather than AEDs. There is no doctrine on duration of AED therapy, and much depends on a patient's age, personal preference, and drug tolerability. However, as a rule of thumb, AED withdrawal can be considered after at least 2 years of seizure freedom, though waiting up to 4 years has been suggested as well [115].

## Experimental Interventions

One of the main goals of PTE studies is to develop a therapeutic strategy which could be delivered during the latent period after TBI in order to prevent epileptogenesis and the development of PTE. Investigators have focused on various mechanistic pathways as potential therapeutic targets. Many studies have attempted to find antioxidant and neuroprotective drugs which prevent the lipid peroxidation of neuronal membranes. Based on the knowledge that magnesium blocks glutamate transmission at NMDA receptors, continuous infusion of magnesium sulfate was carried out within 8 h after moderate or severe TBI. However, this double-blinded RCT did not appear to prevent PTE [23]. The effect of magnesium on PTS could not be assessed because of concomitant use of phenytoin. In a ferrous chloride animal model, tochopherol (vitamin E) use was associated with a delay in the onset of electrical seizures on EEG [116]. The use of adenosine and its derivatives in post-traumatic animal models showed suppression of epileptic discharges through scavenging free radicals such as OH [117]. Subsequently, Malhotra et al. demonstrated that adenosine and its analogues protect against seizures induced by chemical agents through their action on A1 receptors [118].

Although the efficacy of corticosteroids has been established in spinal cord injury, the administration of these agents is controversial in TBI. Previously, Hoeppner had shown that prednisone prevents epileptogenesis in a metallic aluminum-injected animal model [119]. However, in a randomized placebo-controlled trial, the risk of death within 2 weeks after brain injury was higher in the group that received corticosteroids compared with placebo. The prevalence of seizure did not differ significantly between the two groups during this period [120]. In a retrospective study, corticosteroids treatment within the first day of head trauma resulted in increased seizure activity and was not associated with any decrease in PTE [121].

As discussed earlier, TBI initiates a cascade of neuroinflammation in the brain, which may induce epileptogenesis and contribute to development of PTE. As such, recent investigations have attempted to focus on neuroinflammatory agents as the novel therapeutic targets in the post-traumatic phase. Diamond and colleagues demonstrated that patients who developed PTE had a higher ratio of cerebrospinal fluid (CSF)/serum IL-1β and lower levels of serum IL-1β, whereas the difference between CSF IL-1β levels was not significant [122]. Dextromethorphan derivative is an experimental treatment which reduces both neuroinflammation and nonconvulsive seizures in a penetrating ballistic-like brain injury (PBBI) model [123]. Minozac prevents experimental seizure susceptibility by suppression of cytokine upregulation in the hippocampus in a "two-hit" injury model [124]. Most recently, perampanel, an antiepileptic drug, has been shown to have neuroprotective effects through reduced neuronal apoptosis, inhibition of lipid peroxidation, and suppression of pro-inflammatory cytokines such as tumor necrosis factor-α (TNF-α) and IL-1β, as well as increase in the levels of anti-inflammatory cytokines IL-10 and transforming growth factor-β (TGF-β 1) [125] although its prophylactic effect on PTS or PTE has not been studied. Recently, cooling has gained attention as a prophylactic treatment in PTE, possibly via anti-inflammatory mechanisms. Focal mild cooling prevented the onset of epileptic seizures in a rostral parasagittal PFI model both during and after the treatment. Rare remaining seizures were shorter than in controls [126].

Studies have demonstrated that the mTOR signaling pathway is abnormally activated in TBI, and rapamycin, an mTOR inhibitor, suppresses epileptogenesis of dentate gyrus granule cells in the ipsilateral temporal lobe in CCI models [127, 128]. Inhibition of mTOR also showed antiepileptogenic and neuroprotective effect in an organotypic hippocampal culture model of PTE [129]. While exogenous insulin-like growth factor-1 (IGF-1) has neuroprotective effect early after TBI, in long term, it contributes to epileptogenesis through activation of mTOR cascade [130]. In animal epilepsy models, activation of cannabinoid type-1 (CB1) receptor prevents the seizure [131]. Cannabinoid receptors downregulate after TBI, leading to hyperexcitability. This is followed by upregulation in 4 weeks. Despite the protective role of the CB1receptor agonists [131], Echegoyen et al. showed that a single use of a CB1receptor antagonist immediately after TBI could disrupt the epileptogenic process and prevent PTE occurrence [132]. In contrast, Nissinen J and colleagues showed that either immediate single dosage or long-term treatment with SR141716 (a CB1 receptor antagonist) initiated 30 min after injury did not have antiepileptic effect in a lateral FPI model [133]. This difference was attributed to later timepoint assessment, different types of assessment of seizure susceptibility, and the number of included animals.

## Surgical Intervention

The presence of focal cerebral pathology in patients with PTE prompts the consideration of surgical options in medically refractory patients [91]. Indeed, the success rate of surgical resection appears to be comparable to that in the non-traumatic population [77, 134]. Therefore, PTE patients should be worked up similarly to non-traumatic patients with epilepsy in terms of determining surgical candidacy. In an optimal treatment plan, both pharmacological and surgical options should be considered when appropriate, since early surgery prevents progressive secondary injury from recurrent seizures [77]. The likelihood of seizure freedom depends on the ictal onset zone as well as the presence of an identifiable lesion [135]. Rates of seizure freedom in PTE patients with MTLE who undergo temporal lobectomy can be as high as 69–90% [77, 136, 137], compared with 33% in patients with frontal lobe epilepsy, similar to what is seen in the non-traumatic population [77]. While neocortical seizures are less ideal surgical candidates [74, 83], the presence of focal encephalomalacia predicts a good outcome with electrocorticography-guided resections [138].

Nevertheless, in the surgical approach in patients with medically refractory PTE, several challenges might be encountered. Firstly, diffuse cerebral injury induced by TBI can result in multifocal epilepsy which may not be surgically amenable. Secondly, owing to prior craniotomies and breach rhythms, seizure foci might be difficult to localize precisely [139]. In addition, orbitofrontal cortex is commonly involved, impacting accurate localization of the epileptogenic zone [83].

Neuromodulation is a palliative treatment which is reserved for medically refractory patients who are not suitable candidates for conventional resective surgery, either because the seizure onset zone cannot be adequately localized or because it involves eloquent cortex which is not safe to remove. Neuromodulation is believed to provide high-frequency stimulation which desynchronizes the cerebral cortex and prevents seizure. Neuromodulation modalities which are used currently in the treatment of patients with medically refractory epilepsy are deep brain stimulation (DBS), vagal nerve stimulation (VNS), and responsive neurostimulation (RNS).

VNS in post-traumatic patients is thought to be comparable to the non-traumatic population. However, one case-control study indicated that VNS was associated with more than 50% reduction in seizure frequency in 78% of patients with PTE as opposed to 61% in patients with non-traumatic epilepsy at 2-year follow-up, suggesting it may have greater efficacy in this group [140]. Similarly, DBS of the anterior nucleus of the thalamus (ATN) showed a seizure frequency reduction by 40.4% in refractory PTE patients [141]. However, the seizure reduction effect was only significant if the seizures originated from one or both temporal lobes compared with seizures arising from frontal, parietal, and occipital regions or multifocal/diffuse seizures. In addition, the number of responders during the blinded evaluation period was not significantly different between the groups. However, the seizure frequency reduction and responder rates increased significantly in long-term nonblinded follow-up by 56% and 54%, respectively.

Unlike the other two modalities, RNS is a closed-loop system that prevents seizures by detecting epileptiform activities and stimulating the seizure onset zone. Two studies showed a significant difference in seizure frequency reduction (37.9–41.5%) between active and control groups [142, 143]. However, the percentage of the responder was not significant. Similar to DBS, improved efficacy was observed in long-term stimulation. However, there have been no reports of RNS specifically in patients with PTE, and therefore, it is not clear whether efficacy is similar in this population.

## Conclusion

PTE is a serious common complication of TBI, comprising 5% of all epilepsies. Several risk factors have been identified, anticipating the likelihood of developing PTS and PTE. Severe TBI is correlated with an increased risk of developing PTS and PTE. Whether PTS increases the risk of PTE is controversial. Recently, genetic association studies have identified a number of genetic variants predisposing patients with TBI to PTS or PTE. Numerous experimental studies have attempted to identify the nature of hyperexcitability after TBI. The post-traumatic animal models have recently highlighted the putative role of inflammation as one of the underlying pathophysiology of neuronal hyperexcitability. Localization-related epilepsy represents the most common epilepsy occurring after TBI, and there is a high predilection for temporal and frontal lobe epilepsy in this regard. High percentage of recurrence is observed within the first 2 years after injury. Although the role of AEDs in prophylactic treatment of PTS has been well established, they are not able to prevent PTE. Phenytoin is a highly recommended prophylactic therapy within the first week after TBI although levetiracetam has shown comparable effect to phenytoin. No neuroprotective agent has been proved to prevent PTE or PTS in human. Clinical approach and principles of AED selection in PTE are identical to other epilepsy syndromes, and surgery may be indicated in patients who do not respond properly to AEDs.

**Author Disclosures Arezoo Rezazadeh**

This author declares no financial or intellectual conflicts of interest.

**Aylin Reid**

This author declares no financial or intellectual conflicts of interest.

**Danielle M Andrade**

This author declares no financial or intellectual conflicts of interest.

## References


1. Annegers JF, Grabow JD, Groover RV, Laws ER, Elveback LR, Kurland LT. Seizures after head trauma: a population study. Neurology. 1980;30(7 Pt 1):683–9.
2. Annegers JF, Hauser WA, Coan SP, Rocca WA. A population-based study of seizures after traumatic brain injuries. N Engl J Med. 1998;338(1):20–4.
3. Annegers JF, Coan SP. The risks of epilepsy after traumatic brain injury. Seizure. 2000;9(7):453–7.
4. Semah F, Picot M, Adam C, Broglin D, Arzimanoglou A, Bazin B, et al. Is the underlying cause of epilepsy a major prognostic factor for recurrence? Neurology. 1998;51:1256–62.
5. Lowenstein DH. Epilepsy after head injury: an overview. Epilepsia. 2009;50(SUPPL. 2):4–9.
6. Fisher RS, Acevedo C, Arzimanoglou A, Bogacz A, Cross JH, Elger CE, et al. A practical clinical definition of epilepsy. Epilepsia. 2014;55(4):475–82.
7. Frey LC. Epidemiology of posttraumatic epilepsy: a critical review. Epilepsia. 2003;44:11–7.
8. Asikainen I, Kaste M, Sarna S. Early and late posttraumatic seizures in traumatic brain injury rehabilitation patients: brain injury factors causing late seizures and influence of seizures on long-term outcome. Epilepsia. 1999;40(5):584–9.
9. Salazar AM, Jabbari B, Vance SC, Grafman J, Amin D, Dillon JD. Epilepsy after penetrating head injury. I. Clinical correlates: a report of the Vietnam head injury study. Neurology. 1985;35(10):1406–14.
10. Malec JF, Brown AW, Leibson CL, Flaada JT, Mandrekar JN, Diehl NN, et al. The Mayo classification system for traumatic brain injury severity. J Neurotrauma. 2007;24(9):1417–24.
11. Hahn YS, Fuchs S, Flannery AM, Barthel MJ, McLone DG. Factors influencing posttraumatic seizures in children. Neurosurgery. 1988;22(5):864–7.
12. Maganti RK, Rutecki P. EEG and epilepsy monitoring. CONTINUUM Lifelong Learn Neurol. 2013;19:598–622.
13. Vespa PM, Nuwer MR, Nenov V, Ronne-Engstrom E, Hovda DA, Bergsneider M, et al. Increased incidence and impact of nonconvulsive and convulsive seizures after traumatic brain injury as detected by continuous electroencephalographic monitoring. J Neurosurg. 1999;91:750–60.
14. Arndt DH, Lerner JT, Matsumoto JH, Madikians A, Yudovin S, Valino H, et al. Subclinical early posttraumatic seizures detected by continuous EEG monitoring in a consecutive pediatric cohort. Epilepsia. 2013;54(10):1780–8.
15. Ronne-Engstrom E, Winkler T. Continuous EEG monitoring in patients with traumatic brain injury reveals a high incidence of epileptiform activity. Acta Neurol Scand. 2006;114(1):47–53.
16. Waziri A, Claassen J, Morgan Stuart R, Arif H, Michael Schmidt J, Mayer SA, et al. Intracortical electroencephalography in acute brain injury. Ann Neurol. 2009;66(3):366–77.
17. Vespa P, Miller C, McArthur D, Eliseo M, Etchepare M, Hirt D, et al. Nonconvulsive electrographic seizures after traumatic brain injury result in a delayed, prolonged increase in intracranial pressure and metabolic crisis. Crit Care Med. 2007;35(12):2830–6.
18. Vespa PM, McArthur DL, Xu Y, Eliseo M, Etchepare M, Dinov I, et al. Nonconvulsive seizures after traumatic brain injury are associated with hippocampal atrophy. Neurology. 2010;75(9):792–8.
19. Hauser WA, Annegers JF, Kurland LT. Incidence of epilepsy and unprovoked seizures in Rochester, Minnesota: 1935–1984. Epilepsia. 1993;34(3):453–8.
20. Angeleri F, Majkowski J, Cacchio G, Sobieszek A, D'Acunto S, Gesuita R, et al. Posttraumatic epilepsy risk factors: one-year prospective study after head injury. Epilepsia. 1999;40(9):1222–30.
21. Englander J, Bushnik T, Duong TT, Cifu DX, Zafonte R, Wright J, et al. Analyzing risk factors for late posttraumatic seizures: a prospective, multicenter investigation. Arch Phys Med Rehabil. 2003;84(3 SUPPL. 1):365–73.
22. Agrawal A, Timothy J, Pandit L, Manju M. Post-traumatic epilepsy: an overview. Clin Neurol Neurosurg. 2006;108(5):433–9.
23. Temkin NR, Anderson GD, Winn HR, Ellenbogen RG, Britz GW, Schuster J, et al. Magnesium sulfate for neuroprotection after traumatic brain injury: a randomised controlled trial. Lancet Neurol. 2007;6(1):29–38.
24. Temkin NR. Risk factors for posttraumatic seizures in adults. Epilepsia. 2003;44(SUPPL. 10):18–20.
25. Pitkänen A, Lukasiuk K. Molecular and cellular basis of epileptogenesis in symptomatic epilepsy. Epilepsy Behav. 2009;14(1 SUPPL. 1):16–25.
26. Davidson J, Cusimano MD, Bendena WG. Post-traumatic brain injury: genetic susceptibility to outcome. Neurosci. 2015;21(4):424–41.
27. Scheffer IE. Epilepsy genetics revolutionizes clinical practice. Neuropediatrics. 2014;45:70–4.
28. Schaumann BA, Annegers JF, Johnson SB, Moore KJ, Lubozynski MF, Salinsky MC. Family history of seizures in posttraumatic and alcohol-associated seizure disorders. Epilepsia. 1994;35(1):48–52.
29. Christensen J, Pedersen MG, Pedersen CB, Sidenius P, Olsen J, Vestergaard M. Long-term risk of epilepsy after traumatic brain injury in children and young adults: a population-based cohort study. Lancet. 2009;373(9669):1105–10.
30. Hung R, Carroll LJ, Cancelliere C, Cote P, Rumney P, Keightley M, et al. Systematic review of the clinical course, natural history, and prognosis for pediatric mild traumatic brain injury: results of the international collaboration on mild traumatic brain injury prognosis. Arch Phys Med Rehabil. 2014;95(3 Suppl):S174–91.
31. Raymont V, Salazar AM, Krueger F, Grafman J. "Studying injured minds" - the Vietnam head injury study and 40 years of brain injury research. Front Neurol. 2011;2:15.
32. Diaz-Arrastia R, Gong Y, Fair S, Scott KD, Garcia MC, Carlile MC, et al. Increased risk of late posttraumatic seizures associated with inheritance of APOE e4 allele. Arch Neurol. 2003;60:818–22.
33. Cotter D, Kelso A, Neligan A. Genetic biomarkers of posttraumatic epilepsy: a systematic review. Seizure. 2017;46:53–8.

34. Ritter AC, Kammerer CM, Brooks MM, Conley YP, Wagner AK. Genetic variation in neuronal glutamate transport genes and associations with posttraumatic seizure. Epilepsia. 2016;57(6):984–93.
35. Myers KA, Scheffer IE. DEPDC5 as a potential therapeutic target for epilepsy. Expert Opin Ther Targets. 2017;21:591–600.
36. Pitkänen A, McIntosh TK. Animal models of post-traumatic epilepsy. J Neurotrauma. 2006;23(2):241–61.
37. Lifshitz J. Fluid percussion injury model. In: Animal models of acute neurological injuries; 2009. p. 369–84.
38. Bragin A, Li L, Almajano J, Alvarado-Rojas C, Reid AY, Staba RJ, et al. Pathologic electrographic changes after experimental traumatic brain injury. Epilepsia. 2016;57(5):735–45.
39. Reid AY, Bragin A, Giza CC, Staba RJ, Engel J. The progression of electrophysiologic abnormalities during epileptogenesis after experimental traumatic brain injury. Epilepsia. 2016;57(10):1558–67.
40. D'Ambrosio R, Fairbanks JP, Fender JS, Born DE, Doyle DL, Miller JW. Post-traumatic epilepsy following fluid percussion injury in the rat. Brain. 2004;127(Pt 2):304–14.
41. Hunt RF, Scheff SW, Smith BN. Posttraumatic epilepsy after controlled cortical impact injury in mice. Exp Neurol. 2009;215(2):243–52.
42. Edward Dixon C, Clifton GL, Lighthall JW, Yaghmai AA, Hayes RL. A controlled cortical impact model of traumatic brain injury in the rat. J Neurosci Methods. 1991;39(3):253–62.
43. Laurer HL, Lenzlinger PM, McIntosh TK. Models of traumatic brain injury. Eur J Trauma. 2000;26:95–110.
44. Hunt RF, Boychuk JA, Smith BN. Neural circuit mechanisms of post–traumatic epilepsy. Front Cell Neurosci. 2013;7(June):1–14.
45. Mautes AE, Thome D, Steudel WI, Nacimiento AC, Yang Y, Shohami E. Changes in regional energy metabolism after closed head injury in the rat. J Mol Neurosci. 2001;16(1):33–9.
46. Chandel S, Gupta SK, Medhi B. Epileptogenesis following experimentally induced traumatic brain injury - a systematic review. Rev Neurosci. 2016;27(3):329–46.
47. Golarai G, Greenwood a C, Feeney DM, Connor JA. Physiological and structural evidence for hippocampal involvement in persistent seizure susceptibility after traumatic brain injury. J Neurosci. 2001;21(21):8523–37.
48. Reeves TM, Kao CQ, Phillips LL, Bullock MR, Povlishock JT. Presynaptic excitability changes following traumatic brain injury in the rat. J Neurosci Res. 2000;60(3):370–9.
49. Griesemer D, Mautes AM. Closed head injury causes hyperexcitability in rat hippocampal CA1 but not in CA3 pyramidal cells. J Neurotrauma. 2007;24(12):1823–32.
50. Morganti-Kossmann MC, Rancan M, Stahel PF, Kossmann T. Inflammatory response in acute traumatic brain injury: a double-edged sword. Curr Opin Crit Care. 2002;8(2):101–5.
51. Hu S, Sheng WS, Ehrlich LC, Peterson PK, Chao CC. Cytokine effects on glutamate uptake by human astrocytes. Neuroimmunomodulation. 2000;7(3):153–9.
52. Balosso S, Ravizza T, Pierucci M, Calcagno E, Invernizzi R, Di Giovanni G, et al. Molecular and functional interactions between tumor necrosis factor-alpha receptors and the glutamatergic system in the mouse hippocampus: implications for seizure susceptibility. Neuroscience. 2009;161(1):293–300.
53. Pickering M, Cumiskey D, O'Connor JJ. Actions of TNF-alpha on glutamatergic synaptic transmission in the central nervous system. Exp Physiol. 2005;90(5):663–70.
54. Zhu G, Okada M, Yoshida S, Mori F, Ueno S, Wakabayashi K, et al. Effects of interleukin-1?? On hippocampal glutamate and GABA releases associated with Ca2+–induced Ca2+ releasing systems. Epilepsy Res. 2006;71(2–3):107–16.
55. Samuelsson C, Kumlien E, Flink R, Lindholm D, Ronne-Engström E. Decreased cortical levels of astrocytic glutamate transport protein GLT-1 in a rat model of posttraumatic epilepsy. Neurosci Lett. 2000;289(3):185–8.
56. Rao VL, Dogan A, Bowen KK, Todd KG, Dempsey RJ. Antisense knockdown of the glial glutamate transporter GLT-1 exacerbates hippocampal neuronal damage following traumatic injury to rat brain. Eur J Neurosci. 2001;13(1):119–28.
57. Tomkins O, Feintuch A, Benifla M, Cohen A, Friedman A, Shelef I. Blood-brain barrier breakdown following traumatic brain injury: a possible role in posttraumatic epilepsy. Cardiovasc Psychiatry Neurol. 2011;2011:765923.
58. Loscher W, Brandt C. Prevention or modification of Epileptogenesis after brain insults: experimental approaches and translational research. Pharmacol Rev. 2010;62(4):668–700.
59. Gao X, Deng P, Xu ZC, Chen J. Moderate traumatic brain injury causes acute dendritic and synaptic degeneration in the hippocampal dentate gyrus. PLoS One. 2011;6(9):e24566.
60. Robinson S, Berglass JB, Denson JL, Berkner J, Anstine CV, Winer JL, et al. Microstructural and microglial changes after repetitive mild traumatic brain injury in mice. J Neurosci Res. 2017;95(4):1025–35.
61. Shitaka Y, Tran HT, Bennett RE, Sanchez L, Levy MA, Dikranian K, et al. Repetitive closed-skull traumatic brain injury in mice causes persistent multifocal axonal injury and microglial reactivity. J Neuropathol Exp Neurol. 2011;70(7):551–67.
62. Chirumamilla S, Sun D, Bullock MR, Colello RJ. Traumatic brain injury induced cell proliferation in the adult mammalian central nervous system. J Neurotrauma. 2002;19(6):693–703.
63. Griesemer D, Mautes AM. Closed head injury causes Hyperexcitability in rat hippocampal CA1 but not in CA3 pyramidal cells. J Neurotrauma. 2007;24(12):1823–32.
64. Zhang B-L, Chen X, Tan T, Yang Z, Carlos D, Jiang R-C, et al. Traumatic brain injury impairs synaptic plasticity in hippocampus in rats. Chin Med J. 2011;124(5):740–5.
65. Prince DA, Parada I, Scalise K, Graber K, Jin X, Shen F. Epilepsy following cortical injury: cellular and molecular mechanisms as targets for potential prophylaxis. Epilepsia. 2009;50:30–40.
66. Li H, Prince DA. Synaptic activity in chronically injured, epileptogenic sensory-motor neocortex. J Neurophysiol. 2002;88(1):2–12.
67. Cantu D, Walker K, Andresen L, Taylor-Weiner A, Hampton D, Tesco G, et al. Traumatic brain injury increases cortical glutamate network activity by compromising GABAergic control. Cereb Cortex. 2015;25(8):2306–20.
68. Swartz BE, Houser CR, Tomiyasu U, Walsh GO, DeSalles A, Rich JR, et al. Hippocampal cell loss in posttraumatic human epilepsy. Epilepsia. 2006;47(8):1373–82.
69. Atkins CM, Truettner JS, Lotocki G, Sanchez-Molano J, Kang Y, Alonso OF, et al. Post-traumatic seizure susceptibility is attenuated by hypothermia therapy. Eur J Neurosci. 2010;32(11):1912–20.
70. Hu B, Liu C, Bramlett H, Sick TJ, Alonso OF, Chen S, et al. Changes in trkB-ERK1/2-CREB/Elk-1 pathways in hippocampal mossy fiber organization after traumatic brain injury. J Cereb Blood Flow Metab. 2004;24(8):934–43.
71. Hunt RF, Scheff SW, Smith BN. Regionally localized recurrent excitation in the dentate gyrus of a cortical contusion model of posttraumatic epilepsy. J Neurophysiol. 2010;103(3):1490–500.
72. Hunt RF, Haselhorst LA, Schoch KM, Bach EC, Rios-Pilier J, Scheff SW, et al. Posttraumatic mossy fiber sprouting is related to the degree of cortical damage in three mouse strains. Epilepsy Res. 2012;99(1–2):167–70.
73. D'Ambrosio R, Fender JS, Fairbanks JP, Simon EA, Born DE, Doyle DL, et al. Progression from frontal-parietal to mesial-temporal epilepsy after fluid percussion injury in the rat. Brain. 2005;128(1):174–88.

74. Diaz-Arrastia R, Agostini MA, Frol a B, Mickey B, Fleckenstein J, Bigio E, et al. Neurophysiologic and neuroradiologic features of intractable epilepsy after traumatic brain injury in adults. Arch Neurol. 2000;57(11):1611–6.
75. Haltiner AM, Temkin NR, Dikmen SS. Risk of seizure recurrence after the first late posttraumatic seizure. Arch Phys Med Rehabil. 1997;78(8):835–40.
76. Christensen J. The epidemiology of posttraumatic epilepsy epidemiology of traumatic. Brain Inj. 2015;35(3):218–22.
77. Gupta PK, Sayed N, Ding K, Agostini MA, Van Ness PC, Yablon S, et al. Subtypes of post-traumatic epilepsy: clinical, electrophysiological, and imaging features. J Neurotrauma. 2014;31(16):1439–43.
78. Manaka S, Takahashi H, Sano K. The difference between children and adults in the onset of post-traumatic epilepsy. Psychiatry Clin Neurosci. 1981;35(3):301–4.
79. Pohlmann-Eden B, Bruckmeir J. Predictors and dynamics of posttraumatic epilepsy. Acta Neurol Scand. 1997;95(5):257–62.
80. Adams JH, Scott G, Parker LS, Graham DI, Doyle D. The contusion index: a quantitative approach to cerebral contusions in head injury. Neuropathol Appl Neurobiol. 1980;6(4):319–24.
81. Bešenski N, Broz R, Jadro-Šantel D, Pavić D, Mikulić D. The course of the traumatising force in acceleration head injury: CT evidence. Neuroradiology. 1996;38(SUPPL. 1):S36.
82. Curia G, Levitt M, Fender JS, Miller JW, Ojemann J, D'Ambrosio R. Impact of injury location and severity on posttraumatic epilepsy in the rat: role of frontal neocortex. Cereb Cortex. 2011;21(7):1574–92.
83. Marks DA, Kim J, Spencer DD, Spencer SS. Seizure localization and pathology following head injury in patients with uncontrolled epilepsy. Neurology. 1995;4Marks, D(11):2051–7.
84. Jennett B. Posttraumatic epilepsy. Adv Neurol. 1979;22:137–47.
85. Kwan P. The natural history of epilepsy: an epidemiological view. J Neurol Neurosurg Psychiatry. 2004;75(10):1376–81.
86. Ilaria Casetta EC. Post-traumatic epilepsy: review. J Neurol Neurophysiol. 2011;s2(1):009.
87. Hung C, Chen JWY. Treatment of post-traumatic epilepsy. Curr Treat Options Neurol. 2012;14(4):293–306.
88. Chen LLK, Baca CB, Choe J, Chen JW, Ayad ME, Cheng EM, et al. Posttraumatic epilepsy in operation enduring freedom / operation Iraqi freedom veterans. Mil Med. 2014;179(May):492–7.
89. Salinsky M, Storzbach D, Goy E, Evrard C. Traumatic brain injury and psychogenic seizures in veterans. J Head Trauma Rehabil. 2015;30(February):E65–70.
90. Barry E, Krumholz A, Bergey GK, Chatha H, Alemayehu S, Grattan L. Nonepileptic posttraumatic seizures. Epilepsia. 1998;39(4):427–31.
91. Rao V, Parko K. Clinical approach to posttraumatic epilepsy. Semin Neurol. 2015;35(1):057–63.
92. Messori A, Polonara G, Carle F, Gesuita R, Salvolini U. Predicting posttraumatic epilepsy with MRI: prospective longitudinal morphologic study in adults. Epilepsia. 2005;46(9):1472–81.
93. Diaz-Arrastia R, Agostini MA, Madden CJ, Van Ness PC. Posttraumatic epilepsy: the endophenotypes of a human model of epileptogenesis. Epilepsia. 2009;50(SUPPL. 2):14–20.
94. Kou Z, Wu Z, Tong KA, Holshouser B, Benson RR, Hu J, et al. The role of advanced MR imaging findings as biomarkers of traumatic brain injury. J Head Trauma Rehabil. 2010;25(4):267–82.
95. Jennett B, van de Sande J. EEG prediction of post-Traumatic epilepsy. Epilepsia. 1975;16(2):251–6.
96. Steinbaugh LA, Lindsell CJ, Shutter LA, Szaflarski JP. Initial EEG predicts outcomes in a trial of levetiracetam vs. fosphenytoin for seizure prevention. Epilepsy Behav. 2012;23(3):280–4.
97. Heikkinen ER, Ronty HS, Tolonen U, Pyhtinen J. Development of posttraumatic epilepsy. Stereotact Funct Neurosurg. 1990;54–55:25–33.
98. McCrory PR, Bladin PF, Berkovic SF. Retrospective study of concussive convulsions in elite Australian rules and rugby league footballers: phenomenology, aetiology, and outcome. BMJ. 1997;314(7075):171.
99. Temkin NR, Dikmen SS, Wilensky AJ, Keihm J, Chabal S, Winn HR. A randomized, double-blind study of phenytoin for the prevention of post-traumatic seizures. N Engl J Med. 1990;323(8):497–502.
100. Kruer RM, Harris LH, Goodwin H, Kornbluth J, Thomas KP, Slater LA, et al. Changing trends in the use of seizure prophylaxis after traumatic brain injury: a shift from phenytoin to levetiracetam. J Crit Care. 2013;28(5):883.e9.
101. Yang Y, Zheng F, Xu X, Wang X. Levetiracetam versus phenytoin for seizure prophylaxis following traumatic brain injury: a systematic review and meta-analysis. CNS Drugs. 2016; 30(8):677–88.
102. Khan NR, Vanlandingham MA, Fierst TM, Hymel C, Hoes K, Evans LT, et al. Should Levetiracetam or phenytoin be used for posttraumatic seizure prophylaxis? A systematic review of the literature and meta-analysis. Neurosurgery. 2016;79(6):775–81.
103. Szaflarski JP, Sangha KS, Lindsell CJ, Shutter LA. Prospective, randomized, single-blinded comparative trial of intravenous levetiracetam versus phenytoin for seizure prophylaxis. Neurocrit Care. 2010;12(2):165–72.
104. Torbic H, Forni AA, Anger KE, Degrado JR, Greenwood BC. Use of antiepileptics for seizure prophylaxis after traumatic brain injury. Am J Health Syst Pharm. 2013;70:759–66.
105. Jones KE, Puccio AM, Harshman KJ, Falcione B, Benedict N, Jankowitz BT, et al. Levetiracetam versus phenytoin for seizure prophylaxis in severe traumatic brain injury. Neurosurg Focus. 2008;25(4):E3.
106. Glotzner FL, Haubitz I, Miltner F, Kapp G, Pflughaupt KW. Seizure prevention using carbamazepine following severe brain injuries. Neurochirurgia (Stuttg). 1983;26(0028–3819):66–79.
107. Temkin NR, Dikmen SS, Anderson GD, Wilensky AJ, Holmes MD, Cohen W, et al. Valproate therapy for prevention of posttraumatic seizures: a randomized trial. J Neurosurg. 1999;91(4):593–600.
108. Temkin NR. Preventing and treating posttraumatic seizures: the human experience. In: Epilepsia; 2009. p. 10–3.
109. Chadwick D. Seizures and epilepsy after traumatic brain injury. Lancet. 2000;355(9201):334–6.
110. Dikmen SS, Temkin NR, Miller B, Machamer J, Winn HR. Neurobehavioral effects of phenytoin prophylaxis of posttraumatic seizures. JAMA. 1991;265(10):1271–7.
111. Langendorf FG, Pedley TA, Temkin NR. Chapter 253 Posttraumatic Seizures.
112. Burneo JG, Sirven JI, Kiesel LW, Vecht CJ, Jehi L, Chung SS, et al. Managing common complex symptomatic epilepsies: tumors and trauma. Epilepsy Curr. 2013;13:232–5.
113. Hernandez TD. Preventing post-traumatic epilepsy after brain injury: weighing the costs and benefits of anticonvulsant prophylaxis. Trends Pharmacol Sci. 1997;18:59–62.
114. LaFrance WC, Deluca M, MacHan JT, Fava JL. Traumatic brain injury and psychogenic nonepileptic seizures yield worse outcomes. Epilepsia. 2013;54(4):718–25.
115. Camfield P, Camfield C. When is it safe to discontinue AED treatment? Epilepsia. 2008;49:25–8.
116. Levy SL, Burnham WM, Hwang PA. An evaluation of the anticonvulsant effects of vitamin E. Epilepsy Res. 1990;6:12–7.
117. Yokoi I, Toma J, Liu J, Kabuto H, Mori A. Adenosines scavenged hydroxyl radicals and prevented posttraumatic epilepsy. Free Radic Biol Med. 1995;19(4):473–9.
118. Malhotra J, Gupta YK. Effect of adenosine receptor modulation on pentylenetetrazole-induced seizures in rats. Br J Pharmacol. 1997;120(2):282–8.

119. Hoeppner TJ, Morrell F. Control of scar formation in experimentally induced epilepsy. Exp Neurol. 1986;94(3):519–36.
120. Roberts I, Yates D, Sandercock P, Farrell B, Wasserberg J, Lomas G, et al. Effect of intravenous corticosteroids on death within 14 days in 10008 adults with clinically significant head injury (MRC CRASH trial): randomised placebo-controlled trial. Lancet. 2004;364(9442):1321–8.
121. Watson NF, Barber JK, Doherty MJ, Miller JW, Temkin NR. Does glucocorticoid administration prevent late seizures after head injury? Epilepsia. 2004;45(6):690–4.
122. Diamond ML, Ritter AC, Failla MD, Boles JA, Conley YP, Kochanek PM, et al. IL-1β associations with posttraumatic epilepsy development: a genetics and biomarker cohort study. Epilepsia. 2015;56(7):991–1001.
123. Lu X-CM, Shear DA, Graham PB, Bridson GW, Uttamsingh V, Chen Z, et al. Dual therapeutic effects of C-10068, a dextromethorphan derivative, against post-traumatic nonconvulsive seizures and Neuroinflammation in a rat model of penetrating ballistic-like brain injury. J Neurotrauma. 2015;32(20):1621–32.
124. Chrzaszcz M, Venkatesan C, Dragisic T, Watterson DM, Wainwright MS. Minozac treatment prevents increased seizure susceptibility in a mouse "two-hit" model of closed skull traumatic brain injury and electroconvulsive shock-induced seizures. J Neurotrauma. 2010;27(7):1283–95.
125. Chen T, Dai SH, Jiang ZQ, Luo P, Jiang XF, Fei Z, et al. The AMPAR antagonist Perampanel attenuates traumatic brain injury through anti-oxidative and anti-inflammatory activity. Cell Mol Neurobiol. 2017;37(1):43–52.
126. D'Ambrosio R, Eastman CL, Darvas F, Fender JS, Verley DR, Farin FM, et al. Mild passive focal cooling prevents epileptic seizures after head injury in rats. Ann Neurol. 2013;73(2):199–209.
127. Butler CR, Boychuk JA, Smith BN. Differential effects of rapamycin treatment on tonic and phasic GABAergic inhibition in dentate granule cells after focal brain injury in mice. Exp Neurol. 2016;280:30–40.
128. Butler CR, Boychuk JA, Smith BN. Effects of rapamycin treatment on neurogenesis and synaptic reorganization in the dentate gyrus after controlled cortical impact injury in mice. Front Syst Neurosci. 2015;9:163.
129. Berdichevsky Y, Dryer AM, Saponjian Y, Mahoney MM, Pimentel CA, Lucini CA, et al. PI3K-Akt signaling activates mTOR-mediated Epileptogenesis in Organotypic hippocampal culture model of post-traumatic epilepsy. J Neurosci. 2013;33(21):9056–67.
130. Song Y, Pimentel C, Walters K, Boller L, Ghiasvand S, Liu J, et al. Neuroprotective levels of IGF-1 exacerbate epileptogenesis after brain injury. Sci Rep. 2016;6(1):32095.
131. Kozan R, Ayyildiz M, Agar E. The effects of intracerebroventricular AM-251, a CB1-receptor antagonist, and ACEA, a CB1-receptor agonist, on penicillin-induced epileptiform activity in rats. Epilepsia. 2009;50(7):1760–7.
132. Echegoyen J, Armstrong C, Morgan RJ, Soltesz I. Single application of a CB1 receptor antagonist rapidly following head injury prevents long-term hyperexcitability in a rat model. Epilepsy Res. 2009;85(1):123–7.
133. Nissinen J, Andrade P, Natunen T, Hiltunen M, Malm T, Kanninen K, et al. Disease-modifying effect of atipamezole in a model of post-traumatic epilepsy. Epilepsy Res. 2017;136:18–34.
134. Hartzfeld P, Elisevich K, Pace M, Smith B, Gutierrez JA. Characteristics and surgical outcomes for medial temporal post-traumatic epilepsy. Br J Neurosurg. 2008;22(2):224–30.
135. Benbadis SR, Tatum WO, Vale FL. When drugs don't work: an algorithmic approach to medically intractable epilepsy. Neurology. 2000;55(12):1780–4.
136. Elliott RE, Bollo RJ, Berliner JL, Silverberg A, Carlson C, Geller EB, et al. Anterior temporal lobectomy with amygdalohippocampectomy for mesial temporal sclerosis: predictors of long-term seizure control. J Neurosurg. 2013;119:261–72.
137. Spencer S, Huh L. Outcomes of epilepsy surgery in adults and children. Lancet Neurol. 2008;7:525–37.
138. Hakimian S, Kershenovich A, Miller JW, Ojemann JG, Hebb AO, D'Ambrosio R, et al. Long-term outcome of extratemporal resection in posttraumatic epilepsy. Neurosurg Focus. 2012;32(3):E10.
139. Brigo F, Cicero R, Fiaschi A, Bongiovanni LG. The breach rhythm. Clin Neurophysiol. 2011;122:2116–20.
140. Englot DJ, Chang EF, Auguste KI. Vagus nerve stimulation for epilepsy: a meta-analysis of efficacy and predictors of response. J Neurosurg. 2011;115(6):1248–55.
141. Fisher R, Salanova V, Witt T, Worth R, Henry T, Gross R, et al. Electrical stimulation of the anterior nucleus of thalamus for treatment of refractory epilepsy. Epilepsia. 2010;51(5):899–908.
142. Heck CN, King-Stephens D, Massey AD, Nair DR, Jobst BC, Barkley GL, et al. Two-year seizure reduction in adults with medically intractable partial onset epilepsy treated with responsive neurostimulation: final results of the RNS system pivotal trial. Epilepsia. 2014;55(3):432–41.
143. Morrell MJ. Responsive cortical stimulation for the treatment of medically intractable partial epilepsy. Neurology. 2011;77(13):1295–304.

# Traumatic Brain Injury and Electroencephalogram Findings

# 8

Renato Anghinah and Jéssica Natuline Ianof

## History

The discovery of electroencephalography (EEG) in 1929 by the German psychiatrist Hans Berger was a historical advancement that provided a new neurological and psychiatric diagnostic tool at the time, mainly considering the lack of all the exams that are available in daily practice today, such as computed tomography (CT) and magnetic resonance *imaging* (*MRI*), without which the preparation of neurological diagnoses and the planning of neurosurgical operating procedures would not be acceptable [1]. Based on the discovery of Caton and Beck, Danilevsky, Prawdicz-Neminsky, and others that there was a spontaneous (intrinsic) brain electrical current that could be recorded, Berger made the first EEG recording (electrocorticogram) on July 6, 1924, during a neurosurgical operation on a 17-year-old boy. He reported this in 1929, being the first to use the terms alpha and beta [1]. The discovery of electroencephalography was a landmark for the advancement of neuroscience neurological and neurosurgical practice every day, especially for patients with seizures. At a time when lumbar puncture, pneumoencephalography, and ventriculography were the only diagnostic tools to detect and locate "sick sites" in the brain, the EEG revolutionized daily neurological and neurosurgical procedures and exceeded a period of approximately 40 years (1930–1970) until the advent of computed tomography [2]. Its importance, currently, may not be as great as it was before, but it still has its place in the diagnosis of seizures, brain tumors, degenerative brain disorders, and other diseases.

## Introduction

In traumatic brain injury (TBI) patients, diagnosis and treatment are essential for acute patient care and long-term rehabilitation. Cognitive dysfunction (memory impairment, attention, and information processing skill) [3], somatic problems (headache, fatigue, sexual dysfunction, and sleep disorders), mood swings (depression, aggression, emotional liability, and anxiety), and post-traumatic personality changes (self-centered behavior, reduced social awareness, and disinhibited behavior) are some of the several consequences that may occur after TBI.

Electroencephalography (EEG) is important for clinical assessment of consciousness to support diagnosis and prognosis [4, 5]. The electrical activity of brain tissue may have good prognostic value after brain injury. EEG can provide an objective and quantitative measure of the severity of brain injury [6], when performed from 15 days to 4 years after TBI. In addition, EEG can detect early seizure activity and give information about sleep patterns during polysomnography, since sleep disturbances (insomnia, hypersomnia, and altered sleep-wake cycles [7–9]) are common after TBI. The neural mechanisms that contribute to sleep disturbances are multiple – the degree of damage to sleep-wake regulation centers, such as ascending reticular formation and associated pathways or neurotransmitter systems – and may affect sleep [10, 11]. Also, anxiety and depression often occur after TBI, and increased depression is associated with poor sleep quality [12, 13].

Most cognitive disorders have a primary diagnosis that is clinically based, but the EEG plays a role in evaluation, classification, and follow-up of some of these disorders. The EEG is a widely accepted method for evaluating cortical information processing and neurophysiologic changes that occur during unconsciousness and the different states of conscious awareness [14]. In addition, it is now possible to increase EEG sensitivity through the use of digital EEG (dEEG) and the mathematical procedures implemented in quantitative EEG (qEEG).

R. Anghinah (✉)
Department of Neurology – Cognitive Rehabilitation after TBI, Clinics Hospital – School of Medicine – University of São Paulo, São Paulo, Brazil

Center of Excellence in Neurology – Americas Serviços Médicos, São Paulo, Brazil

J. N. Ianof
Department of Neurology – Cognitive Rehabilitation after TBI, Clinics Hospital – School of Medicine – University of São Paulo, São Paulo, Brazil


R. Anghinah et al. (eds.), *Topics in Cognitive Rehabilitation in the TBI Post-Hospital Phase*,
https://doi.org/10.1007/978-3-319-95376-2_8

Clinical electrophysiologic techniques are frequently used in the evaluation of cerebral function following TBI [15]. These tools enables noninvasive recording of the electrical or magnetic activity of the brain. Conventional EEG is the prototypic clinical electrophysiological assessment and was the first neurodiagnostic tool to allow characterization of disturbances in cerebral physiology produced by TBI [16, 17]. The digital recording of cerebral function is acquired from 21 electrodes arranged on the scalp, according to the International 10–20 System, and generates waveform tracings suitable for visual inspection by a qualified electroencephalographer [18, 19].

The electroencephalogram (EEG) records the electrical potential difference between brain electrical activities recorded between two electrodes [20]. EEG records the average membrane potential of apical dendrites of cortical pyramidal neurons, which tends to oscillate. It detects the synchronous occurrence of dendritic synaptic potentials – excitatory and inhibitory postsynaptic [21].

The physiological basis of these oscillations is a manifestation of both intrinsic properties of neurons (ionic conductances) and network interactions (connectivity). Different frequency oscillations are guided principally by cortico-cortical connections and thalamocortical connections to varying degrees depending on the specific oscillation. EEG oscillations exist in a broad range of frequencies from below 1 Hz to several hundred hertz. The physiology is best understood for several "classic" frequency bands including delta (0.5–4 Hz), theta (4–7 Hz), alpha (8–13 Hz), beta (14–30 Hz), and gamma (30–100 Hz). These frequency ranges [22] represent different oscillatory phenomena with unique underlying physiological mechanisms, cortical topographies, and functions. Different combinations of frequency bands in different quantities represent different states of the brain – attentive wakefulness, drowsiness, and stages of sleep.

EEG clinical assessment usually involves a visual inspection of the electrical activity of the brain in a variety of brain states and the evaluation of the topography and amount of appropriate oscillatory activity of the state, as well as examination for the presence of pathological potentials. For the detection of epileptiform activity, the human eye actually exceeds computerized waveform analysis despite decades of attempts to automate EEG interpretation [23]. But when it comes to the evaluation of topography and the amount of oscillating activity and what constitutes a normal or abnormal distribution of this activity, visual inspection fails considerably, and the use of computerized algorithms is needed.

For example, to obtain a quantitative evaluation of the amount of oscillatory activity at any and all frequencies in a specific region of the brain, the qEEG frequency analysis transforms the original EEG data over a period of time into a representation of its frequency content, generating a continuous EEG "force spectrum."

## Utility of EEG

EEGs enhance conventional medical approaches to imaging the structure and function of the brain. EEG as a neuroimaging modality holds several advantages over more conventional medical approaches. Nowadays, computed tomography (CT) and MRI are the current "gold standards" for imaging assessment of neurophysiological trauma. They have an excellent spatial resolution for easily identifying lesions; but both approaches require very large and expensive equipment, special facilities for their use, and dedicated technicians for operation and are not available everywhere. CT uses small doses of radiation, which can carry potential risks for long-term side effects if patients are scanned frequently and MRI uses an extremely strong magnetic field, and needs a careful operating room. Also, it has a lot of limitations – its use has contraindication of medical devices, implants, and any foreign ferrous metal objects in the patient's body. Equipment used for EEG is more portable and cheaper and requires no special facilities. These characteristics lead to field ability and a broader operational effectiveness [24].

The data derived from EEG are also essentially distinct as compared to CT and MRI data. In particular, while CT and MRI have excellent spatial resolution, the resulting images (which may take several minutes to acquire) are temporally static and thus provide no direct measurement of functional, ongoing brain activity. Even the best current methods of "functional MRI" are limited to multiple seconds for the acquisition of whole-brain images. In contrast, EEG is extremely high-resolution in the time domain (EEG can be sub-millisecond) and, as described above, is a direct measurement of neuronal activity. This enables a great number of analyses, which capitalize on direct responses to stimuli, cognitive responses, interrelatedness of continuous signals, and the oscillation of both discrete and cross-regional networks of brain areas [20].

## EEG in TBI

Electrical activity is a relatively sensitive index of the pathophysiological response of the brain to the immediate and secondary damage of the TBI, and that is why it is intimately related to the outcome of the patient's situation [25].

Glasgow Coma Scale, duration of loss of consciousness, and duration of post-traumatic amnesia (PTA) are considered important clinical predictors of the severity and long-term prognosis of brain damage. However, these assessments are often unknown or unregistered. Therefore, there is a need to develop an objective and quantitative measure of the severity of brain injury using the EEG tests [26].

Immediately after TBI, EEG initially shows epileptiform activity [27], followed by suppressed cortical activity – which can last from seconds to about 1 min [28]. Many patients return to normal within 1 h, while others continue to have focal or generalized EEG slowing – that can last from weeks to months. The posterior alpha frequency is on average 0.7 Hz lower and gradually returns to baseline frequency over a period of time ranging from weeks to a few months [29]. The theta/alpha ratio increases after mild TBI and tends to return to normal within weeks to months [30].

In general, high-frequency EEG (beta and gamma) rhythms are produced by cortical generators, whereas lower-frequency rhythms (delta) are the product of corticothalamic synchrony and may be more prominent when the choro-thalamic connections are interrupted [31].

EEG abnormalities are more common than clinical symptoms in the early months after mild TBI. Later, after the injury, there is little correspondence between EEG and clinical signs, symptoms, results of images, or psychometric tests [29].

Quantitative EEG (qEEG) also shows immediate reduction in mean alpha frequency and increase in slow theta activity. These changes usually take weeks to months to resolve. Improvement is associated with symptom reduction [29]. Theta/beta ratio is increased. Compared to healthy controls, there are more slow waves in patients with mild TBI [32].

## Mild TBI

Electroencephalography (EEG) was the first clinical neurodiagnostic assessment that revealed abnormal brain function following traumatic brain injury [17, 33, 34]. EEG may be more sensitive than clinical neurological examination to detect brain injury. After mild traumatic TBI (mTBI), most patients (86%) with an abnormal neurological examination had an abnormal EEG. But only 23% of abnormal EEGs were accompanied by an abnormal neurological examination [35]. EEG changes are not uniform in all individuals, due to differences in the severity of head injury. Some people have a clinically normal EEG as early as 15 min after concussion [36].

EEG abnormalities are more frequent in patients with durations of unconsciousness lasting more than 2 min (56%) than in patients with briefer periods of unconsciousness (17%) [37].

It is important to emphasize that there are no clear EEG or qEEG features unique to mild traumatic brain injury.

- *Acute EEG changes*
- Immediately after mTBI, there is epileptiform activity (high-amplitude sharp waves or high-frequency discharges), followed by diffuse suppression of cortical activity that usually last for 1–2 min, then there is a diffuse slowing of the EEG, and brain activity returns to the normal baseline within 10 min to 1 h [27, 38, 39]. qEEG often shows immediate reduction in mean alpha frequency [40], with increased theta [41, 42], increased delta [43], or increased theta/alpha ratio [44, 45].
- *Subacute EEG changes*
- Weeks to months after mTBI, there is a 1–2 Hz increase in the frequency of the posterior alpha rhythm – it represents a return to the original baseline from the post-traumatic slowing [29, 35]. The majority of the acute EEG abnormalities resolve by 3 months – 90% resolve within 1 year of the head trauma [29].
- *Chronic EEG changes*
- Lewine et al. (2007) studied a group of 30 patients with persistent psychiatric, somatic, or cognitive complaints (lasting >1 year) that was developed within the first few weeks of mTBI. The magnetoencephalography (MEG) revealed epileptiform abnormalities in 16% and slow-wave abnormalities in 63% [46]. They found a higher power in the delta band (1.5–5 Hz) and a lower power in the alpha band (8.5–12 Hz) in postconcussive syndrome patients compared with matched controls.

## Improving EEG Analysis

Digital EEG (dEEG) is not recorded on paper, like the conventional EEG. The collected data is presented in video monitor and its storage is in digital format, which allows flexibility in the analysis. The qEEG represents the mathematical processing of the digital EEG. Often, it is not possible through visual analysis to recognize changes in the electroencephalographic record. In addition, despite the presence of neurological disorders, the visual analysis of the EEG tracing may be normal. The use of the qEEG allows a more in-depth analysis of the base activity, slow or fast focal activities, subtle asymmetries, waves, and spicules [47].

The routine EEG (up to 32 electrodes) has a high temporal resolution (on the order of milliseconds) but poor spatial resolution. This limits the use of conventional EEG in mapping and distributing brain electrical activity spatially [48]. One way to improve spatial resolution is through the use of a larger number of electrodes. The low-resolution brain electromagnetic tomography (LORETA) method helps to solve the inverse EEG problem – problem in calculating the distribution of currents for a given electrical potential – since the electrical activity found in the exam is distributed in a CT scan image that corresponds to an average brain of the population. The functional images of LORETA represent the electrical activity in each voxel as power of the spectral density [49].

LORETA is a mathematical algorithm that estimates the sources of EEG recorded on the scalp [50] and is widely used in EEG studies. New improved versions of LORETA have been developed – standardized low-resolution brain electromagnetic tomography (sLORETA) and exact low-resolution brain electromagnetic tomography (eLORETA). sLORETA [51] and eLORETA [52] have the same low spatial resolution, with zero localization error, but the eLORETA provides better localization of the signal source in the presence of noise [53].

Leon-Carrion et al. (2008) performed a study with 16 patients with TBI, among them 7 subjects had minimally conscious state, and 9 had severe neurocognitive disorders. The presence of slow waves was twice as large in the first group. They also found differences in LORETA in relation to the theta frequency in the middle occipital cortex [54].

The study of Tomkins et al. (2011) included 37 patients, of whom 19 suffered from post-traumatic epilepsy. They found, through sLORETA, that TBI patients had slower delta waves than controls, regardless of whether or not they had post-trauma epilepsy [55].

Corradini and Persinger (2013) noted, through the use of sLORETA, a decrease in parahippocampal electrical activity and in regions adjacent to the temporal lobe in individuals with mild TBI [56].

The study of Ledwidge and Molfese (2016) used sLORETA to compare athletes with concussion and control athletes and found that those with concussion had higher electrical current density in the lower parietal gyrus than controls. These findings support the hypothesis that individuals with a past concussion recruited compensatory neural resources to meet the demands of executive functioning [57].

The study of Ianof et al. (2017) compared 19 patients with diffuse axonal injury (DAI) –type of TBI that results from acceleration/deceleration or rotational injuries to the brain – and 17 healthy adults submitted to high-resolution EEG with 128 channels. Cortical sources of EEG rhythms were estimated by exact low-resolution electromagnetic tomography (eLORETA) analysis. The mean alpha frequency peak was 10.23 Hz (±0.90 SE) for the control participants and 9.73 Hz (±1.02 SE) for the DAI group. No statistically significant difference was found between the control and DAI groups (Mann-Whitney U test, $p > 0.125$). In comparison to the control, the DAI group had increased theta activity in the limbic, occipital, sublobar, and temporal areas [58].

## Post-traumatic Epilepsy: An Overview

Epilepsy is a disorder of the brain characterized by a predisposition to generate epileptic seizures with neurobiological, cognitive, psychological, and social consequences [59]. It can also be defined as unprovoked recurrent seizures that occur 24 h apart, at least [60].

Seizures are a frequent consequence of TBI, and its incidence is of 15–22% in TBI patients [61]. Post-traumatic epilepsy (PTE) and post-traumatic seizures (PTS) are terms used to describe seizures that occur after head trauma that are believed to be causally related to the trauma itself [62]. PTS are seizures that occur in the first week after TBI and are considered to be provoked by head injury. PTE is defined as one or more unprovoked seizures that occur at least a week after TBI [63].

The occurrence of seizures after head injury is a lifelong complication of TBI and has been demonstrated to worsen functional outcome significantly [64].

Seizures begin, in approximately half of PTE cases, within the first year and in 80%, within the first 2 years. One population-based study estimated that 86% of patients with one seizure, occurring at least 1 week after TBI, had a second seizure within 2 years [65].

There has been significant focus on computed tomography, EEG, and MRI after TBI to evaluate risk of PTE. Angeleri et al. (1999) performed a 12-month prospective study evaluating clinical progress, EEG, and computed tomography at four scheduled intervals. Some of the patients in this study also underwent MRI. Their study showed correlation of PTE with early seizures, frontal or temporal lesions on acute computed tomography, development of an EEG focus 1 month after TBI, and cortical MRI hyperintense areas [66]. It is recommended to obtain neuroimaging and EEG after PTS.

## EEG and Sleep

Electrophysiologic changes in sleep may be present in both the acute and chronic stages of TBI and vary according to the severity of the injury. Cognitive dysfunctions may be caused by sleep disturbances and may aggravate impairment in patients with TBI. Sleep disturbances can include hypersomnia, insomnia, altered sleep-wake cycles, periodic limb movements during sleep, disorders of rapid eye movement during sleep, and respiratory disorders of fast sleep in the movement of the eyes, such as obstructive sleep apnea or central apnea. In patients with obstructive sleep apnea, there is a greater impairment of neurocognitive function, mostly memory and sustained attention, than patients who do not present disordered breathing during sleep [67].

After the acute stage of TBI, sleep disorders are common [67]. Mild TBI patients may show longer sleep latency and lower sleep efficiency. Also they have a lower delta power (but higher alpha and beta power) during non-REM (NREM) sleep [68, 69]. This EEG pattern of fast frequencies intruding into deep NREM sleep has been described in insomnia patients and may represent a deficit in turning off arousal [70].

After severe TBI, EEG patterns in the acute stage may have prognostic implications. A retrospective study of 64 adults with severe TBI admitted to the intensive care unit revealed that sleep features seen on continuous EEG monitoring were associated with significantly better functional outcomes [71].

In patients with TBI, sleep architecture findings are inconsistent and may include no change at all, increase of slow wave, and changes in rapid eye movement (REM) during sleep – decreased REM sleep, increased REM sleep during the second half of the night, no change in the REM sleep, or decreased onset latency of REM sleep. The sleep-wake regulation centers and associated pathways are damaged in the TBI, and these damages are the cause of disturbances of the sleep architecture. Sleep disturbances lead to fatigue that may be associated with mental retardation and slower processing of information [72]. Sleep disorders also contribute to anxiety and depression. Patients with TBI may have disrupted circadian regulation of melatonin synthesis, including lower levels of melatonin production at night [12].

Chronic changes in sleep architecture have also been described after TBI. A review of 105 polysomnograms (PSG) in patients with severe TBI identified lack of deep sleep and increased sleep fragmentation in those more severely affected [73]. PSG 6 months after TBI revealed consolidated NREM sleep and a trend toward a higher amount of delta power compared with controls [74].

Reduced sleep quality induces depression. Early diagnosis is important, and treatment may involve modafinil, melatonin light therapy, lifestyle modifications, and improving alertness and mood [67].

Due to the association between TBI and sleep disturbances, it is important to analyze the qEEG during sleep. There seems to be an interference of sleep disturbances with rehabilitation contributing to long-term disability [75–77].

## Conclusion

Quantitative EEG is promising as a diagnostic assessment for TBI and postconcussive symptoms. Further scientific studies are needed to provide a better understanding of the pathophysiology and elucidate how EEG can aid in the care of patients who have sustained a TBI.

**Conflict of Interest** There is no conflict of interest to declare.

## References


1. Berger H. Über das Elektrenkephalogramm des Menschen. Arch Psychiatr Nervenkr. 1929;87:527–43.
2. Tudor M, Tudor L, Tudor KI. Hans Berger (1873-1941) – the history of electroencephalography. Acta Med Croatica. 2005;59(4):307–13.
3. Schacter DL, Crovitz HF. Memory function after closed head injury: a review of the quantitative research. Cortex. 1977;13:150–76.
4. Thatcher RW, Walker RA, Gerson I, Geisler FH. EEG discriminant analyses of mild head trauma. Electroencephalogr Clin Neurophysiol. 1989;73:94–106.
5. Dockree PM, Robertson IH. Electrophysiological markers of cognitive deficits in traumatic brain injury: a review. Int J Psychophysiol. 2011;82:53–60.
6. Thatcher RW, North DM, Curtin RT, Walker RA, Biver CJ, et al. An EEG severity index of traumatic brain injury. J Neuropsychiatry Clin Neurosci. 2001;13:77–87.
7. Castriotta RJ, Wilde MC, Lai JM, Atanasov S, Masel BE, et al. Prevalence and consequences of sleep disorders in traumatic brain injury. J Clin Sleep Med. 2007;3:349–56.
8. Orff HJ, Ayalon L, Drummond SP. Traumatic brain injury and sleep disturbance: a review of current research. J Head Trauma Rehabil. 2009;24:155–65.
9. Castriotta RJ, Murthy JN. Sleep disorders in patients with traumatic brain injury: a review. CNS Drugs. 2011;25:175–85.
10. Parcell DL, Ponsford JL, Redman JR, Rajaratnam SM. Poor sleep quality and changes in objectively recorded sleep after traumatic brain injury: a preliminary study. Arch Phys Med Rehabil. 2008;89:843–50.
11. Frieboes RM, Müller U, Murck H, von Cramon DY, Holsboer F, et al. Nocturnal hormone secretion and the sleep EEG in patients several months after traumatic brain injury. J Neuropsychiatry Clin Neurosci. 1999;11:354–60.
12. Shekleton JA, Parcell DL, Redman JR, Phipps-Nelson J, Ponsford JL, et al. Sleep disturbance and melatonin levels following traumatic brain injury. Neurology. 2010;74:1732–8.
13. Rao V, Spiro J, Vaishnavi S, Rastogi P, Mielke M, et al. Prevalence and types of sleep disturbances acutely after traumatic brain injury. Brain Inj. 2008;22:381–6.
14. Kotchoubey B, Lang S, Mezger G, et al. Information processing in severe disorders of consciousness: vegetative state and minimally conscious state. Clin Neurophysiol. 2005;116:2441–53.
15. Arciniegas DB. Clinical electrophysiologic assessments and mild traumatic brain injury: state-of-the-science and implications for clinical practice. Int J Psychophysiol. 2011;82:41–52.
16. Glaser MA, Sjaardema H. The value of the electroencephalogram in craniocerebral injuries. West J Surg Obstet Gynecol. 1940;48:684–96.
17. Jasper HH, Kershman J, Elvidge A. Electroencephalographic studies of injury to the head. Arch Neurol Psychiatr. 1940;44:328–48.
18. Nuwer M. Assessment of digital EEG, quantitative EEG, and EEG brain mapping: report of the American Academy of Neurology and the American clinical neurophysiology society. Neurology. 1997;49(1):277–92.
19. Nuwer MR, Comi G, Emerson R, Fuglsang-Frederiksen A, Guérit JM, Hinrichs H, Ikeda A, Luccas FJ, Rappelsberger P. IFCN standards for digital recording of clinical EEG. The International Federation of Clinical Neurophysiology. Electroencephalogr Clin Neurophysiol Suppl. 1999;52:11–4.
20. Rapp PE, Keyser DO, Albano A, Hernandez R, Gibson DB, Zambon RA, Hairston WD, Hughes JD, Krystal A, Nichols AS. Traumatic brain injury detection using electrophysiological methods. Front Hum Neurosci. 2015;9:11.
21. Berridge MJ, Rapp PE. A comparative survey of the function, mechanism and control of cellular oscillators. J Exp Biol. 1979;81:217–79.
22. Penttonen M, Buzsáki G. Natural logarithmic relationship between brain oscillators. Thalamus Relat Syst. 2003;2:145–15210.
23. Harner R. Automatic EEG spike detection. Clin EEG Neurosci. 2009;40(4):262–70.
24. McDowell K, Chin-Teng L, Oie KS, Tzyy-Ping J, Gordon S, Whitaker KW, et al. Real-world neuroimaging technologies. IEEE. 2013;1:131–49.
25. Bricolo A. Electroencephalography in neurotraumatology. Clin Electroencephalogr. 1976;7:184–97.

26. Urakami Y. Relationship between, sleep spindles and clinical recovery in patients with traumatic brain injury: a simultaneous EEG and MEG study. Clin EEG Neurosci. 2012;43:39–47.
27. Walker AE, Kollros JJ, Case TJ. The physiological basis of concussion. J Neurosurg. 1944;1:103–16.
28. Shaw NA. The neurophysiology of concussion. Prog Neurobiol. 2002;67:281–344.
29. Nuwer MR, Hovda DA, Schrader LM, Vespa PM. Routine and quantitative EEG in mild traumatic brain injury. Clin Neurophysiol. 2005;116:2001–25.
30. McCrea M, Prichep L, Powell MR, Chabot R, Barr WB. Acute effects and recovery after sport-related concussion: a neurocognitive and quantitative brain electrical activity study. J Head Trauma Rehabil. 2010;25:283–92.
31. Olejniczak P. Neurophysiologic basis of EEG. J Clin Neurophysiol. 2006;23(3):186–9.
32. Modarres M, Kuzma NN, Kretzmer T, Pack AI, Lim MM. EEG slow waves in traumatic brain injury: convergent findings in mouse and man. Neurobiol Sleep Circadian Rhythms. 2016;1:1.
33. Glaser MA, Sjaardema H. The value of the electroencephalograph in craniocerebral injuries. West J Surg. 1940;48:689–96.
34. Williams D. The electro-encephalogram in acute head injuries. J Neurol Psychiatry. 1941;4:107–30.
35. Koufen H, Dichgans J. Frequency and course of posttraumatic EEG-abnormalities and their correlations with clinical symptoms a systematic follow up study in 344 adults. Fortschr Neurol Psychiatr Grenzgeb. 1978;46:165–77.
36. Dow RS, Ulett G, Raaf J. Electroencephalographic studies immediately following head injury. Am J Psychiatry. 1944;101:174–83.
37. Geets W, Louette N. Early EEG in 300 cerebral concussions.( Fre). Rev Electroencephalogr Neurophysiol Clin. 1985;14:333–8.
38. Meyer JS, Denny-Brown D. Studies of cerebral circulation in brain injury II Cerebral concussion. Electroencephalogr Clin Neurophysiol. 1955;7:529–44.
39. Hayes RL, Katayama Y, Young HF, Dunbar JG. Coma associated with flaccidity produced by fluid-percussion concussion in the cat I: is it due to depression of activity within the brainstem reticular formation? Brain Inj. 1988;2:31–49.
40. Tebano MT, Cameroni M, Gallozzi G, Loizzo A, Palazzino G, Pezzini G, Ricci GF. EEG spectral analysis after minor head injury in man. Electroencephalogr Clin Neurophysiol. 1988;70:185–9.
41. McClelland RJ, Fenton GW, Rutherford W. The postconcussional syndrome revisited. J R Soc Med. 1994;87:508–10.
42. Fenton G. The postconcussional syndrome reappraised. Clin Electroencephalogr. 1996;27:174–82.
43. Gosselin N, Lassonde M, Petit D, Leclerc S, Mongrain V, Collie A, Montplaisir J. Sleep following sport-related concussions. Sleep Med. 2009;10:35–46.
44. Watson MR, Fenton GW, McClelland RJ, Lumsden J, Headley M, Rutherford WH. The post-concussional state neurophysiological aspects. Br J Psychiatry. 1995;167:514–21.
45. Chen XP, Tao LY, Chen AC. Electroencephalogram and evoked potential parameters examined in Chinese mild head injury patients for forensic medicine. Neurosci Bull. 2006;22:165–70.
46. Lewine JD, Davis JT, Bigler ED, Thoma R, Hill D, Funke M. Objective documentation of traumatic brain injury subsequent to mild head trauma multimodal brain imaging with MEG, SPECT, and MRI. J Head Trauma Rehabil. 2007;22:141–55.
47. Kanda PAM, Anghinah R, Schmidt MT, Jorge MS. The clinical use of quantitative EEG in cognitive disorders. Dement Neuropsychol. 2009;3(3):195–203.
48. Zhang X, van Drongelen W, Hecox K, Towle V, Frim D, McGee A, et al. High-resolution EEG: cortical potential imaging of interictal spikes. Clin Neurophysiol. 2003;114:1963–73.
49. Pascual-Marqui RD, Michel CM, Lehmann D. Low resolution electromagnetic tomography: a new method for localizing electrical activity in the brain. Int J Psychophysiol. 1994;18:49965.
50. Babiloni C, Frisoni G, Pievani M, Vecchio F, Lizio R, Buttiglione M, et al. Hippocampal volume and cortical sources of EEG alpha rhythms in mild cognitive impairment and Alzheimer disease. NeuroImage. 2009;44(1):123–35.
51. Pascual-Marqui RD. Standardized low-resolution brain electromagnetic tomography (sloreta): technical details. Methods Find Exp Clin Pharmacol. 2002;24.(Suppl D:5–12.
52. Pascual-Marqui R. Discrete, 3D distributed, linear imaging methods of electric neuronal activity. Part 1: exact, zero error localization. 2007.
53. Canuet L, Tellado I, Couceiro V, Fraile C, Fernandez-Novoa L, Ishii R, et al. Resting-state network disruption and APOE genotype in Alzheimer's disease: a lagged functional connectivity study. PLoS One. 2012;7:e46289.
54. Leon-Carrion J, Martin-Rodriguez JF, Damas-Lopez J. Barroso y Martin JM, Dominguez-Morales MR. brain function in the minimally conscious state: a quantitative neurophysiological study. Clin Neurophysiol. 2008;119(7):1506–14.
55. Tomkins O, Feintuch A, Benifla M, Cohen A, Friedman A, Shelef I. Blood-brain barrier breakdown following traumatic brain injury: a possible role in posttraumatic epilepsy. Cardiovasc Psychiatry Neurol. 2011;2011:765923.
56. Corradini PL, Persinger MA. Standardized low resolution electromagnetic tomography (sLORETA) is a sensitive Indicator of protracted neuropsychological impairments following "mild" (concussive) traumatic brain injury. J Neurol Neurophysiol. 2013;4:176.
57. Ledwidge PS, Molfese DL. Long-term effects of concussion on electrophysiological indices of attention in varsity college athletes: an event-related potential and standardized low-resolution brain electromagnetic tomography approach. J Neurotrauma. 2016;33(23):2081–90.
58. Ianof JN, Fraga FJ, Ferreira LA, et al. Comparative analysis of the electroencephalogram in patients with Alzheimer's disease, diffuse axonal injury patients and healthy controls using LORETA analysis. Dement Neuropsychol. 2017;11(2):176–85.
59. Fisher RS, van Emde BW, Blume W, et al. Epileptic seizures and epilepsy: definitions proposed by the international league against epilepsy (ILAE) and the International Bureau for Epilepsy (IBE). Epilepsia. 2005;46:470–2.
60. Hauser WA, Annegers JF, Kurland LT. Prevalence of epilepsy in Rochester, Minnesota: 1940–1980. Epilepsia. 1991;32:429–45.
61. Friedman D, Claassen J, Hirsch LJ. Continuous electroencephalogram monitoring in the intensive care unit. Anesth Analg. 2009;109(2):506–23.
62. Frey LC. Epidemiology of posttraumatic epilepsy: a critical review. Epilepsia. 2003;44(Suppl 10):11–7. Thorough epidemiological review of post-traumatic epilepsy (PTE) that provides important information on incidence and risk factors for developing PTE in both civilian and military populations, as well as the working definitions involved in PTE
63. Jennett B. Early traumatic epilepsy. Incidence and significance after nonmissile head injuries. Arch Neurol. 1974;30(5):394–8.
64. Asikainen I, Kaste M, Sarna S. Early and late posttraumatic seizures in traumatic brain injury rehabilitation patients: brain injury factors causing late seizures and influence of seizures on long-term outcome. Epilepsia. 1998;40:584–9.
65. Haltiner AM, Temkin NR, Dikmen SS. Risk of seizure recurrence after the first late posttraumatic seizure. Arch Phys Med Rehabil. 1997;78:835–40.
66. Angeleri F, Majkowski J, Cacchio G, et al. Posttraumatic epilepsy risk factors: one-year prospective study after head injury. Epilepsia. 1999;40:1222–30.

67. Urakami Y. Electrophysiologic evaluation of diffuse axonal injury after traumatic brain injury. J Neurol Neurophysiol. 2013;4:157.
68. Rao V, Bergey A, Hill H, et al. Sleep disturbance after mild traumatic brain injury: indicator of injury? J Neuropsychiatry Clin Neurosci. 2011;23:201.
69. Khoury S, Chouchou F, Amzica F, et al. Rapid EEG activity during sleep dominates in mild traumatic brain injury patients with acute pain. J Neurotrauma. 2013;30:633.
70. Feige B, Baglioni C, Spiegelhalder K, et al. The microstructure of sleep in primary insomnia: an overview and extension. Int J Psychophysiol. 2013;89:171.
71. Sandsmark DK, Kumar MA, Woodward CS, et al. Sleep features on continuous electroencephalography predict rehabilitation outcomes after severe traumatic brain injury. J Head Trauma Rehabil. 2016;31:101.
72. Ponsford JL, Ziino C, Parcell DL, Shekleton JA, Roper M, et al. Fatigue and sleep disturbance following traumatic brain injury--their nature, causes, and potential treatments. J Head Trauma Rehabil. 2012;27:224–33.
73. Harada M, Minami R, Hattori E, et al. Sleep in brain-damaged patients. An all night sleep study of 105 cases. Kumamoto Med J. 1976;29:110.
74. Imbach LL, Valko PO, Li T, Maric A, Symeonidou ER, Stover JF, Bassetti CL, Mica L, Werth E, Baumann CR. Increased sleep need and daytime sleepiness 6 months after traumatic brain injury: a prospective controlled clinical trial. Brain. 2015;138(Pt 3):726–35.
75. Nakase-Richardson R, Yablon SA, Sherer M. Prospective comparison of acute confusion severity with duration of post-traumatic amnesia in predicting employment outcome after traumatic brain injury. J Neurol Neurosurg Psychiatry. 2007;78(8):872–6.
76. Nakase-Richardson R, Sherer M, Barnett SD, Yablon SA, Evans CC, Kretzmer T, Schwartz DJ, Modarres M. Prospective evaluation of the nature, course, and impact of acute sleep abnormality after traumatic brain injury. Arch Phys Med Rehabil. 2013;94(5):875–82.
77. Sherer M, Yablon SA, Nakase-Richardson R, Nick TG. Effect of severity of post-traumatic confusion and its constituent symptoms on outcome after traumatic brain injury. Arch Phys Med Rehabil. 2008;89(1):42–7.

# Mild Traumatic Brain Injury and Postconcussion Syndrome

9

Marcia Mitie Nagumo, Daniele Vieira da Silva, and Robson Luis Oliveira de Amorim

## Abbreviations

| | |
|---|---|
| ACRM | American Congress of Rehabilitation Medicine |
| DALY | Disability-adjusted life year |
| DSM-IV | *Diagnostic and Statistical Manual of Mental Disorders*, fourth edition |
| GCS | Glasgow Coma Scale |
| ICD-10 | International Classification of Diseases, 10th revision |
| LOC | Loss of consciousness |
| mTBI | Mild traumatic brain injury |
| N/A | Not applicable |
| PCS | Postconcussion syndrome |
| PPCS | Persistent postconcussion syndrome |
| PTA | Posttraumatic amnesia |
| SCAT3 | Sport Concussion Assessment Tool V.3 |
| TBI | Traumatic brain injury |

## Introduction

Mild traumatic brain injury (mTBI) continues to be a major concern worldwide, and despite favorable recovery rates, overall a subset of individuals experience symptoms months to years post-injury. Patients often experience a wide range of cognitive, emotional, and physical symptoms such as headache, dizziness, irritability, sleep disorders, or difficulty concentrating. Those symptoms are commonly referred to as postconcussion syndrome (PCS). In this chapter, we will discuss about mTBI and PCS and how a transdisciplinary team can work together in the rehabilitation of those patients.

M. M. Nagumo
Department of Neurology – Neurosurgery – Clinics Hospital – School of Medicine – University of São Paulo, São Paulo, Brazil

D. V. da Silva
Nursing School – University of São Paulo, São Paulo, Brazil

R. L. O. de Amorim (✉)
Department of Neurology – Neurosurgery – Clinics Hospital – School of Medicine – University of São Paulo, São Paulo, Brazil

Department of Neurology – Neurosurgery – Amazonas State University, Amazonas, Brazil

## Mild Traumatic Brain Injury

### Definition and Classification

The definition of mTBI as per the American Congress of Rehabilitation Medicine (ACRM) [1] consists of one or more of the following criteria:

1. Any period of loss of consciousness.
2. Any loss of memory for events immediately before or after the accident.
3. Any alteration in mental status at the time of the accident (e.g., feeling dazed, disoriented, or confused).
4. Focal neurological deficit(s) that may or may not be transient but where the severity of the injury does not exceed the following: loss of consciousness of approximately 30 min or less; after 30 min, an initial Glasgow Coma Scale (GCS) of 13–15 points; and posttraumatic amnesia (PTA) not greater than 24 h.

This definition includes the head being struck, the head striking an object, and the brain undergoing an acceleration/deceleration movement (i.e., whiplash) without direct external trauma to the head. Radiological findings may be normal with this class of injuries. Tables 9.1 and 9.2 show the Glasgow Coma Scale and TBI classification.

### Focal and Diffuse Brain Injury

Brain injuries may be considered predominantly focal or diffuse, but most injuries are heterogeneous with both focal and diffuse components.


R. Anghinah et al. (eds.), *Topics in Cognitive Rehabilitation in the TBI Post-Hospital Phase*,
https://doi.org/10.1007/978-3-319-95376-2_9

**Table 9.1** Glasgow Coma Scale

| Glasgow Coma Scale | | |
|---|---|---|
| Eye opening | Verbal response | Motor response |
| 4 = spontaneous<br>3 = to speech<br>2 = to pain<br>1 = none | 5 = oriented<br>4 = confused conversation<br>3 = inappropriate words<br>2 = incomprehensible sounds<br>1 = none | 6 = obeys commands<br>5 = localizes pain<br>4 = withdraw<br>3 = abnormal flexion (decorticate)<br>2 = extension (decerebrate)<br>1 1 = none |

Adapted from Teasdale and Jennett [2]

**Table 9.2** Glasgow Coma Scale and TBI severity

| GCS score | TBI classification |
|---|---|
| 13–15 points | Mild |
| 9–12 points | Moderate |
| <9 points | Severe |

*GCS* Glasgow Coma Scale, *TBI* traumatic brain injury

- Focal injury: injury occurs in a specific location and usually is a result of external mechanical force applied to the cranium and the intracranial contents. Examples of focal injuries: cerebral contusion, cerebral laceration, subdural hematoma, epidural hematoma, intracerebral hemorrhage, and intraventricular hemorrhage [3].
- Diffuse injury: injury usually occurs from acceleration/deceleration injuries or rotational forces. Examples of diffuse injuries: axonal injury, hypoxic-ischemic injury, and microvascular injury that affect widely distributed anatomic regions [3].

## Primary and Secondary Injuries

Primary injuries occur at the moment of the trauma. They are the result of direct external mechanical forces that produce deformation of the skull and brain tissue and disruption of normal brain function. Secondary injuries are due to further cellular damage and inflammatory or metabolic alterations from the effects of primary injuries. Secondary injury may develop over a period of hours or days following the primary injury.

It has been hypothesized that PCS is caused by microstructural damage to the brain due to shearing injury, which is not detectable with conventional image exams and may be responsible for a functional deficit [4, 5]. The region affected by mTBI seems to especially involve the mesial region of the brain, as well as deeper regions such as the hippocampus. This "preference" would justify the deficits found in postconcussion patients who basically have memory complaints. Another area that is frequently involved is the prefrontal cortex which would explain the executive deficits that may persist even after 3 months post trauma.

Cognitive dysfunction is characterized by impairment of attention/concentration, memory, and/or executive function. Patients may have difficulties performing preinjury tasks and jobs or following instructions that would ordinarily be routine before the trauma [6].

Although some brain lesions may not be detected through image exam, patients often present cognitive deficits and behavioral disorders. The pathological mechanism involved in all those altered neuronal functions and in the recovery process is not fully understood and remains still uncertain.

## Mild TBI and Concussion

The terms mTBI and concussion have been used interchangeably. The term concussion is from the Latin "concutere" which means "to shake violently" [7] and is more commonly used in sports medicine. Although the definition of mTBI is associated with the concussion phenomenon, the exclusive use of the term concussion should not be used as a synonym in clinical practice. Concussion is a mental state occurring after trauma, which may or may not include loss of consciousness, and the symptoms reflect a functional disturbance rather than structural injury. Box 9.1 summarizes the most common scales to describe the severity of concussion.

When a concussion is suspected, the athlete must be immediately removed from play for a neurological examination that includes cognitive and balance testing [11]. If the athlete is diagnosed with a concussion, they should not return to play that day and should be managed by a healthcare professional with competence in the treatment of concussion. The Zurich Symposium on Concussion in Sport in 2012 [12] placed emphasis on symptoms and signs of acute concussion (Table 9.3) and an on-field or sideline evaluation (Table 9.4).

## Mortality

In 2013, only in the United States occurred around 2.8 million of TBI-related emergency department visits, hospitalizations, and deaths. Individuals older than 75 years old have higher rates of TBI mortality, and the main cause is the fall. TBI contributes to about 30% of all injury deaths and is associated with an increased risk of death especially in the elderly [13].

TBI is the most frequent cause of mortality in the United States among children and adolescents. Approximately one third of all pediatric injury cases are TBI. Falls are also the leading causes of TBI in the range between 0 and 4 years old.

Although the association of TBI with increased risk of death has been noted, the relationship of mild TBI to death is

**Box 9.1 Concussion rating scales**

| | Grade | Altered mental status | PTA | LOC |
|---|---|---|---|---|
| Cantu | I | N/A | <30 min | No LOC |
| | II | N/A | >30 min and <24 h | <5 min |
| | III | N/A | >24 h | >5 min |
| American Academy of Neurology | I | Transient confusion (<15 min) | N/A | No LOC |
| | II | Transient confusion (>15 min) | N/A | No LOC |
| | III | Any transient confusion | N/A | Any loss of consciousness, brief or prolonged |
| Colorado Medical Society School and Sports Medicine Committee | I | Present | No PTA | No LOC |
| | II | Present | Present | No LOC |
| | III | Present | Present | Present |

Adapted from Cantu [8], Colorado Medical Society School and Sports Medicine Committee [9], American Academy of Neurology [10]

*PTA* posttraumatic amnesia, *LOC* loss of consciousness, *N/A* not applicable

**Table 9.3** Symptoms and signs of acute concussion

| | |
|---|---|
| Somatic | Headache |
| Cognitive | Feeling like being in a fog |
| Emotional symptoms | Lability |
| Physical signs | Loss of consciousness, amnesia |
| Behavioral changes | Irritability |
| Cognitive impairment | Slowed reaction times |
| Sleep disturbance | Insomnia |

Adapted from Consensus statement on concussion in sport: the 4th International Conference on Concussion in Sport, Zurich, November 2012

**Table 9.4** On-field or sideline evaluation of acute concussion

| |
|---|
| 1.The player should be evaluated by a physician or other licensed healthcare provider on-site using standard emergency management |
| 2. If no healthcare provider is available, the player should be safely removed from practice or play and urgently referred to a physician |
| 3. Once the first aid issues are addressed, an assessment of the concussive injury should be made using the sport concussion assessment tool V.3 (SCAT3) or other sideline assessment tools |
| 4. The player should not be left alone following the injury and serial monitoring for deterioration is essential over the initial few hours following injury |
| 5. A player diagnosed with concussion should not be allowed to return to play on the day of injury |

Adapted from Consensus statement on concussion in sport: the 4th International Conference on Concussion in Sport, Zurich, November 2012

still inconclusive. A cohort study with elderly patients have found that those with a single mild TBI have a higher risk of death later in their liver when compared to the general population [14].

## Disability

The symptoms that affect the individuals post TBI, especially those related to memory and cognitive impairment, render the patient unable to perform his/her daily activities that, until then, were done independently. Very often those symptoms are referred by the patients as "usual" or "normal" and may be seen as a onset of a neurodegenerative diseases when the patient is elderly. The disability-adjusted life year (DALY) is higher in low-income countries due to the lack of education and adequate diagnostics resources. It is estimated that 80,000 to 90,000 people that suffer a TBI may develop some permanent disability [15].

## Demographics

### Causes

Common causes include road traffic accidents (60%), falls (20–30%), assault and violence (10%), and sport injuries or work-related injuries (10%) [16]. In non-sport injuries, alcohol and/or drug influence is a key contributory factor. In 2013, falls were the leading cause of TBI in the United States; being struck by or against an object was the second cause of TBI, and among all ages groups, motor vehicle crashes were the third overall leading cause [17].

## Postconcussion Syndrome

Postconcussion syndrome (PCS) is characterized by a set of cognitive, emotional, and physical symptoms that occur after days or weeks after a traumatic brain injury. Although there is no universally accepted definition of PCS, the World Health Organization's International Classification of Diseases [18], 10th revision (ICD-10), defines PCS as:

> a syndrome that occurs following head trauma (usually sufficiently severe to result in loss of consciousness) and includes a number of disparate symptoms such as headache, dizziness, fatigue, irritability, difficulty in concentration and performing mental tasks, impairment of memory, insomnia, and reduced tolerance to stress, emotional excitement, or alcohol.

The *Diagnostic and Statistical Manual of Mental Disorders*, fourth edition (DSM-IV), has established the following criteria for the diagnosis of PCS:

1. A history of head trauma that causes "significant cerebral concussion".
2. Objective evidence of deficits in attention or memory.
3. A minimum of three of the following symptoms must be present and persist for at least 3 months: easily fatigued, headache, dizziness, disordered sleep, easily provoked irritability or aggression, anxiety, depression or emotional lability, apathy, personality changes, or inappropriate behavior.
4. Symptoms must begin or worsen after the brain injury.
5. Significant decline from previous level of functioning (social, occupational, or academic functioning).
6. Symptoms do not meet criteria for dementia due to head trauma and are not better accounted by another disorder.

The natural course after mTBI is the resolution of symptoms within 3 months and a return to preinjury functioning, which is the outcome for the majority of patients. However, a considerable proportion of them will experience postconcussion symptoms (Table 9.5) for a prolonged period after injury, diagnosed as persistent postconcussion syndrome (PPCS) [19]. Cognitive deficit is common following mTBI, particularly in attention and executive functioning. These multiple cognitive deficits, coupled with other frequently associated neuropsychiatric symptoms, most often in the form of anxiety and depression [20, 21], have an effect on functional status and may lead to disability and reduced quality of life [22]. Much of the disability (and costs) associated with mTBI is hidden, as survivors may have no physical evidence of their injury. Despite this, the consequences of mTBI can permanently change a person's life, resulting in family disruption, loss of income and earning potential, and considerable expense over a lifetime [23].

**Table 9.5** Common postconcussion symptoms

| Physical | Cognitive | Emotional |
|---|---|---|
| Headache | Difficultly concentrating | Irritability |
| Nausea | Poor memory | Anxiety |
| Vomiting | Difficulty learning new things | Depression |
| Dizziness | Difficulty sustaining attention | Nervousness |
| Fatigue | Impaired problem-solving skills | Apathy |
| Balance problems | Problems in planning or organizing | Poor frustration tolerance |
| Visual problems (blurred/double vision) | Difficulty making decisions | Personality changes |
| Sensitivity to sound | Impaired judgment | Disinhibition |
| Sensitivity to light | | |
| Sleep disturbances | | |

## Management of mTBI

There is no specific treatment for mTBI and its sequelae. Currently the best practice model includes [24]:

1. Early identification of mTBI by emergency medical staff, physician, and other health professionals.
2. Early treatment of symptoms should be provided for physical-medical problems such as dizziness, nausea, or vomiting, and pain or psychological assessment and counseling should be provided if the injury event triggers an acute stress reaction.
3. Provide information to all patients and family members about typical symptoms that can follow after mTBI as part of natural recovery process, recommendations for gradual return to regular activities, and cautions about incurring another head injury.
4. Symptomatic patients should be followed up every 2 to 4 weeks from the time of initial contact until they are no longer symptomatic.
5. Interdisciplinary assessment and treatment for those who have not returned to work or are still symptomatic after 3 to 4 months post-injury.

## Rehabilitation Post mTBI

TBI may or may not cause long-term physical disability, but it is the complex neurobehavioral sequelae that may produce a drastic reduction of patient's quality of life, months or years of impairment affecting occupational, social, and emotional functioning. The cognitive and behavioral changes and difficulties maintaining personal relationships and coping with school and/or work can be more disabling than any residual physical deficits. Box 9.2 presents a suggestion of a transdisciplinary rehabilitation team.

**Box 9.2 Transdisciplinary rehabilitation team**

- Patients and their family
- Physiatrist
- General practitioner
- Neurosurgeon/neurologist
- Rehabilitation nurse
- Neuropsychologist
- Physical therapist
- Occupational therapist
- Speech/language pathologist
- Social worker

The transdisciplinary approach to care delivery is performed by a team with different professions that come together from the beginning, exchange ideas, discuss each case, and work together to come up with a holistic rehabilitation plan for each patient. The goals of rehabilitation post TBI need to be holistic and individualized to each patient and his/her family needs. Given the high predominance of young adults sustaining TBI, it is essential that the outcomes following injury are properly documented as a basis for developing rehabilitation guidelines for professionals, families, and educators.

It is essential that patients and their family understand the effects of the injury and their limitations, and as with all rehabilitations, the main goal is to help the patient achieve the maximum degree of return to their previous level of functioning.

## Conclusion

In view of the importance of the theme discussed in this chapter, the complexity of mTBI and PCS is due to several heterogeneous factors. Even if the TBI is mild and closed, it may be associated with a variety of psychological and physical symptoms. Indeed it is important for patients experiencing prolonged symptoms to have a particular need for a knowledgeable and coordinated management with a transdisciplinary rehabilitation team. The fast symptom recognition and proper diagnoses of PCS are expected to increase considerably as health professionals and patient's families become more aware of its existence, magnitude, and extent.

## References


1. Kay T, Harrington DE, Adams R, Andersen T, Berrol S, Cicerone K, et al. Definition of mild traumatic brain injury. J Head Trauma Rehabil. 1993;8(3):86–7.
2. Teasdale G, Jennett B. Assessment of coma and impaired consciousness. A practical scale. Lancet. 1974;2:81–4.
3. Andrade AF, Paiva WS, Amorim RLO, Figueiredo EG, Rusafa Neto E, Teixeira MJ. The pathophysiological mechanisms following traumatic brain injury. Rev Assoc Med Bras [Internet]. 2009;55(1):75–81. Available from: http://www.scielo.br/scielo.php?script=sci_arttext&pid=S0104-42302009000100020&lng=en.
4. Bigler ED. Distinguished Neuropsychologist Award Lecture 1999. The lesion(s) in traumatic brain injury: implications for clinical neuropsychology. Arch Clin Neuropsychol. 2001;16:95–131.
5. King N. Mild head injury neuropathology, sequelae, measurement and recovery. Br J Clin Psychol. 1997;36(Part 2):161–84.
6. Riggio S, Wong M. Neurobehavioral sequelae of traumatic brain injury. Mt Sinai J Med. 2009;76:163–72.
7. Pearce JMS. Observations on concussion: a review. Eur Neurol. 2008;58:113–9.
8. Cantu RC. Return to play guidelines after a head injury. Clin Sports Med. 1998;17:45–60.
9. Colorado Medical Society School and Sports Medicine Committee. Guidelines for the management of concussion in sports. Colo Med. 1900;87:4.
10. Reports of the Quality Standards Subcommittee. Practice parameter: the management of concussion in sports (summary statement). Neurology. 1997;48:581–5.
11. MullallyWJ.Concussion.AmJMed.2017;pii:S0002-9343(17)30482-5. https://doi.org/10.1016/j.amjmed.2017.04.016.
12. McCrory P, Meeuwisse WH, Aubry M, Cantu RC, Dvorak J, Echemendia RJ, Engebretsen RJ, Johnston K, Kutcher JS, Raftery M, et al. Consensus statement on concussion in sport: the 4th International Conference on Concussion in Sport, Zurich, November 2012. J Athl Train. 2013;48(4):554–75.
13. McIntyre A, Mehta S, Aubut J, Dijkers M, Teasell RW. Mortality among older adults after a traumatic brain injury: a meta-analysis. Brain Inj. 2013;27(1):31–40.
14. Cheng PL, Lin HY, Lee YK, Hsu CY, Lee CC, Su YC. Higher mortality rates among the elderly with mild traumatic brain injury: a nationwide cohort study. Scand J Trauma Resusc Emerg Med. 2014 Jan 28;22:7. https://doi.org/10.1186/1757-7241-22-7.
15. Thurman DJ, Alverson C, Dunn KA, Guerrero J, Sniezek JE. Traumatic brain injury in the United States: a public health perspective. J Head Trauma Rehabil. 1999;14(6):602–15.
16. Gururaj G. An epidemiological approach to prevention – prehospital care and rehabilitation in neurotrauma. Neurol India. 1995;43(3):95–105.
17. Centers for Disease Control and Prevention (CDC), National Center for Injury Prevention and Control. Report to Congress on mild traumatic brain injury in the United States: steps to prevent a serious public health problem. Atlanta (GA): Centers for Disease Control and Prevention; 2003.
18. WHO (World Health Organization). International statistical classification of diseases and related health problems. 2010. [January 30, 2016]. (10th Revision. [Online version.]). http://apps.who.int/classifications/icd10/browse/2010/en.
19. Ahman S, Saverman BI, Styrke J, Bjornstig U, Stalnacke BM. Long term follow up of patients with mild traumatic brain injury: a mixed-methods study. J Rehabil Med. 2013;45:758–64.
20. Ponsford J, Willmott C, Rothwell A, et al. Factors influencing outcome following mild traumatic brain injury in adults. J Inte Neuropsychol Soc. 2000;6:568–79.
21. Rogers JM, Read CA. Psychiatric comorbidity following traumatic brain injury. Brain Inj. 2007;21:1321–33.
22. Pagulayan KF, Hoffman JM, Temkin NR, Machamer JE, Dikmen SS. A longitudinal study of health-related quality of life after traumatic brain injury. Arch Phys Med Rehabil. 2006;87:611–8.
23. U.S. National Institutes of Health. Rehabilitation of persons with traumatic brain injury: NIH consensus statement. JAMA. 1999;282(10):974–83.
24. Marshall S, Bayley M, McCullagh S, Velikonja D, Berrigan L. Clinical practice guidelines for mild traumatic brain injury and persistent symptoms. Can Fam Physician. 2012;58:257–67.

# Traumatic Brain Injury in the National Football League

# 10

Renata Areza-Fegyveres

## Introduction

The present chapter is going to encompass a different perspective of concussion and chronic traumatic encephalopathy (CTE) linked to the National Football League (NFL).

## Brief History of NFL

The National Football League (NFL) was founded in 1920 as the American Professional Football Association (APFA). It included ten teams from four states; all of them existed in some form as participants of regional leagues in their respective territory. It took on its current name in 1922 [1]. The NFL was the first professional football league to successfully establish a nationwide presence, after several decades of failed attempts. League membership progressively stabilized throughout the 1920s and 1930s as the league adopted more formal organization.

During World War II, NFL football activity declined. After that the rival American Football League was founded in 1960. At a certain point, there was a merge with NFL that resulted in a greatly expanded league and the creation of Super Bowl, which has become the most watched annual sporting event in USA. At that time, its current size had 32 teams. A series of agreements have helped the league to be one of the most profitable and the only major league in the USA since the 1990s.

## Local and National US Policies [Adapted from 2]

During the last decade, laws, policies, and action plans on concussion were created.

**State Laws** In 2009, the State of Washington was the first to create a law about concussion in sports, the Zackery Lystedt Law [3]. One month later, Max's law [4] was passed in Oregon. In total, between 2009 and 2012, 43 states, and the District of Columbia, passed laws on concussion in sports for youth and/or high school athletes, often called Return to Play Laws. So far in 2013, four additional states have also passed Return to Play Laws. Some organizations, such as the National Conference of State Legislatures, have created online maps to track and update concussion in sports laws by state [5].

Most concussion in sports laws includes three action steps:

1. Inform and educate coaches and athletes and their parents and guardians about concussion through training and/or a concussion information sheet.
2. Remove athlete from play: an athlete who is believed to have a concussion is to be removed from play right away.
3. Obtain permission to return to play: an athlete can only return to play or practice after at least 24 h and with permission from a health-care professional.

These action steps are based on recommendations presented in the international concussion consensus statement [6]. First created in 2002 and most recently updated in 2008, the consensus statement was developed by experts in the field and includes the latest science available on concussion in sports.

**Local Policies and Action Plans** Along with the three action steps listed above, some school and league concussion policies include additional strategies in their policies or implementation plans. Research is needed to learn if including these additional strategies can help protect children and teens from concussion and other serious brain injuries. Based on interviews by the Centers for Disease Control and Prevention (CDC) with nine states, below is a list of some examples of additional strategies in local policies and action plans.

R. Areza-Fegyveres (✉)
University of São Paulo, School of Medicine – University of São Paulo, São Paulo, Brazil


R. Anghinah et al. (eds.), *Topics in Cognitive Rehabilitation in the TBI Post-Hospital Phase*,
https://doi.org/10.1007/978-3-319-95376-2_10

- *Be ready for an emergency* by creating a concussion emergency medical action plan. These plans often include contact information for local emergency medical responders and the location of trauma centers, if available. Identify appropriate health professional(s) for games and practices to help assess and manage concussion among their athletes.
- *Ensure Safer Play* by:
  (a) Limiting contact during sports practices (when appropriate for the sport).
  (b) Putting in place rule changes and/or banning or limiting the use of certain drills or techniques to help reduce the chances of injury.
  (c) Checking sports equipment often. This includes making sure the equipment fits the athletes well, is in good condition, is stored properly, and is repaired and replaced based on instructions from the equipment companies.
- *Build the Science* by:
  (a) Collecting data from schools on the number of concussions reported by athletes during the season
  (b) Studying changes in concussion knowledge and awareness among coaches and parents before and after the policy is put in place
- *Focus on Education* by:
  (a) Posting information for parents, coaches, and athletes at schools and on the field or sidelines. Posted information often includes concussion signs and symptoms, as well as what to do if a concussion occurs.
  (b) Hosting or requiring regular trainings for athletes, parents, coaches, and school and health-care professionals about concussion.
- *Manage Return to School* by:
  (a) Providing information on returning to school. It includes creating a concussion management team to check on students with concussion for any changes in behavior or increased problems with schoolwork and a plan that includes special support or help for students during the school day to help with their recovery.

  A National Concussion Surveillance System was created in the CDC [7] in order to inform, prevent, and guide the population and the amateur and professional teams (coach, sports official, physician, others) on this issue.

## NFL Policies and Rules [Adapted from 8]

The NFL implemented the concussion protocol in 2009 and has adjusted it in the last 7 years. The league has instituted protocol to address the diagnosis and management of concussions.

The NFL made changes to the protocol after completing investigations in the way two teams handled head injuries to players during the 2017 season. The Seahawks were fined $100,000 when the league found they did not follow the protocol with quarterback Russell Wilson. The Texans were cleared by the league regarding their process with quarterback Tom Savage, but those two investigations pushed the league to refine the protocol to better protect players.

After the Seahawks investigation concluded, the league added a rule that requires teammates, coaches, or officials to take the player directly to a member of the medical team for evaluation. The changes after the Savage investigation were more sweeping. Among other things, the NFL has added an additional unaffiliated neurotrauma consultant to each post-season game, including the Super Bowl, to identify, monitor, and evaluate players for head injuries. Players also must be removed from the field of play and taken to the locker room for evaluation after the update.

In September 2016, the NFL announced the initiative "Play Smart, Play Safe" to continue to strive for a healthier game. The "NFL Game Day Concussion Protocol" was first implemented in 2009, adjusted in 2011, and tweaked in the last 5 years, including the introduction of disciplinary action in 2016 for teams that do not adhere properly.

## NFL's Concussion Protocol

In addition to the team medical staff and an unaffiliated neurological consultant, the league employs two medical spotters in the booth who watch the game with binoculars and video replay to identify injuries that others missed. The league added a rule in 2015 allowing for the medical spotters to stop the game with a medical timeout to remove an injured player.

## "Observable Symptoms"

The following are the seven observable symptoms used to identify players with concussions:

- Any loss of consciousness
- Slow to get up following a hit to the head ("hit to the head" may include secondary contact with the playing surface)
- Motor coordination/balance problems (stumbles, trips/falls, slow/labored movement)
- Blank or vacant look
- Disorientation (e.g., unsure of where he is on the field or location of bench)
- Clutching of head after contact
- Visible facial injury in combination with any of the above

When spotters or other medical personnel see those signs, that's when the protocol goes into effect.

## Return to Play Process

In addition to the in-game protocol, there is also a "Return-to-Participation Protocol" that can keep players out of action for more practices or games until they pass and are cleared to return.

It is a five-step process without any set timeline for a full return from a concussion:

1. *Rest and recovery*: Until a player returns to the "baseline level of signs and symptoms and neurological examination," only limited stretching and balance activities are recommended. Electronics, social media, and team meetings are all to be avoided.
2. *Light aerobic exercise*: The NFL recommends 10–20 min on a stationary bike or treadmill without resistance training or weight training. The cardiovascular activity is monitored by an athletic trainer to "determine if there are any recurrent concussion signs or symptoms."
3. *Continued aerobic exercise and introduction of strength training*: Increased duration and intensity of aerobic exercise with strength training added. An athletic trainer will supervise to watch for recurrent concussions signs or symptoms.
4. *Football-specific activities*: The cognitive load of playing football will be added and players will participate in non-contact activities for the typical duration of a full practice.
5. *Full football activity/clearance*: A player returns to full participation in practice, including contact without restriction.

During the off-season this year, the NFL added a measure that would punish teams that failed to properly enforce the concussion protocols. Any violation—either in-game or return-to-participation—could cost a team fines or even the forfeiture of draft picks.

The decision to add an unaffiliated neurotrauma consultant was stationed at the command center that has been used primarily for game-replay review [9].

- A central UNC will be stationed in the NFL's command center to assist in oversight of each game via broadcasts.
- Any sign of impact seizure will be considered the same as loss of consciousness, and the player will be taken out of the game and may not return.
- A referee who removes a player from the game for suspected head trauma must notify the medical staff.
- A player who exhibits gross motor instability or significant loss of balance must be taken to the locker room for evaluation if it is not diagnosed as an orthopedic injury.
- A player who is evaluated for a concussion must be re-evaluated within 24 h, even if the player has an off day.
- A third unaffiliated neurotrauma consultant will be on site for the playoffs and the Super Bowl, in addition to the two already assigned to each regular-season game.

The adjustments were implemented by the league's head, neck, and spine committee and communicated in two conference calls headed by Sills and Dr. Thom Mayer, the medical director for the NFL Players Association, with an estimated 400 people involved in the concussion process, including every team physician, every athletic trainer, every unaffiliated neurotrauma consultant, and every booth spotter [9].

The reason to add an extra unaffiliated neurotrauma consultant (UNC) for the playoffs and the Super Bowl is to allow a UNC to still be present if another is occupied when a player is taken to the locker room. This practice will be re-evaluated in the next season.

## Future Directions

History of sports concussion and chronic traumatic repetitive injury in sports had changed a lot in the last two decades. Significant literature contributions were made and the knowledge is transcending science and coming to the general public. The issue is being diffused and broadcasted by the media in order to inform people and prevent lesions. Several laws and policies have already been created and will be continuously updated in order to turn our football games safer.

## References


1. www.footballresearch.com/articles.
2. www.cdc.gov "Get a Heads Up on Concussion in Sports Policies". Information for Parents, Coaches, and School & Sports Professionals. CDC National Center for Injury Prevention and Control. Division of Unintentional Injury Prevention.
3. Washington State. Engrossed House Bill 1824, Chapter 475, Laws of 2009, 61st Legislature, 2009 Regular Session. Effective July 26, 2009. Available from: http://apps.leg.wa.gov/documents/billdocs/2009-10/pdfbills/session%20law%202009/1824. SL.pdf. Accessed 3 Jan 2011.
4. Oregon State. Senate Bill 348. 75th Oregon Legislative Assemble-2009 Regular Session. Avaiable from: http://www.leg.state.or.us/09reg/measures/sb0300.dir/sb0348.en.html. Accessed 3 July 2011.
5. Map of Concusssion in Sports Legislation. National Conference of State Legislatures. http://www.ncsl.org/issues-research/health/traumatic-brain-injury-legislation.aspx. Accessed 13 May 2013.
6. McCrory P, Meeuwisse W, Johnston K, Dvorak J, Aubry M, Molloy M, Cantu R. Consensus Statement on concussion in sport – The 3rd International Conference on Concussion in Sport, held in Zurich, November 2008. J Clin Neurosci. 2009;16:755–63.
7. www.cdc.gov/traumaticbraininjury.
8. www.sbnatio.com/nfe-concussion-protocol-explained, by Adan Stites, February 4th 2018.
9. http://www.espn.com/nfl/story/_/id/21864620/nfl-making-significant-changes-concussion-protocol.

# Traumatic Brain Injury in Fighting Sports

# 11

Renato Anghinah and Jéssica Natuline Ianof

## Introduction

Although millions of individuals suffer a traumatic brain injury (TBI) worldwide each year, it is only recently that TBI has been recognized as a major public health concern. There is growing recognition that a single severe TBI (sTBI) or repeated mild TBIs (rTBIs) can also induce insidious neurodegenerative processes, which may be associated with chronic traumatic encephalopathy (CTE) [1].

The objective of a boxing match is to render an opponent temporarily unconscious through blunt head injury, with subsequent intermittent loss of consciousness (knockout, KO). Prolonged exposure to repetitive head trauma can result in chronic traumatic encephalopathy (CTE), a neurological syndrome characterized by progressive impairments in cognitive, behavioral, and motor function [2].

Mixed martial arts (MMA), sometimes called "ultimate fighting," is used to describe full-contact combat sport activities utilizing a combination of Oriental martial arts (karate, judo, jiujitsu, and taekwondo) and Western combat sports (boxing, Greco-Roman wrestling, and kickboxing) [3]. It is a combative sport between two athletes that has undergone considerable growth and expansion in the United States over the past 15 years [4]. Bouts typically are 5 min in duration and consist of 3 to 5 rounds. Winners often are declared by judges' decision, technical knockout (TKO), referee stoppage, submission, knockout (KO), physician stoppage, or disqualification [5].

R. Anghinah (✉)
Department of Neurology – Cognitive Rehabilitation after TBI, Clinics Hospital – School of Medicine – University of São Paulo, São Paulo, Brazil

Center of Excellence in Neurology – Americas Serviços Médicos, São Paulo, Brazil

J. N. Ianof
Department of Neurology – Cognitive Rehabilitation after TBI, Clinics Hospital – School of Medicine – University of São Paulo, São Paulo, Brazil

Kickboxing is a combat sport which involves two competitors directing full-force strikes with the hands, elbows, knees, shins, and feet at each other. It is one of the modern combat sports and requires athletes to achieve high thresholds of several aspects of physical fitness [6].

## History

Martland introduced the term "punch drunk," in 1928, to describe neurological symptoms, like confusion, tremors, slowed speech, and the gait disturbances, seen in boxers suffering from repeated blows to the head [7].

Millspaugh coined the term "dementia pugilistica" to describe similar cases, in 1937 [8]. Courville introduced the term, "psychopathic deterioration of pugilists" [9]. In 1957, Critchley reported on 69 cases of progressive neurological disease in boxers and proposed "chronic progressive traumatic encephalopathy of boxers" [10].

The neuropathology of CTE was first described by Brandenburg and Hallervorden and later by Corsellis who found several characteristic areas of damage: septum pellucidum, adjacent periventricular gray, frontal and temporal lobes, substantia nigra, cerebellar scarring, and diffuse neuronal loss [11–13].

Although originally described in boxers, CTE is also found in other contact sports (football, hockey, wrestling), as well as in individuals suffering repetitive brain trauma who were not athletes [11, 12], such as military blast victims and people who suffered physical abuse and epilepsy [11].

## Pathophysiology

Catastrophic brain injuries refer to severe brain trauma associated with cerebral contusions or intracranial hemorrhage, and it can lead to long-term neurological sequelae or even death. The most common cause of death in sports-related



R. Anghinah et al. (eds.), *Topics in Cognitive Rehabilitation in the TBI Post-Hospital Phase*,
https://doi.org/10.1007/978-3-319-95376-2_11

TBI, especially in boxers, is subdural hematoma [14, 15]. Each year in boxing, about ten deaths occur, most of which following knockout or technical knockout [16]. Deaths are more common in lower weight classes in boxing.

A knockout is associated with concussion and loss of consciousness. Concussion occurs more frequently in professional boxing than in amateur boxing or other contact sports [17]. Concussion can also happen in other martial arts like karate [18], taekwondo [17], and kickboxing [19, 20]. The work of Koh and Cassidy [21] showed that in a Korean taekwondo tournament, the incidence of head blows and concussions was 226 – there were 2328 competitors. The younger participants had a higher the incidence of head blows and concussions [21].

Cognitive impairment often persists beyond the subjectively symptomatic time in boxers following mild TBI or a knockout, as revealed by the neuropsychological tests – it can be impaired for days following a knockout in amateur boxers [22].

Subconcussion refers to a mild head injury that causes these subtle subjective and objective neuropsychiatric deficits [23].

Rapid acceleration and deceleration forces, either linear or rotational, on the brain are the primary mechanism in which concussion and subconcussion occur. When subjected to these forces, the brain – including its neurons, glial cells, and blood vessels – is stretched. And that may disrupt their normal functions. Axons are particularly susceptible to stretching, which can lead to diffuse axonal injury [24]. Blows to the head by hook punches (rotational acceleration) in boxing results in concussion more often than linear acceleration caused by straight head blows and head contacts, common in other sports such as American football [25].

## Acute Brain Injury

The study of Matser et al. [26] evaluated 38 amateur boxers before and after a bout. Concussion was observed in 13 percent of cases after the fight. Porter (92) observed 281 amateur fights, and 12% of them ended in a knockout (KO) or in the intervention of the referee following blows to the head [26].

## Chronic Brain Injury

In 1969, Roberts examined 224 former professional boxers from the United Kingdom for neurological abnormalities. Signs of brain injury were found in roughly half the subjects. The study reported a CTE prevalence of 17%. Longer duration of exposure to sport (measured as the number of bouts), older age at retirement from boxing, and longer length of boxing career are important variables that can increase an individual's risk of developing CTE [27].

Eighteen former and active boxers were evaluated by Casson et al. [28]. They conducted neurological and neuropsychological tests and performed EEGs and computed tomographic (CT) scans. In 13 of the 15 professional boxers (87%), at least two of the four tests revealed abnormal findings, suggestive of chronic brain injury. All the professional boxers and the three amateurs boxers had abnormal scores in at least one of the neuropsychological tests [28].

Jordan et al. [29] performed brain CT scans in 338 active professional boxers. Definite abnormalities were observed in 7% (25 boxers) and possible abnormalities in over 49% of the sample (75 boxers). There was no difference between boxers with clear abnormalities and the rest of the group in terms of age, in terms of number of bouts fought, won or lost, or in terms of type of EEG abnormality. Of the boxers with defined CT abnormalities, 68% suffered one or more KOs, compared with 49% of people with possible abnormalities and only 37% of those without abnormalities [29]. Jordan et al. [30], in another study, tested 30 professional boxers using neurological and neuropsychological evaluations. Chronic abnormalities of a mild to severe nature were observed in 19 of the subjects (63% of the sample). The severity of the abnormalities was related to the number of bouts [30].

## Biomarkers

In lumbar cerebrospinal fluid (CSF) in boxers 4–10 days after a bout and in boxers who have not been knockout total tau protein levels are elevated and the level normalize within the 8–12 weeks if the boxers are not subjected to further bouts [31, 32].

In amateur boxers with mild TBI after a bout, levels of neurofilament light polypeptide (NFL) in lumbar CSF are also raised [31, 32]. NFL in lumbar CSF is probably the most sensitive biomarker of axonal injury and represents the susceptibility of long myelinated axons to mild TBI [33]. Exposure to head trauma – including number of blows to the head – is correlated with NFL levels in lumbar CSF in amateur boxers [31, 32].

## Chronic Traumatic Encephalopathy in Boxing

CTE includes a latent period of 8–10 years followed by onset of behavioral disturbance, characterized by impulsivity and depression. Cognitive symptoms include disturbance of attention and memory [34]. Post-traumatic parkinsonism is also related to extensive boxing exposure [35].

Advances in brain imaging provide an opportunity to characterize in vivo neurodegeneration in athletes. The findings of frequent magnetic resonance imaging (MRI) in professional boxers include hippocampal atrophy, cavum septum pellucidum, dilated perivascular spaces, indications of diffuse axonal injury (DAI), pituitary gland atrophy, and ventricular enlargement [36].

Diffusion tensor imaging (DTI) is an advanced MRI technique that measures the microstructural integrity of brain tissue using metrics such as fractional anisotropy (FA) and apparent diffusion coefficient (ADC). FA measures, indirectly, white matter microstructure by assessing the tendency of water molecules to move parallel to structural components of axons (anisotropic diffusion) that act as barriers to diffusion rather than across them. Higher FA is commonly associated with a structural environment characterized by higher fiber density and organization, homogeneity of the direction of the fibers, axonal diameter, and degree of myelination. ADC assesses how freely water moves inside the brain tissue (isotropic diffusion or diffusivity) and is usually negatively correlated with the components of the structural environment described above. Moderate and severe traumatic brain injury (TBI) frequently results in decreased FA and increased ADC in the chronic stage [37, 38]. In acute mild TBI, the directionality of FA has been reported as elevated in some studies and reduced in others, and the reason for that is not clearly understood [39]. DTI is of great importance because it can detect changes in white matter tracts that are not observed on conventional MRI, including potential DAI associated with CTE [34].

Previous DTI studies on the chronic effects of boxing showed lower FA and greater diffusivity in professional boxers in comparison with a control group [40–42].

Chappell and colleagues compared DTI in 81 professional boxers with 12 control subjects using a voxel-based analysis, and the analysis revealed regions of white matter that presented lower FA and increased ADC, including the midbrain, medial temporal lobe, lower fronto-occipital fasciculus, inferior longitudinal fasciculus, and cerebral peduncles [40]. Zhang and colleagues [42] found lower FA in the genu, splenium, and posterior internal capsule of boxers who also had greater diffusivity in the anterior and posterior limbs of the internal capsule, and for that they used a DTI region of interest (ROI) analysis. However, the comparison groups of these studies were composed of healthy individuals and did not control participation in sports.

Researchers also examined subject variables and boxing history in relation to DTI. Chappell et al. [40] found that diffusivity in subcortical structures increased with age in both boxers and the control group, but the correlation between diffusion parameters such as ADC or mean diffusivity and age in boxers (mean age of 28 years) was significantly higher than in the control group [40]. This indicates that although diffusion parameters generally increase with age, they do so at a higher rate in boxers, possibly suggesting a neurodegenerative process. The exposure to boxing is frequently estimated by the number of boxing matches and years of boxing. Shin and colleagues studied the relationship between AF, diffusion measures, and knockouts (KOs) in boxers. These researchers found a positive correlation between KOs and diffusion and a negative correlation between KOs and FA in the corpus callosum, isthmus of the cingulum bundle, pericalcarine region, precuneus, and amygdala [43].

It is important to emphasize that most DTI studies have imaged professional boxers [40–42]. Even though several studies using conventional MRI suggested that amateur boxers also exhibit chronic and neurobehavioral effects of repetitive head trauma [44, 45], an investigation of boxers and amateur boxers who have recently become professionals reported negative MRI scans and neurobehavioral findings that did not differ from a control group of athletes engaged in contactless sports [46]. In addition, the rate of chronic traumatic brain injury among amateur boxers has been viewed as insignificant [35]. The gaps in the boxing literature include sparse DTI-related data and MRI imaging for cognitive performance and history of exposure. In addition, not all studies included a comparison group with similar demographic characteristics and participation in noncontact sports.

Davis et al. [47] *studied the* effect of the rules change in 2013 on amateur boxing strategy, technique, and safety. Pre-2013 and post-2013 3 × 3 min elite-level amateur boxing was compared from video footage of 29 Olympic (pre-2013) and 50 World Championship bouts (post-2013), totaling 99 male boxers. *They found that several* techniques that were dominant pre-2013 were used less post-2013, including total punches thrown, rear hand punches, and hook rear hand, while defensive movements were higher post-2013. Boxers have increased their foot movement by 20%, post-2013, to move in and then away from their opponent, combined with long-range punches and deliberate defensive movements. Pre-2013, 1.7% of bouts did not last the full duration due to referee stoppage, while post-2013, this increased to 4.2% as a result of two knockouts and eight technical knockouts. An increase in skin splits and technical knockouts is apparent. It is likely that boxers believe head guard removal has made them more prone to knockouts [47].

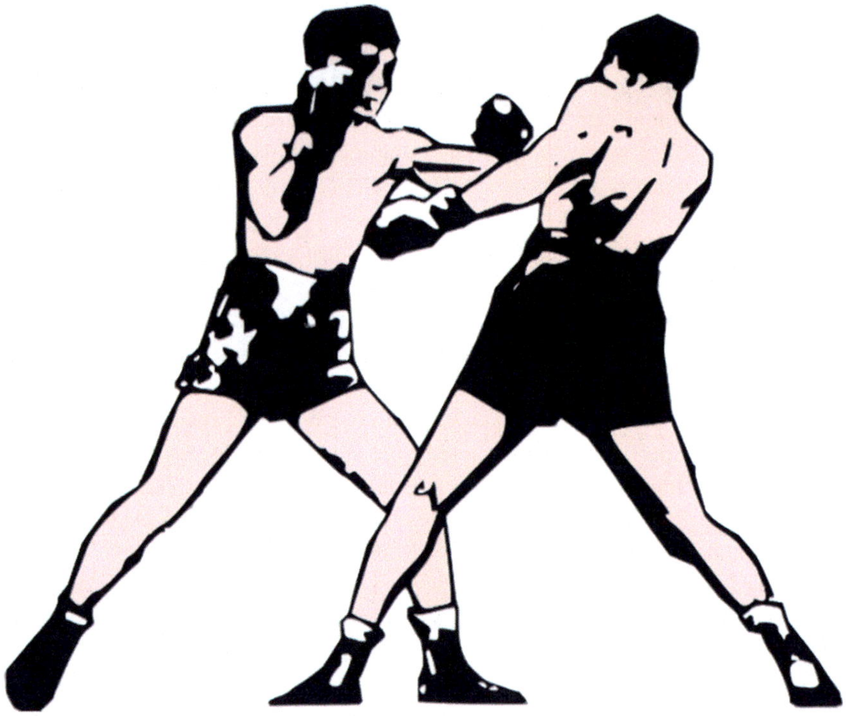

**Fonte: Pixabay**

## Mixed Martial Arts

The review of Lystad et al. [48] revealed that the head was the most commonly injured anatomic region, ranging from 66.8% to 78.0%. The most common type of injury was laceration/abrasion, ranging from 36.7% to 59.4%, followed by fracture, ranging from 7.4% to 43.3%, and concussion, ranging from 3.8% to 20.4%. There is a very high proportion of head injuries in MMA and professional boxing where punches to the bare head are allowed. The high proportion of head injuries in MMA is a cause for concern, since continued repetitive head trauma is associated with degeneration in brain structures such as the bilateral hippocampi, basal ganglia, and thalamus, which can lead to cognitive impairment [48].

Published rates of injury are similar between boxing (17–25%) and MMA (24%), and therefore many studies assume that MMA injury patterns will be similar to other combat sports such as boxing and wrestling, but given the different components of each one used in MMA, it may not be possible to extrapolate exactly that data. In fact, a review of the MMA literature reveals considerable variation in observed injury patterns, limiting the generalization of boxing and wrestling analysis to this population. A notable difference is that the lighter gloves used in MMA (4–6 oz) versus boxing (16 oz) serve only to protect the hands of competitors and do not decrease attack forces compared to wearing no gloves at all [49, 50].

Some of the available studies reviewed video evidence to evaluate head trauma but it is complicated to determine the incidence of concussion on the basis of video evidence of head trauma alone.

The study of Buse (2006) revealed (after he reviewed video footage of 1284 men competing in 642 matches from 1993 to 2003) that the proportion of matches ending by head trauma was higher in MMA (28%) compared with boxing (9%) and kickboxing (8%). An important limitation of Buse's review was that it was simply a video review of televised matches [51].

Ngai observed severe concussion – a loss of consciousness resulting from a KO – as an injury in 3.3% of matches. He reported this incidence to be similar to what has been demonstrated in taekwondo competitions [52]. The study of Scoggin evaluated 116 bouts in Hawaii, and he reported that 11 of the 55 injuries were concussions. Of the 55 fighters, 7 who had concussions had loss of consciousness, 4 had retrograde amnesia, and 5 reported facial injuries. Concussions occurred in 4.7% of exposures, and facial injuries occurred in 2.2% of exposures [53].

Heath and Callahan studied a sample of MMA athletes ($n = 19$) that reported concussive symptoms, training routines, and medical histories through an online survey. Almost 15% of the MMA athletes reported history of a knockout, and nearly one-third reported a technical knockout [54].

## Kickboxing

Chronic TCE can be caused by knockout (KO) with loss of consciousness or by the cumulative effect of punching or kicking the head. Kickboxers with long experience or kickboxers with limited defense skills who repeatedly suffered heavy blows are at the highest risk of developing this condition [20]. Kickboxing is associated with chronic repeated chronological trauma that can cause brain injuries [20, 55], unconsciousness, and neurological abnormalities, mainly hypopituitarism [65]. Some studies have investigated pituitary function in amateur kickboxers and demonstrated that kickboxing is a cause of TBI, and growth hormone (GH) deficiency and insufficient adrenocorticotropic hormone (ACTH) were also very common (22.7% and 9.1%, respectively) among the 22 amateur kickboxers [56]. Consequently, Tanriverdi et al. [57] reported that GH is the most common hormone lost after TBI, followed by ACTH, gonadotropin (luteinizing hormone (LH) and follicle-stimulating hormone (FSH)), and thyroid-stimulating hormone (TSH). The mechanisms responsible for pituitary dysfunction after BIT are not entirely clear, but genetic predisposition and autoimmunity may play a role.

As in Muay Thai, all body targets are permissible in both amateur and professional kickboxing except for the groin [19]. Thus, the head, arms, and trunk would be expected to be the primary targets/injury sites for kickboxers [20, 58]. Head injuries were found as the second most frequent injury in amateur and professional kickboxers [59]. Zazryn et al. [20] reported that the head, neck, and face, followed by the lower extremities, were the most common body regions injured. The latter authors also reported that Australian kickboxers suffered more head injuries than those in the United Kingdom and the Netherlands (51.6% vs. 42.5%) but fewer lower extremity injuries (39.8% vs. 53.4%).

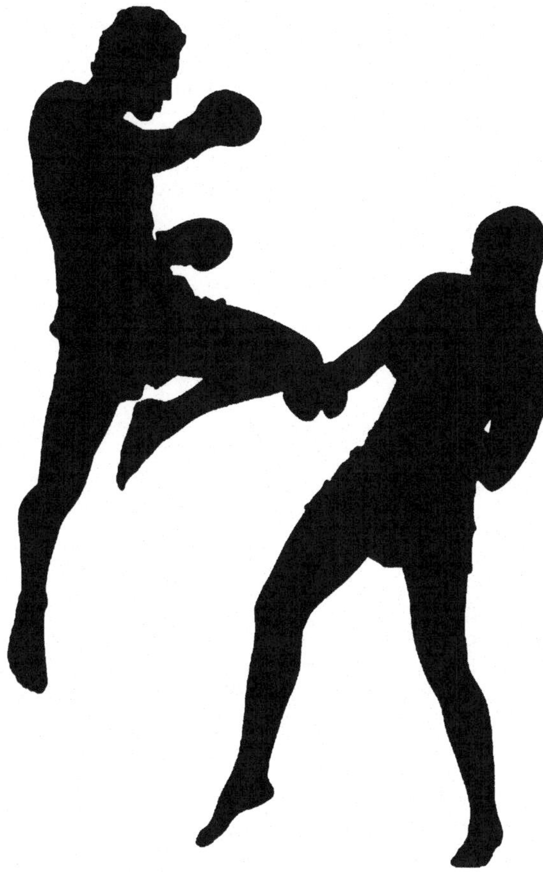

**Fonte: Pixabay**

## Boxing x Martial Arts

In the study of Lee et al. [60], a conventional 3 T RM image was used to evaluate 499 fighters (boxers, mixed martial artists, and martial artists) and 62 controls for nonspecific white matter changes, cerebral hemorrhage, cavum septum pellucidum, and cavum vergae. The prevalence of non-specific white matter changes was similar between the groups. Fighters had a prevalence of cerebral hemorrhage (4.2% vs. 0% for controls, $P = 0.152$) and a higher prevalence of cavum septum pellucidum versus controls (53.1% versus 17.7%, $P < 0.001$) and cavum vergae versus controls (14.4% versus 0%, $P < 0.001$). The lengths of the cavum septum pellucidum plus the cavum septum pellucidum for the septum pellucidum length ratio ($P = 0.009$) were higher in the fighters than in controls. They found that the number of combats was slightly correlated with the length of the septum of the cavum septum pellucidum plus cavum vergae ($R = 0.306$; $P < 0.001$) and the length of the cavum septum and pellucidum ($R = 0.278$; $P < 0.001$). When the fighters were subdivided into boxers, mixed martial artists, and martial artists, the results were similar to those of the whole-group analysis. Although brain microhemorrhages were greater in fighters than in controls, this finding was not statistically significant, possibly due in part to insufficient study [60].

## Conclusion

The objective of fighting sports, like boxing, kickboxing, and mixed martial arts, is to render an opponent temporarily unconscious through blunt head injury, with subsequent intermittent loss of consciousness (knockout, KO). Prolonged exposure to repetitive head trauma can result in chronic traumatic encephalopathy (CTE), a neurological syndrome characterized by progressive impairments in cognitive, behavioral, and motor function.

Increasing data supporting the link of repetitive TBI and long-term neurodegenerative consequence has had significant implications in sports which is leading to changes in the sports' rules.

**Conflict of Interest** There is no conflict of interest to declare.

## References


1. Johnson VE, Stewart W, Arena JD, Smith DH. Traumatic brain injury as a trigger of neurodegeneration. Adv Neurobiol. 2017;15:383–400.
2. Parker H. Traumatic encephalopathy of professional pugilists. J Neurol Psychopathol. 1934;15:20–8.
3. Sáchez Garcia R, Malcolm D. Decivilizing, civilizing or informalizing? The international development of mixed martial arts. Int Rev Sociol Sport. 2010;45:39–58.
4. Stuart JI, Hudson IL, Sarkisian SA, Simpson MP, Donham BP. Injuries sustained during modern Army Combatives tournaments. Mil Med. 2018;
5. Walrod B. Current review of injuries sustained in mixed martial arts competition. Curr Sports Med Rep. 2011;10(5):288–9.
6. Slimani M, Chaabene H, Miarka B, Franchini E, Chamari K, Cheour F. Kickboxing review: anthropometric, psychophysiological and activity profiles and injury epidemiology. Biol Sport. 2017;34(2):185–96.
7. Martland HS. Punch drunk. JAMA. 1928;91:1103–7.
8. Millspaugh JA. Dementia pugilistica. US Nav Med Bull. 1937;35:297–303.
9. Courville CB. Punch drunk. Its pathogenesis and pathology on the basis of a verified case. Bull Los Angel Neurol Soc. 1962;27:160–8.
10. Critchley M. Medical aspects of boxing, particularly from a neurological standpoint. Br Med J. 1957;1(5015):357–62.
11. McKee AC, Cantu RC, Nowinski CJ, Hedley-Whyte ET, Gavett BE, Budson AE, Santini VE, Lee HS, Kubilus CA, Stern RA. Chronic traumatic encephalopathy in athletes: progressive tauopathy after repetitive head injury. J Neuropathol Exp Neurol. 2009;68:709–35.
12. Corsellis JAN, Bruton CJ, Freeman-Browne D. The aftermath of boxing. Psychol Med. 1973;3:270–303.
13. Brandenburg W, Hallervorden J. Dementia pugilistica with anatomical findings Virchows arch, vol. 325; 1954. p. 680–709.
14. Guterman A, Smith RW. Neurological sequelae of boxing. Sports Med. 1987;4(3):194–210.
15. Unterharnscheidt F. A neurologist's reflections on boxing. I: impact mechanics in boxing and injuries other than central nervous system damage. Rev Neurol. 1995;23(121):661–74.
16. Svinth JR. Death under the spotlight: the Manuel Velazquez boxing fatality collection. J. Combat Sport. 2011:1–28.
17. Koh JO, Cassidy JD, Watkinson EJ. Incidence of concussion in contact sports: a systematic review of the evidence. Brain Inj. 2003;17(10):901–17.
18. Stricevic MV, Patel MR, Okazaki T, Swain BK. Karate: historical perspective and injuries sustained in national and international tournament competitions. Am J Sports Med. 1983;11(5):320–4.
19. Gartland S, Malik MH, Lovell ME. Injury and injury rates in Muay Thai kick boxing. Br J Sports Med. 2001;35(5):308–13.
20. Zazryn TR, Finch CF, McCrory P. A 16 year study of injuries to professional kickboxers in the state of Victoria, Australia. Br J Sports Med. 2003;37(5):448–51.
21. Koh JO, Cassidy JD. Incidence study of head blows and concussions in competition taekwondo. Clin J Sport Med. 2004;14(2):72–9.
22. Bleiberg J, Cernich AN, Cameron K, Sun W, Peck K, Ecklund PJ, Reeves D, Uhorchak J, Sparling MB, Warden DL. Duration of cognitive impairment after sports concussion. Neurosurgery. 2004;54(5):1073–8.
23. Guskiewicz KM, Mihalik JP, Shankar V, Marshall SW, Crowell DH, Oliaro SM, Ciocca MF, Hooker DN. Measurement of head impacts in collegiate football players: relationship between head impact biomechanics and acute clinical outcome after concussion. Neurosurgery. 2007;61(6):1244–52.
24. McKee AC, Daneshvar DH, Alvarez VE, Stein TD. The neuropathology of sport. Acta Neuropathol. 2014;127(1):29–51.
25. Ohhashi G, Tani S, Murakami S, Kamio M, Abe T, Ohtuki J. Problems in health management of professional boxers in Japan. Br J Sports Med. 2002;36(5):346–52.
26. Matser EJ, Kessels AG, Lezak MD, Troost J, Jordan BD. Acute traumatic brain injury in amateur boxing. Phys Sportsmed. 2000;28(1):87–92.
27. Roberts AH. Brain damage in boxers: a study of the prevalence of traumatic encephalopathy among ex-professional boxers. London: Pitman Medical and Scientific Publishing Co; 1969.
28. Casson IR, Siegel O, Sham R, Campbell EA, Tarlau M, DiDomenico A. Brain damage in modern boxers. JAMA. 1984;251(20):2663–7.
29. Jordan BD, Jahre C, Hauser WA, Zimmerman RD, Zarrelli M, Lipsitz EC, Johnson V, Warren RF, Tsairis P, Folk FS. CT of 338 active professional boxers. Radiology. 1992;185(2):509–12.
30. Jordan BD, Relkin NR, Ravdin LD, Jacobs AR, Bennett A, Gandy S. Apolipoprotein E epsilon4 associated with chronic traumatic brain injury in boxing. JAMA. 1997;278(2):136–40.
31. Neselius S, Brisby H, Theodorsson A, Blennow K, Zetterberg H, Marcusson J. CSF-biomarkers in Olympic boxing: diagnosis and effects of repetitive head trauma. PLoS One. 2012;7(4):e33606.
32. Zetterberg H, Hietala MA, Jonsson M, Andreasen N, Styrud E, Karlsson I, Edman A, Popa C, Rasulzada A, Wahlund LO, Mehta PD, Rosengren L, Blennow K, Wallin A. Neurochemical aftermath of amateur boxing. Arch Neurol. 2006;63(9):1277–80.
33. Zetterberg H, Smith DH, Blennow K. Biomarkers of mild traumatic brain injury in cerebrospinal fluid and blood. Nat Rev Neurol. 2013;9(4):201–10.
34. McKee AC, Stern RA, Nowinski CJ, Stein TD, Alvarez VE, Daneshvar DH, Lee HS, Wojtowicz SM, Hall G, Baugh CM, Riley DO, Kubilus CA, Cormier KA, Jacobs MA, Martin BR, Abraham CR, Ikezu T, Reichard RR, Wolozin BL, Budson AE, Goldstein LE, Kowall NW, Cantu RC. The spectrum of disease in chronic traumatic encephalopathy. Brain. 2013;136(Pt 1):43–64.
35. Jordan BD. The clinical spectrum of sport-related traumatic brain injury. Nat Rev Neurol. 2013;9(4):222–30.
36. Orrison WW, Hanson EH, Alamo T, Watson D, Sharma M, Perkins TG, Tandy RD. Traumatic brain injury: a review and high-field MRI findings in 100 unarmed combatants using a literature-based checklist approach. J Neurotrauma. 2009;26(5):689–701.
37. Huisman TA, Schwamm LH, Schaefer PW, Koroshetz WJ, Shetty-Alva N, Ozsunar Y, Wu O, Sorensen AG. Diffusion tensor imaging as potential biomarker of white matter injury in diffuse axonal injury. AJNR Am J Neuroradiol. 2004;25(3):370–6.
38. Hulkower MB, Poliak DB, Rosenbaum SB, Zimmerman ME, Lipton ML. A decade of DTI in traumatic brain injury: 10 years and 100 articles later. AJNR Am J Neuroradiol. 2013;34(11):2064–74.
39. Shenton ME, Hamoda HM, Schneiderman JS, Bouix S, Pasternak O, Rathi Y, Vu MA, Purohit MP, Helmer K, Koerte I, Lin AP, Westin CF, Kikinis R, Kubicki M, Stern RA, Zafonte R. A review of magnetic resonance imaging and diffusion tensor imaging findings in mild traumatic brain injury. Brain Imaging Behav. 2012;6(2):137–92.
40. Chappell MH, Uluğ AM, Zhang L, Heitger MH, Jordan BD, Zimmerman RD, Watts R. Distribution of microstructural damage

in the brains of professional boxers: a diffusion MRI study. J Magn Reson Imaging. 2006;24(3):537–42.
41. Zhang L, Ravdin LD, Relkin N, Zimmerman RD, Jordan B, Lathan WE, Uluğ AM. Increased diffusion in the brain of professional boxers: a preclinical sign of traumatic brain injury? AJNR Am J Neuroradiol. 2003;24(1):52–7.
42. Zhang L, Heier LA, Zimmerman RD, Jordan B, Ulug AM. Diffusion anisotropy changes in the brains of professional boxers. AJNR Am J Neuroradiol. 2006;27(9):2000–4.
43. Shin W, Mahmoud SY, Sakaie K, Banks SJ, Lowe MJ, Phillips M, Modic MT, Bernick C. Diffusion measures indicate fight exposure-related damage to cerebral white matter in boxers and mixed martial arts fighters. AJNR Am J Neuroradiol. 2014;35(2):285–90.
44. Zazryn T, Cameron P, McCrory P. A prospective cohort study of injury in amateur and professional boxing. Br J Sports Med. 2006;40(8):670–4.
45. Hähnel S, Stippich C, Weber I, Darm H, Schill T, Jost J, Friedmann B, Heiland S, Blatow M, Meyding-Lamadé U. Prevalence of cerebral microhemorrhages in amateur boxers as detected by 3T MR imaging. AJNR Am J Neuroradiol. 2008;29(2):388–91.
46. Levin HS, Lippold SC, Goldman A, Handel S, High WM Jr, Eisenberg HM, Zelitt D. Neurobehavioral functioning and magnetic resonance imaging findings in young boxers. J Neurosurg. 1987;67(5):657–67.
47. Davis P, Waldock R, Connorton A, Driver S, Anderson S. Comparison of amateur boxing before and after the 2013 rules change and the impact on boxers' safety. Br J Sports Med. 2018;52(11):741–46. https://doi.org/10.1136/bjsports-2017-097667. Epub 2017 Sep 27.
48. Lystad RP, Gregory K, Wilson J. The epidemiology of injuries in mixed martial arts: a systematic review and meta-analysis. Orthop J Sports Med. 2014;2(1):2325967113518492.
49. Seidenberg P. Mixed martial arts: injury patterns and issues for the ringside physician. Curr Sports Med Rep. 2011;1003:147–50.
50. Schwartz ML, Hudson AR, Fernie GR, Hayashi K, Coleclough AA. Biomechanical study of full-contact karate contrasted with boxing. J Neurosurg. 1986 Feb;64(2):248–52.
51. Buse GJ. No holds barred sport fighting: a 10 year review of mixed martial arts competition. Br J Sports Med. 2006;40(2):169–72. https://doi.org/10.1136/bjsm.2005.021295.
52. Ngai KM, Levy F, Hsu EB. Injury trends in sanctioned mixed martial arts competition: a 5-year review from 2002 to 2007. Br J Sports Med. 2007;42:686–9.
53. Scoggin JF 3rd, Brusovanik G, Pi M, et al. Assessment of injuries sustained in mixed mixed martial arts competition. Am J Orthop (Belle Mead NJ). 2010;39:247–51.
54. Heath CJ, Callahan JL. Self-reported concussion symptoms and training routines in mixed martial arts athletes. Res Sports Med. 2013;21(3):195–203.
55. Lystad RP. Injuries to professional and amateur kickboxing contestants: a 15-year retrospective cohort study. Orthop J Sports Med. 2015;3(11):2325967115612416.
56. Tanriverdi F, Unluhizarci K, Coksevim B, Selcuklu A, Casanueva FF, Kelestimur F. Kickboxing sport as a new cause of traumatic brain injury-mediated hypopituitarism. Clin Endocrinol. 2007;66(3):360–6.
57. Tanriverdi F, Schneider HJ, Aimaretti G, Masel BE, Casanueva FF, Kelestimur F. Pituitary dysfunction after traumatic brain injury: a clinical and pathophysiological approach. Endocr Rev. 2015;36(3):305–42.
58. Shimoyama T, Masuda I, Numa T, Horie N. Mandibular fracture with a mouth formed mouthguard in kickboxing. Dent Traumatol. 2009;25(2):242–4.
59. Gartland S, Malik MH, Lovell M. A prospective study of injuries sustained during competitive Muay Thai kickboxing. Clin J Sport Med. 2005;15(1):34–6.
60. Lee JK, Wu J, Banks S, et al. Prevalence of traumatic findings on routine MRI in a large cohort of professional fighters. Am J Neuroradiol. 2017;38:1303–10.

# 12 Neuropsychiatric Symptoms of Post-concussion Syndrome (PCS) and Chronic Traumatic Encephalopathy (CTE)

Anna Vasilevskaya and Maria Carmela Tartaglia

## Abbreviations

| | |
|---|---|
| AD | Alzheimer's disease |
| ALS | Amyotrophic lateral sclerosis |
| CTE | Chronic traumatic encephalopathy |
| DSM-IV | *Diagnostic and Statistical Manual of Mental Disorders*, Fourth Edition |
| DSM-V | *Diagnostic and Statistical Manual of Mental Disorders*, Fifth Edition |
| fMRI | Functional magnetic resonance imaging |
| GABA | gamma-aminobutyric acid |
| ICD-10 | *International Classification of Diseases*, Tenth Revision |
| MDD | Major depressive disorder |
| mTBI | mild traumatic brain injury |
| NFL | National Football League |
| OCD | Obsessive-compulsive disorder |
| PCS | Post-concussion syndrome |
| PD | Parkinson's disease |
| TBI | Traumatic brain injury |

A. Vasilevskaya (✉)
Institute of Medical Science, University of Toronto, Toronto, ON, Canada

Centre for Research in Neurodegenerative Diseases, University of Toronto, Toronto, ON, Canada
e-mail: hanna.vasileuskaya@mail.utoronto.ca

M. C. Tartaglia
Institute of Medical Science, University of Toronto, Toronto, ON, Canada

Centre for Research in Neurodegenerative Diseases, University of Toronto, Toronto, ON, Canada

Division of Neurology, University Health Network, Toronto, ON, Canada

## Concussion (Mild Traumatic Brain Injury)

Concussion (also known as mild traumatic brain injury, or mTBI) has gained considerable attention in recent years, following the findings that mTBIs are more common than previously thought and can have enduring consequences and possibly lead to neurodegeneration [10]. Global estimates suggest ten million new TBI cases each year with the vast majority being mild TBIs (concussions) [41]. Concussion can have many causes, with the most common being motor vehicle accidents, falls, sports, and blast injuries in a military setting [41]. Concussions used to be regarded as trivial, but recent evidence suggests they result from a brain injury leading to neuropathological, neurophysiological, and neuropsychological changes [24]. The symptoms associated with concussions fall into three clusters:

- Somatic (includes neurological symptoms like headaches, nausea, dizziness, etc.)
- Affective (refers to changes in the affective state like irritability, depression, and anxiety)
- Cognitive (changes in cognitive functioning like impaired memory and concentration) [44, 92]

Research shows that most patients with mTBIs (80–90%) see their symptoms resolve within 7–10 days. In the remaining 10–20%, the symptoms may persist for months following the head trauma, with 25–33% of those patients moving on to develop persistent post-concussion symptoms [41], which is referred to as a post-concussion syndrome (PCS) [87].

In recent years, there is a growing concern that repeated concussions can be associated with delayed neurodegeneration including a number of neurodegenerative diseases such as Alzheimer's disease, Parkinson's disease, and more specifically chronic traumatic encephalopathy (CTE). CTE is the pathological correlate of the largely behavioral and cognitive impairments that have been reported for the most


R. Anghinah et al. (eds.), *Topics in Cognitive Rehabilitation in the TBI Post-Hospital Phase*,
https://doi.org/10.1007/978-3-319-95376-2_12

part in a few former professional athletes playing contact sports.

The aim of this chapter is to review the neuropsychiatric symptoms associated with the clinical syndrome of PCS and the pathological entity of CTE.

## Diagnosis of PCS

When symptoms of concussion persist, then the diagnosis of PCS needs to be considered. In the absence of confirmed imaging or molecular biomarkers, current diagnosis of PCS is subjective and includes self-reported symptoms [41]. The first proposed diagnostic criteria for PCS was published in the *International Classification of Diseases*, Tenth Revision (ICD-10), in 1992. ICD-10 requires a clinical history of TBI and the presence of three or more of the following symptoms for at least 4 weeks: headache, dizziness, fatigue, irritability, insomnia, concentration, memory difficulty, and intolerance of stress, emotion, or alcohol [10, 41]. The second widely accepted clinical criteria used for PCS diagnosis is that of the *Diagnostic and Statistical Manual of Mental Disorders*, Fourth Edition (DSM-IV). The main differences between ICD-10 and DSM-IV are that the latter requires the person to have memory or attention difficulties, without dementia related to head injury, and the symptoms should last for at least 3 months and interfere with social functioning [10]. The term "post-concussion syndrome" has been changed to "Neurocognitive symptoms associated with traumatic brain injury" in DSM-V [41]. The fifth edition of DSM also brought upon the following changes in PCS diagnosis: the patient needs to meet the criteria for mild or moderate neurocognitive disorder, which should present itself immediately after the injury or recovery of consciousness following injury, and last beyond the acute posttraumatic phase of the injury. The list of possible symptoms also included posttraumatic amnesia, loss of consciousness, disorientation, and confusion [2]. The most recent consensus statement on concussion in sport highlighted the need for a standard definition of a PCS diagnosis and proposed that persistent post-concussion symptoms should be diagnosed if they last for longer than 10–14 days in adults [66].

## Post-concussion Syndrome and Chronic Traumatic Encephalopathy

Chronic traumatic encephalopathy (CTE) is a neurodegenerative disease that currently can only be diagnosed pathologically. It has been associated with repeated concussions and presents with distinctive tau pathology [34, 70]. At the moment, the relationship between PCS and CTE is not entirely clear. There is some symptom overlap between the two conditions, and although there is evidence to support that CTE is not just a cumulative effect of PCS-related changes [5, 34], there may be pathological changes that predate overt clinical signs as in other neurodegenerative diseases [53].

The first scientific account of deficits resulting from multiple head injuries was documented by Martland in 1928. In his paper, Martland described the symptoms seen in boxers with repetitive head trauma and called this punch-drunk syndrome. These symptoms included unsteadiness and sluggish movement. In some cases, there was mild mental confusion, however, many symptoms remained mild in nature and insufficient to interfere with fighting. The most severe cases, conversely, showed pronounced Parkinsonism and marked mental deterioration [61]. The term punch-drunk was later changed to dementia pugilistica [76] and then renamed once again by Critchley [19] to chronic traumatic encephalopathy. Roberts [85] in his study revisited the boxers' data and, according to Corsellis [17], found the brains contained a "widespread deposition of β-protein in the cortex." Miller [75] in his article notes that concussed patients often reported numerous neuropsychiatric symptoms including irritability, anxiety, bouts of depression, and nightmares about the accident. Retrospective analysis of previous case studies on presumptive CTE (called "punch drunk" at the time) [16, 63] in boxers suggests two different clinical presentations. The first presentation was believed to have a younger onset (mean age about 35 years old) with behavioral and mood disturbances (i.e., depression, aggression, mood lability, and suicidality) but very little cognitive or motor changes. The second presentation had an older onset (mean age about 60 years old) with pronounced cognitive features (i.e., impaired executive function, memory and concentration problems) and motor disturbances [5, 54, 94]. The most advanced CTE stages are associated with dementia [54, 90, 94].

Most neuropathologically confirmed cases of CTE to date had a history of repeated mild head traumas, with the vast majority coming from contact sports [70, 77]. Omalu et al. [81] studied autopsy brain tissue of 14 professional players of contact sports and 10 (71%) of them were positive for CTE. The biggest case study by Mez et al. [74] examined the brains of 202 players of American football with histories of multiple concussions. The evidence of CTE pathology was found in 87% of these cases. Interestingly, out of 111 former National Football League (NFL) players included in this study, 110 had confirmed CTE pathology. Out of these same 110 confirmed cases, 95 were severe – suggesting a possible link between the disease burden and the highest level of play [74].

There has been increasing awareness that CTE can also be found in people who have never played a contact sport but may have suffered head injuries in other contexts such as the military [62, 70, 83]. The noted neuropsychiatric and behavioral symptoms observed in the military personnel found to have CTE included emotional instability, aggression, irritability, depression, suicidal thoughts, and poor judgment [91].

## Controversies in CTE Autopsy Results

The incidence of CTE among all those having suffered multiple head injuries, in particular those playing contact sports, remains unknown. A very limited number of people involved in contact sports or in the military have been examined postmortem. Many of those examined had significant behavioral/cognitive changes prior to death leading to a biased referral [33, 60]. Although there is a very high number of CTE reported in some cases series [74], this isn't observed by all. Bieniek et al. [9] examined 1721 brains in their brain bank, and in the brains of 66 men with a history of contact sports, only 21 (32%) had tau pathology consistent with CTE. A study by Hazrati et al. [45] examined six brains of former professional football players with a history of multiple concussions and found that dementia symptomatology is not always correlated with a postmortem CTE diagnosis. Many CTE symptoms also closely resemble those of other neurodegenerative conditions – particularly Alzheimer's disease (AD), Parkinson's disease (PD), and frontotemporal dementia [96]. This, and the range of symptoms between patients, poses challenges for diagnosing the clinical correlate of CTE [22, 31, 32].

Currently, multiple concussions are believed to be the only risk factor for CTE, but a recent case report of a single patient with clinical diagnosis of amyotrophic lateral sclerosis (ALS) and no known history of head trauma had CTE-consistent neuropathology upon autopsy. The patient was never involved in contact sports and had no psychiatric symptoms at any point throughout his life [30]. This is the first confirmed case of CTE pathology in someone with no known history of head trauma of any severity. This recent discovery highlights the need for more research in this area. The subjective nature of patient histories, collected from family members or self-reported by patients, remains a limiting factor in CTE research [30, 70, 82].

Despite multiple studies looking into potential in vivo biomarkers of CTE, currently CTE remains a postmortem diagnosis [32]. This is a significant obstacle to better understanding how prevalent CTE is in people who have suffered multiple concussions.

## Neuropsychiatric Symptoms Following Concussion: PCS and CTE

Due to the heterogeneity of symptoms, the absence of a unified PCS diagnosis, and the inability to diagnose CTE during the patient's lifetime, the neuropsychiatric symptoms of PCS and CTE are difficult to characterize with certainty. The neuropsychiatric symptoms of PCS are usually self-reported and the most common include irritability, depression, and anxiety [1, 36]. Less common symptoms include obsessive-compulsive disorder (OCD) [8, 25, 71], mania [55, 93], psychosis [11, 29], and personality disorder [79]. Symptoms associated with CTE, on the other hand, are usually collected from the patient's family after the person's death. Postmortem retrospective review of neuropsychiatric symptoms associated with CTE has shown a variety of neuropsychiatric symptoms including impulsivity, aggression, depression, apathy, anxiety, and suicidal ideation [45, 70, 82]. Depression and anxiety often co-occur in both PCS and CTE cases and are the most common symptoms reported [1]. Until now, suicidal ideation has only been documented in CTE patients; however, the relationship between head trauma and suicidal thoughts is still unknown [50].

## Overview and Rates of Neuropsychiatric Symptoms Following Concussions

Depression appears to be the most well-studied symptom following a sport-related concussion [84]. A cross-sectional study by Guskiewicz et al. [40] reported on 2552 retired professional football players. Out of 884 athletes that self-reported one or two previous concussions, 9.74% had a clinical diagnosis of depression. Of the 595 athletes that reported three or more concussions, 20.17% had a clinical diagnosis of depression. Decq et al. [21] noted a similar frequency with retired players of other sports, where 17 (12.32%) out of 138 players self-reported having depressive episodes. A significant relationship was found between depression and a number of self-reported concussions, regardless of the sport played [21]. The exact rates of symptoms other than depression in concussed patients are not entirely clear. A previous study found that at long-term follow-up, concussed individuals self-report worse anxiety and behavioral dyscontrol [72], and those with three or more concussions are more aggressive and impulsive than their peers with no concussion history [56].

The rates of neuropsychiatric symptoms in patients with postmortem CTE come from retrospective case series. Mez et al. [74] report on the clinical features of 111 autopsy confirmed CTE cases. Out of those, 101 had informant-reported behavioral or mood symptoms. Some of the noted symptoms included impulsivity, depression, anxiety, behavioral dyscontrol (i.e., verbal violence or social inappropriateness), paranoia, suicidality, or mania. The most frequent symptoms were impulsivity, depression, and explosivity which were found in 88 (79%), 64 (58%), and 56 (50%) of 111 cases, respectively. Suicidality was very frequent and was seen in 36 (32%) of 111 patients [74]. In a case series by Hazrati et al. [45], all of the three examined CTE cases showed apathy. Irritation, aggression, and delusions were each present in two out of three cases, while depression and anxiety were each seen in one person. An older paper by Omalu et al. [82]

presented five CTE cases of people who committed suicides and parasuicides. All five exhibited depression, paranoia, aggression, and violent and criminal behaviors.

## Depression

Major depression is the most frequent psychiatric symptom in those with a history of concussion. The studies have shown that at least 60% of patients will meet criteria for a diagnosis of depression at some point following their injury [4, 46, 69]. Guskiewicz et al. [40] report that patients with three or more concussions are three times more likely to be clinically diagnosed with depression than people with no or limited history of concussion. Their findings support previous results that the lifetime prevalence of depression and depressive symptoms significantly correlates with the number of concussions [23]. Many of the psychiatric conditions following TBIs co-occur together, with depression and anxiety showing comorbidity with substance abuse [4].

There has been a long-standing debate whether the depressive symptoms in athletes were present pre-injury or are an emotional reaction to ongoing PCS, rather than resulting from an underlying concussion-related pathology [15]. A number of studies have noted that the diagnostic criteria for depression is quite similar to some of the symptoms observed in PCS, which makes misdiagnosis possible [51, 97]. One study examined the prevalence of post-concussion-like symptoms in patients with depression and found that at least half of all participants met the criteria for PCS diagnosis [51]. Another study by Gunstad and Suhr [39] reported that depressed people without prior head injuries had higher levels of PCS-like symptoms than did controls. The same trend was found for people receiving treatment for either depression or headache with no prior history of TBIs. This suggests possible non-neurological- or non-concussion-related factors contributing to self-reported levels of PCS symptoms. More importantly, these findings raise doubts on the efficacy of self-report measures in the clinical diagnosis of PCS [39]. There is, however, a growing body of research showing a direct relationship between post-concussive brain changes and ensuing depressive symptoms in patients. Chen et al. [15] observed distinct differences including less gray matter volume in the medial frontal and temporal regions and in the rostral anterior cingulate cortex in patients with co-occurring depression symptoms. The rostral anterior cingulate volume was negatively related to severity of depressive state. The concussed athletes from Chen's study were young with no medical history of mood disorders [15]. This corroborates previous findings [64] and makes it less likely that depression was pre-existing in those athletes and more likely was a consequence of head trauma.

## Aggression and Irritability

Posttraumatic irritability and its associated symptoms (i.e., annoyance, impatience) are common during the acute phase of concussion and are seen in response to nearly any stressor but tend to resolve over time. In the cases where symptoms are prolonged enough to obtain a diagnosis of PCS, the irritable behavior persists and is triggered even by trivial causes that are unpredictable in nature [3, 26]. Irritability often co-occurs with aggressive behavior in patients with TBIs of all severities [3]. Previous studies have reported that the anger subsequent to concussions differs from ordinary emotions. Patients with concussions describe their experiences as sudden waves of explosive rage in short outbursts that they are not always able to control. These sudden behavioral and mood changes can be a complete change in personality [27, 48]. The attacks can last anywhere from minutes to hours, followed by remorse. On occasion, the guilt a person experiences is strong enough to result in suicide attempts [59]. Aggression and irritability have been widely documented in PCS patients, as well as patients discovered to have CTE upon death [36, 70, 82]; however, overall rates for these symptoms in people who have been concussed are unknown.

## Suicidal Ideation

Suicidality among former athletes has gained significant media attention in recent years due to a number of high-profile cases. CTE was diagnosed in former athletes who had suffered repetitive concussions and committed suicide; however, no causal relationship between multiple concussions and suicide has yet been established. One case series of postmortem CTE described five cases of former professional contact sport athletes who committed suicides and parasuicides. All five cases were found to have CTE upon autopsy, and all five had neuropsychiatric impairments prior to their death [82]. Unfortunately, the small sample size does not allow for conclusive remarks. One of the limitations of postmortem studies is that patients with significant cognitive, emotional, and behavioral abnormalities are the ones most likely to end up with a brain autopsy. This introduces significant biases into data collection and provides challenges for studying the true incidence of CTE within suicide victims as well as within the population that has suffered recurrent concussions.

Current epidemiological data shows that former NFL players have lower mortality than the general population and specifically lower suicide rates [50, 100]. A systematic review completed by Wortzel et al. [100] examined 85 unique articles related to CTE and suicide. After taking a closer look, only two case studies fit the selection criteria.

Both of the chosen studies had very low quality of evidence and high risk of bias. Iverson [52] elaborates on known risk factors that might play a role in suicide ideation among CTE patients. The number one risk factor for suicide is depression [2]. Chronic pain, which is also common in former NFL players [18, 43], is bidirectionally associated with depression. In other words, people with chronic pain are much more likely to experience depression, and vice versa. Both conditions also have a magnifying effect on each other [12]. It has been reported that people with chronic pain are at an increased risk of suicide ideation [49]. Previous studies have found that the rate of chronic pain and depression is high among former NFL players and that those same players report more life stress and financial difficulties [18, 88]. This means that former players with chronic pain, depression, financial problems, and stressors may be at a higher risk of suicide [52]. In fact, an anonymous survey of 763 retired NFL players reported that most players had difficulty adjusting to life after their NFL career and had financial struggles, among other things [65]. Overall, not enough evidence currently exists to make any conclusive claims about the link between CTE and suicide among athletes, and much more prospective research is needed in this area. Suicides among athletes should be looked at in a broader sense, including evaluation of other risk factors such as lack of meaningful relationships, physical abuse, financial difficulties, and stressful life events [52].

## Pathophysiology of Neuropsychiatric Symptoms Following Concussions

Previous fMRI studies offer a possible explanation for the persistent depressive symptoms following a sport-related concussion [13, 14, 67]. The pathophysiological abnormality within the limbic-frontal system is the proposed neural correlate of depression in concussed patients [67]. Cerebral blood flow and glucose metabolism changes within the frontal and cingulate cortex have been previously established to play a role in major depressive disorder (MDD) [89]. These brain regions are believed to be involved in emotion-processing and cognitive control of affective states, which are dysfunctional in depression [58]. A more recent study examining concussed patients with depressive symptoms reported similar findings, consistent with the limbic-frontal model of depression [15]. Specifically, the severity of depressive symptoms in concussed athletes was correlated with reduced activation in the prefrontal region and the striatum and attenuated deactivation in medial frontal and temporal regions [15]. Previous studies on neurotransmitters involved in depression showed increased levels of serotonin transporter binding in the prefrontal cortex, anterior cingulate cortex, putamen, and thalamus. These changes are believed to be the cause behind dysfunctional attitudes among people with depressive symptoms [73]. Other papers noted a possible causative relationship between altered serotonin, norepinephrine, and dopamine neurotransmitter systems in the brain and MDD [86].

The loss of control associated with emotional (annoyance and irritability) and behavioral (aggression and impulsivity) symptoms in PCS and CTE is believed to arise from frontal lobe damage [98]. In fact, frontal and temporal lobes are particularly vulnerable to damage as a result of mechanical forces during the TBI event [78]. Previous studies using fMRI techniques found significant changes in activation patters of frontal, occipitoparietal, and temporal regions of the brain following a mTBI [38]. Dean et al. [20] in their study on mTBI patients found reduced gray matter volume in frontal and temporal cortices 1 year post-injury. Other studies have also reported correlations between structural damage to frontal and temporal lobes and aggression, violent behavior, and altered decision-making [35, 37, 80]. This collective evidence suggests that concussed patients are more likely to overreact and misperceive stimuli and lack the communication skills to negotiate conflict [98]. The aggression has been previously linked to three major neurotransmitter systems – serotonergic, dopaminergic, and gamma-aminobutyric acidergic (GABAergic). Serotonin is believed to be responsible for inhibition of aggressive behavior. Dopamine and GABA, on the other hand, are related to initiation and appraisal of aggression-related cues, respectively [42, 99].

Not much is known about the neural correlates of suicidal thoughts, but they may result from an association between mood changes due to amygdala pathology and impulsivity due to orbitofrontal pathology [34]. Serotonin transporter genes are believed to be implicated in suicidal behavior; however, results are still inconclusive [28, 57].

## Final Remarks

A substantial number of concussed patients develop persistent somatic, affective, and cognitive symptoms. Although PCS is uncommon after concussion, it represents a significant economic burden on the health-care system [7]. The unemployment rate of PCS patients ranges from 12% at 2 months following injury to 20% at 1 year. Early identification and timely treatment of symptoms associated with PCS would reduce post-mTBI disability and patient morbidity [6]. Research in PCS and CTE is still in its infancy. The heterogeneity of symptoms, inconsistent diagnostic criteria, and lack of a diagnostic biomarker for PCS and in vivo CTE hinder research into the pathophysiology of this syndrome. As well, the relationship between PCS and CTE is unknown. More research is currently needed to examine the relationship between concussions, PCS, and CTE. The scientific community is in dire need of in vivo biomarkers for diagnosing PCS and CTE. The lack of these diagnostic markers impedes research into the pathophysiology as well as treatment of both PCS and CTE.

## References


1. Alexander MP. Mild traumatic brain injury: pathophysiology, natural history, and clinical management. Neurology. 1995;45:1253.
2. American Psychiatric Association. Diagnostic and statistical manual of mental disorders (DSM-5®): American Psychiatric Pub.; 2013.
3. Arciniegas DB, Wortzel HS. Emotional and behavioral dyscontrol after traumatic brain injury. Psychiatric Clin. 2014;37(1):31–53.
4. Ashman TA, Gordon WA, Cantor JB, Hibbard MR. Neurobehavioral consequences of traumatic brain injury. Mt Sinai J Med. 2006;73(7):999–1005.
5. Baugh CM, Robbins CA, Stern RA, McKee AC. Current understanding of chronic traumatic encephalopathy. Curr Treat Options Neurol. 2014;16(9):306.
6. Bazarian JJ, Atabaki S. Predicting postconcussion syndrome after minor traumatic brain injury. Acad Emerg Med. 2001;8(8):788–95.
7. Begaz T, Kyriacou DN, Segal J, Bazarian JJ. Serum biochemical markers for post-concussion syndrome in patients with mild traumatic brain injury. J Neurotrauma. 2006;23(8):1201–10.
8. Berthier ML, Kulisevsky J, Gironell A, López OL. Obsessive-compulsive disorder and traumatic brain injury: behavioral, cognitive, and neuroimaging findings. Cogn Behav Neurol. 2001;14(1):23–31.
9. Bieniek KF, Ross OA, Cormier KA, Walton RL, Soto-Ortolaza A, Johnston AE, DeSaro P, Boylan KB, Graff-Radford NR, Wszolek ZK, Rademakers R. Chronic traumatic encephalopathy pathology in a neurodegenerative disorders brain bank. Acta Neuropathol. 2015;130(6):877–89.
10. Boake C, McCauley SR, Levin HS, Pedroza C, Contant CF, Song JX, Brown SA, Goodman H, Brundage SI, Diaz-Marchan PJ. Diagnostic criteria for postconcussional syndrome after mild to moderate traumatic brain injury. J Neuropsychiatry Clin Neurosci. 2005;17(3):350–6.
11. Buckley P, Stack JP, Madigan C, O'Callaghan E, Larkin C, Redmond O, Ennis JT, Waddington JL. Magnetic resonance imaging of schizophrenia-like psychoses associated with cerebral trauma: clinicopathological correlates. Am J Psychiatry. 1993.
12. Campbell LC, Clauw DJ, Keefe FJ. Persistent pain and depression: a biopsychosocial perspective. Biol Psychiatry. 2003;54(3):399–409.
13. Chen JK, Johnston KM, Collie A, McCrory P, Ptito A. A validation of the post concussion symptom scale in the assessment of complex concussion using cognitive testing and functional MRI. J Neurol Neurosurg Psychiatry. 2007;78(11):1231–8.
14. Chen JK, Johnston KM, Frey S, Petrides M, Worsley K, Ptito A. Functional abnormalities in symptomatic concussed athletes: an fMRI study. NeuroImage. 2004;22(1):68–82.
15. Chen JK, Johnston KM, Petrides M, Ptito A. Neural substrates of symptoms of depression following concussion in male athletes with persisting postconcussion symptoms. Arch Gen Psychiatry. 2008;65(1):81–9.
16. Corsellis JA, Bruton CJ, Freeman-Browne D. The aftermath of boxing1. Psychol Med. 1973;3(3):270–303.
17. Corsellis JA. Boxing and the brain. BMJ Br Med J. 1989;298(6666):105.
18. Cottler LB, Abdallah AB, Cummings SM, Barr J, Banks R, Forchheimer R. Injury, pain, and prescription opioid use among former National Football League (NFL) players. Drug Alcohol Depend. 2011;116(1):188–94.
19. Critchley M. Punch-drunk syndromes: the chronic traumatic encephalopathy of boxers. Hommage a Clovis Vincent. 1949:131–41.
20. Dean PJ, Sato JR, Vieira G, McNamara A, Sterr A. Long-term structural changes after mTBI and their relation to post-concussion symptoms. Brain Inj. 2015;29(10):1211–8.
21. Decq P, Gault N, Blandeau M, Kerdraon T, Berkal M, ElHelou A, Dusfour B, Peyrin JC. Long-term consequences of recurrent sports concussion. Acta Neurochir. 2016;158(2):289–300.
22. DeKosky ST, Blennow K, Ikonomovic MD, Gandy S. Acute and chronic traumatic encephalopathies: pathogenesis and biomarkers. Nat Rev Neurol. 2013;9(4):192–200.
23. Didehbani N, Munro Cullum C, Mansinghani S, Conover H, Hart J. Depressive symptoms and concussions in aging retired NFL players. Arch Clin Neuropsychol. 2013;28(5):418–24.
24. Dikmen SS, Levin HS. Methodological issues in the study of mild head injury. J Head Trauma Rehabil. 1993;8(3):30–7.
25. Drummond LM, Gravestock S. Delayed emergence of obsessive-compulsive neurosis following head injury. Case report and review of its theoretical implications. Br J Psychiatry. 1988;153(6):839–42.
26. Eames PG. Distinguishing the neuropsychiatric, psychiatric, and psychological consequences of acquired brain injury. Neurobehavioural disability and social handicap following traumatic brain injury; 2001. p. 29–45.
27. Elliott FA. Neurological factors in violent behavior (the dyscontrol syndrome). J Am Acad Psychiatry Law Online. 1976;4(4):297–315.
28. Fatemi AB, de Luca V, Kennedy J, Mulsant BH, Lenze E, Reynolds CF. Association of Serotonin Genes with history of suicide attempt in late life depression. Am J Geriatr Psychiatry. 2017;25(3):S116.
29. Fujii DE, Ahmed I. Psychosis secondary to traumatic brain injury. Cogn Behav Neurol. 1996;9(2):133–8.
30. Gao AF, Ramsay D, Twose R, Rogaeva E, Tator C, Hazrati LN. Chronic traumatic encephalopathy-like neuropathological findings without a history of trauma. Int J Pathol Clin Res. 2017;3:050.
31. Gardner RC, Yaffe K. Epidemiology of mild traumatic brain injury and neurodegenerative disease. Mol Cell Neurosc. 2015;66:75–80.
32. Gardner A, Iverson GL, McCrory P. Chronic traumatic encephalopathy in sport: a systematic review. Br J Sports Med. 2014:bjsports-2014.
33. Gardner A, Iverson GL, McCrory P. Chronic traumatic encephalopathy in sport: a systematic review. Br J Sports Med. 2013:bjsports-2013.
34. Gavett BE, Cantu RC, Shenton M, Lin AP, Nowinski CJ, McKee AC, Stern RA. Clinical appraisal of chronic traumatic encephalopathy: current perspectives and future directions. Curr Opin Neurol. 2011;24(6):525–31.
35. Goswami R, Dufort P, Tartaglia MC, Green RE, Crawley A, Tator CH, Wennberg R, Mikulis DJ, Keightley M, Davis KD. Frontotemporal correlates of impulsivity and machine learning in retired professional athletes with a history of multiple concussions. Brain Struct Funct. 2016;221(4):1911–25.
36. Gouvier WD, Cubic B, Jones G, Brantley P, Cutlip Q. Postconcussion symptoms and daily stress in normal and head-injured college populations. Arch Clin Neuropsychol. 1992;7(3):193–211.
37. Grafman J, Schwab K, Warden D, Pridgen A, Brown HR, Salazar AM. Frontal lobe injuries, violence, and aggression a report of the Vietnam head injury study. Neurology. 1996;46(5):1231.

38. Guay JL, Lebretore BM, Main JM, DeFrangesco KE, Taylor JL, Amedoro SM. The era of sport concussion: evolution of knowledge, practice, and the role of psychology. Am Psychol. 2016;71(9):875.
39. Gunstad J, Suhr JA. Cognitive factors in postconcussion syndrome symptom report. Arch Clin Neuropsychol. 2004;19(3):391–405.
40. Guskiewicz KM, Marshall SW, Bailes J, McCrea M, Harding HP, Matthews A, Mihalik JR, Cantu RC. Recurrent concussion and risk of depression in retired professional football players. Med Sci Sports Exerc. 2007;39(6):903.
41. Hadanny A, Efrati S. Treatment of persistent post-concussion syndrome due to mild traumatic brain injury: current status and future directions. Expert Rev Neurother. 2016;16(8):875–87.
42. Hagenbeek FA, Kluft C, Hankemeier T, Bartels M, Draisma HH, Middeldorp CM, Berger R, Noto A, Lussu M, Pool R, Fanos V. Discovery of biochemical biomarkers for aggression: a role for metabolomics in psychiatry. Am J Med Genet B Neuropsychiatr Genet. 2016;171(5):719–32.
43. Halchin LE. Former NFL players: disabilities, benefits, and related issues. Federal Publications. 2008:525.
44. Hall RC, Hall RC, Chapman MJ. Definition, diagnosis, and forensic implications of postconcussional syndrome. Psychosomatics. 2005;46(3):195–202.
45. Hazrati LN, Tartaglia MC, Diamandis P, Davis KD, Green RE, Wennberg R, Wong JC, Ezerins L, Tator CH. Absence of chronic traumatic encephalopathy in retired football players with multiple concussions and neurological symptomatology. Front Hum Neurosci. 2013;7.
46. Hibbard MR, Uysal S, Kepler K, Bogdany J, Silver J. Axis I psychopathology in individuals with traumatic brain injury. J Head Trauma Rehabil. 1998;13(4):24–39.
47. Hof PR, Knabe R, Bovier P, Bouras C. Neuropathological observations in a case of autism presenting with self-injury behavior. Acta Neuropathol. 1991;82(4):321–6.
48. Hooper RS, McGregor JM, Nathan PW. Explosive rage following head injury. Br J Psychiatry. 1945;91(385):458–71.
49. Ilgen MA, Zivin K, McCammon RJ, Valenstein M. Pain and suicidal thoughts, plans and attempts in the United States. Gen Hosp Psychiatry. 2008;30(6):521–7.
50. Iverson GL. Chronic traumatic encephalopathy and risk of suicide in former athletes. Br J Sports Med. 2014;48(2):162–4.
51. Iverson GL. Misdiagnosis of the persistent postconcussion syndrome in patients with depression. Arch Clin Neuropsychol. 2006;21(4):303–10.
52. Iverson GL. Suicide and chronic traumatic encephalopathy. J Neuropsychiatry Clin Neurosci. 2016;28(1):9–16.
53. Jack CR, Knopman DS, Jagust WJ, Petersen RC, Weiner MW, Aisen PS, Shaw LM, Vemuri P, Wiste HJ, Weigand SD, Lesnick TG. Tracking pathophysiological processes in Alzheimer's disease: an updated hypothetical model of dynamic biomarkers. Lancet Neurol. 2013;12(2):207–16.
54. Jordan BD. The clinical spectrum of sport-related traumatic brain injury. Nat Rev Neurol. 2013;9(4):222–30.
55. Jorge RE, Robinson RG, Starkstein SE, Arndt SV, Forrester AW, Geisler FH. Secondary mania following traumatic brain injury. Am J Psychiatry. 1993;150:916.
56. Kerr ZY, Evenson KR, Rosamond WD, Mihalik JP, Guskiewicz KM, Marshall SW. Association between concussion and mental health in former collegiate athletes. Injury Epidemiol. 2014;1(1):28.
57. Lee HY, Hong JP, Hwang JA, Lee HJ, Yoon HK, Lee BH, Kim YK. Possible association between serotonin transporter gene polymorphism and suicide behavior in major depressive disorder. Psychiatry Investig. 2015;12(1):136–41.
58. Liao C, Feng Z, Zhou D, Dai Q, Xie B, Ji B, Wang X. Dysfunction of fronto-limbic brain circuitry in depression. Neuroscience. 2012;201:231–8.
59. Mark VH, Ervin FR. Violence and the brain. Oxford, UK: Harper & Row; 1970.
60. Maroon JC, Winkelman R, Bost J, Amos A, Mathyssek C, Miele V. Chronic traumatic encephalopathy in contact sports: a systematic review of all reported pathological cases. PLoS One. 2015;10(2):e0117338.
61. Martland HS. Punch drunk. J Am Med Assoc. 1928;91(15):1103–7.
62. Matser JT, Kessels AG, Jordan BD, Lezak MD, Troost J. Chronic traumatic brain injury in professional soccer players. Neurology. 1998;51(3):791–6.
63. Mawdsley C, Ferguson FR. Neurological disease in boxers. Lancet. 1963;282(7312):795–801.
64. McAllister TW, Flashman LA, McDonald BC, Saykin AJ. Mechanisms of working memory dysfunction after mild and moderate TBI: evidence from functional MRI and neurogenetics. J Neurotrauma. 2006;23(10):1450–67.
65. McCarthy TC. Life after football. Newsday. http://data.newsday.com/projects/sports/football/life-football/. 2015. Accessed 17 Oct 2017.
66. McCrory P, Meeuwisse W, Dvorak J, Aubry M, Bailes J, Broglio S, Cantu RC, Cassidy D, Echemendia RJ, Castellani RJ, Davis GA. Consensus statement on concussion in sport—the 5th international conference on concussion in sport held in Berlin, October 2016. Br J Sports Med. 2017:bjsports-2017.
67. McCrory P, Meeuwisse W, Johnston K, Dvorak J, Aubry M, Molloy M, Cantu R. Consensus statement on concussion in sport–the 3rd international conference on concussion in sport held in Zurich, November 2008. S Afr J Sports Med. 2009;21(2).
68. McKee AC, Cairns NJ, Dickson DW, Folkerth RD, Keene CD, Litvan I, Perl DP, Stein TD, Vonsattel JP, Stewart W, Tripodis Y. The first NINDS/NIBIB consensus meeting to define neuropathological criteria for the diagnosis of chronic traumatic encephalopathy. Acta Neuropathol. 2016;131(1):75–86.
69. McKee AC, Cantu RC, Nowinski CJ, Hedley-Whyte ET, Gavett BE, Budson AE, Santini VE, Lee HS, Kubilus CA, Stern RA. Chronic traumatic encephalopathy in athletes: progressive tauopathy after repetitive head injury. J Neuropathol Exp Neurol. 2009;68(7):709–35.
70. McKee AC, Stein TD, Nowinski CJ, Stern RA, Daneshvar DH, Alvarez VE, Lee HS, Hall G, Wojtowicz SM, Baugh CM, Riley DO. The spectrum of disease in chronic traumatic encephalopathy. Brain. 2012;136(1):43–64.
71. McKeon JO, McGuffin P, Robinson P. Obsessive-compulsive neurosis following head injury. A report of four cases. Br J Psychiatry. 1984;144(2):190–2.
72. Meehan WP III, Taylor AM, Berkner P, Sandstrom NJ, Peluso MW, Kurtz MM, Pascual-Leone A, Mannix R. Division III collision sports are not associated with neurobehavioral quality of life. J Neurotrauma. 2016;33(2):254–9.
73. Meyer JH. Imaging the serotonin transporter during major depressive disorder and antidepressant treatment. J Psychiatry Neurosci. 2007;32(2):86.
74. Mez J, Daneshvar DH, Kiernan PT, Abdolmohammadi B, Alvarez VE, Huber BR, Alosco ML, Solomon TM, Nowinski CJ, McHale L, Cormier KA. Clinicopathological evaluation of chronic traumatic encephalopathy in players of American football. JAMA. 2017;318(4):360–70.
75. Miller H. Mental after-effects of head injury. J R Soc Med. 1966;59(3):257–61.
76. Millspaugh JA. Dementia pugilistica. US Naval Med Bull. 1937;35(297):e303.

77. Montenigro PH, Stein TD, Cantu RC, Stern RA. Chronic traumatic encephalopathy: historical origins and current perspective. Annu Rev Clin Psychol. 2015;11:309.
78. Moy S. Concussion in athletes: from pathophysiology to current guidelines and recommendations. Osteopathic Family Physician. 2013.
79. Oder W, Goldenberg G, Spatt J, Podreka I, Binder H, Deecke L. Behavioural and psychosocial sequelae of severe closed head injury and regional cerebral blood flow: a SPECT study. J Neurol Neurosurg Psychiatry. 1992;55(6):475–80.
80. Okuda J, Fujii T, Ohtake H, Tsukiura T, Tanji K, Suzuki K, Kawashima R, Fukuda H, Itoh M, Yamadori A. Thinking of the future and past: the roles of the frontal pole and the medial temporal lobes. NeuroImage. 2003;19(4):1369–80.
81. Omalu B, Bailes J, Hamilton RL, Kamboh MI, Hammers J, Case M, Fitzsimmons R. Emerging histomorphologic phenotypes of chronic traumatic encephalopathy in American athletes. Neurosurgery. 2011;69(1):173–83.
82. Omalu BI, Bailes J, Hammers JL, Fitzsimmons RP. Chronic traumatic encephalopathy, suicides and parasuicides in professional American athletes: the role of the forensic pathologist. Am J Forensic Med Pathol. 2010;31(2):130–2.
83. Omalu BI, DeKosky ST, Minster RL, Kamboh MI, Hamilton RL, Wecht CH. Chronic traumatic encephalopathy in a National Football League player. Neurosurgery. 2005;57(1):128–34.
84. Rice SM, Parker AG, Rosenbaum S, Bailey A, Mawren D, Purcell R. Sport-related concussion and mental health outcomes in elite athletes: a systematic review. Sports Med. 2017:1–9.
85. Roberts AH. Brain damage in boxers: a study of the prevalence of traumatic encephalopathy among ex-professional boxers. Pitman Medical & Scientific Publishing Co. Ltd.; 1969.
86. Ruhe HG, Mason NS, Schene AH. Mood is directly related to serotonin, norepinephrine and dopamine levels in humans: a meta-analysis of monoamine depletion studies. Mol Psychiatry. 2007;12(4):331–59.
87. Ryan LM, Warden DL. Post concussion syndrome. Int Rev Psychiatry. 2003;15(4):310–6.
88. Schwenk TL, Gorenflo DW, Dopp RR, Hipple E. Depression and pain in retired professional football players. Med Sci Sports Exerc. 2007;39(4):599–605.
89. Seminowicz DA, Mayberg HS, McIntosh AR, Goldapple K, Kennedy S, Segal Z, Rafi-Tari S. Limbic–frontal circuitry in major depression: a path modeling metanalysis. NeuroImage. 2004;22(1):409–18.
90. Shively S, Scher AI, Perl DP, Diaz-Arrastia R. Dementia resulting from traumatic brain injury: what is the pathology? Arch Neurol. 2012;69(10):1245–51.
91. Smith DH, Johnson VE, Stewart W. Chronic neuropathologies of single and repetitive TBI: substrates of dementia? Nat Rev Neurol. 2013;9(4):211–21.
92. Smith-Seemiller L, Fow NR, Kant R, Franzen MD. Presence of post-concussion syndrome symptoms in patients with chronic pain vs mild traumatic brain injury. Brain Inj. 2003;17(3):199–206.
93. Starkstein SE, Mayberg HS, Berthier ML, Fedoroff P, Price TR, Dannals RF, Wagner HN, Leiguarda R, Robinson RG. Mania after brain injury: neuroradiological and metabolic findings. Ann Neurol. 1990;27(6):652–9.
94. Stern RA, Daneshvar DH, Baugh CM, Seichepine DR, Montenigro PH, Riley DO, Fritts NG, Stamm JM, Robbins CA, McHale L, Simkin I. Clinical presentation of chronic traumatic encephalopathy. Neurology. 2013;81(13):1122–9.
95. Stern RA, Riley DO, Daneshvar DH, Nowinski CJ, Cantu RC, McKee AC. Long-term consequences of repetitive brain trauma: chronic traumatic encephalopathy. PM&R. 2011;3(10):S460–7.
96. Tartaglia MC, Hazrati LN, Davis KD, Green RE, Wennberg R, Mikulis D, Ezerins LJ, Keightley M, Tator C. Chronic traumatic encephalopathy and other neurodegenerative proteinopathies. Front Hum Neurosci. 2014;8:30.
97. Trahan DE, Ross CE, Trahan SL. Relationships among postconcussional-type symptoms, depression, and anxiety in neurologically normal young adults and victims of mild brain injury. Arch Clin Neuropsychol. 2001;16(5):435–45.
98. Turkstra L, Jones D, Toler HL. Brain injury and violent crime. Brain Inj. 2003;17(1):39–47.
99. Willner P. The neurobiology of aggression: implications for the pharmacotherapy of aggressive challenging behaviour by people with intellectual disabilities. J Intellect Disabil Res. 2015;59(1):82–92.
100. Wortzel HS, Shura RD, Brenner LA. Chronic traumatic encephalopathy and suicide: a systematic review. Biomed Res Int. 2013;2013:1.

# Functional Neuroimage

# 13

Celi Santos Andrade, Leandro Tavares Lucato,
Carlos Alberto Buchpiguel, and Claudia da Costa Leite

## Abbreviations

| | |
|---|---|
| $^{1}$H-MRS | Proton magnetic resonance spectroscopy |
| AD | Axial diffusivity |
| ASL | Arterial spin labeling |
| BIAA | Brain Injury Association of America |
| BOLD | Blood-oxygen-level-dependent |
| CBF | Cerebral blood flow |
| CBV | Cerebral blood volume |
| Cho | Choline |
| Cr | Creatine |
| CT | Computed tomography |
| CTE | Chronic traumatic encephalopathy |
| DAI | Diffuse axonal injury |
| DSC | Dynamic susceptibility contrast imaging |
| DTI | Diffusion tensor imaging |
| FA | Fractional anisotropy (FA) |
| FDG | [18F]fluorodeoxyglucose |
| FLAIR | Fluid-attenuated inversion recovery |
| fMRI | Functional MRI |
| GCS | Glasgow coma scale |
| GLx | Glutamate/glutamine |
| Ins | Myoinositol |
| Lac | Lactate |
| MD | Mean diffusivity |
| MRI | Magnetic resonance imaging |
| MTT | Mean transit time |
| NAA | N-acetyl aspartate |
| PET | Positron-emission tomography |
| PIB | 11C-Pittsburgh compound B |
| rCBV | Regional cerebral blood flow |
| RD | Radial diffusivity |
| ROI | Region of interest |
| RS-fMRI | Resting-state fMRI |
| SPECT | Single photon emission computed tomography |
| SWI | Susceptibility-weighted imaging |
| T2*-GRE | T2*-weighted gradient-recalled echo |
| TBI | Traumatic brain injury |
| TBSS | Tract-based spatial statistics |
| WM | White matter |

C. S. Andrade · C. A. Buchpiguel
Department of Radiology and Oncology, School of Medicine – University of São Paulo, São Paulo, Brazil

L. T. Lucato · C. da Costa Leite (✉)
Department of Radiology and Oncology, School of Medicine – University of São Paulo, São Paulo, Brazil

LIM 44-Laboratory of Magnetic Resonance Imaging in Neuroradiology, São Paulo, Brazil
e-mail: claudia.leite@hc.fm.usp.br

## Introduction

Traumatic brain injury (TBI) remains an important cause of morbidity and mortality and is a major public health problem worldwide [1, 2]. Survivors may present with severe disability and commonly have persistent deficits in cognition, behavior, and executive functions [3–6].

Under this wide nomenclature, TBI comprises a large range of distinct clinical conditions and pathological findings. The Glasgow Coma Scale (GCS) assesses the level of consciousness after TBI, and it has been historically used as the primary clinical parameter for estimating the severity and prognosis of trauma. Patients are typically classified into the broad categories of mild, moderate, and severe injury. There are several limitations of this scoring categorization, such as the elapsed time from injury, use of drugs and toxic substances, and hemodynamic parameters [7, 8]. Furthermore, this classification system does not give any clue about the pathophysiologic mechanisms or the anatomic features underlying the neurological deficits.

For instance, a patient with severe TBI may present with several distinct or concurrent pathologic features, such as extra-axial hematomas (epidural and subdural hematomas), subarachnoid and intraventricular hemorrhages, brain contusions and lacerations, diffuse swelling, herniations, and



R. Anghinah et al. (eds.), *Topics in Cognitive Rehabilitation in the TBI Post-Hospital Phase*,
https://doi.org/10.1007/978-3-319-95376-2_13

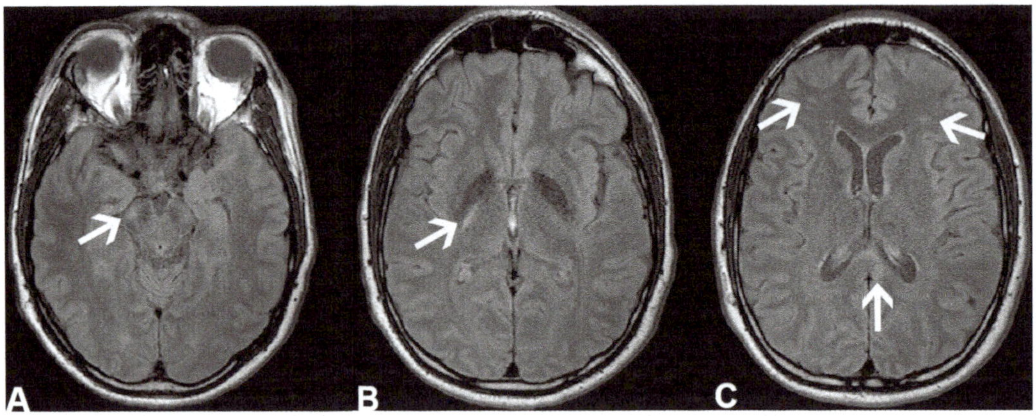


**Fig. 13.1** A 27-year-old male patient with moderate TBI due to a motorcycle accident. Axial FLAIR images show hyperintense lesions (arrows) in the lateral aspect of the right cerebral peduncle (**a**), right internal capsule (**b**), and splenium of the corpus callosum, as well as subtle lesions in the subcortical bilateral frontal white matter (**c**)

diffuse axonal injury [8]. In this setting, neuroimaging tools play an important role to help differentiate the multiple types of brain injury and give further information to assist in the clinical management and follow-up of patients.

In the acute setting of trauma, especially at higher levels of injury severity, patients are usually initially scanned with computed tomography (CT). CT guides decision-making process during the acute phase by showing hemorrhagic lesions, mass effect, brain swelling, midline shifts, brain herniation, ventricular distortion, skull fractures, displaced bone fragments, and intracranial air [9]. CT is widely available and highly reliable and is a low-cost imaging method. On the other hand, one major concern related to CT overuse is radiation exposure. Moreover, CT scans may depict only minor lesions or even no lesions in some unconscious patients despite the severity of the clinical picture [10, 11]. In such cases, diffuse axonal injury (DAI) may be suspected, especially if there is no history of drug abuse and if other conditions like hypoxia and hypotension are ruled out.

DAI typically occurs during high-speed trauma that generates rotational, acceleration, and deceleration forces, with ultimate shear injuries in the cortico-subcortical interfaces. The axons are torn or stretched, thus impairing axoplasmic transport and the electrical neural network [12–14]. As the intensity of the DAI increases, deeper areas of the brain are involved in a sort of centripetal progression: in milder cases, the gray-white matter interfaces are affected, and then the corpus callosum and finally the brain stem may be injured in more severe cases [10, 15].

Therefore, many advocate magnetic resonance imaging (MRI) as the preferable imaging modality in the evaluation of patients with TBI. Multiplanar T1-weighted images provide excellent resolution of the more striking anatomic findings, such as mass effect, midline shift, and ventricular distortion. The addition of gadolinium-based contrast offers no significant advantage for lesion detection or characterization in patients with head injury. In the spectrum of DAI, fluid-attenuated inversion recovery (FLAIR) and T2 sequences are sensitive for non-hemorrhagic lesions (Fig. 13.1). T2*-weighted gradient-recalled echo (T2*-GRE) and susceptibility-weighted imaging (SWI) are more sensitive sequences for blood product detection [8, 11].

Still, CT and conventional MRI may underestimate the extent of DAI and poorly correlate with long-term outcomes. Some patients present progressive cerebral atrophy and persistent cognitive deficits despite the fact that initial imaging failed to show gross pathology or exhibited only discrete findings [16, 17]. Consequently, there is considerable interest in developing more sensitive diagnostic tools. Further advances in neuroimaging may help to elucidate the underlying pathological mechanisms and the natural history of TBI. Modern imaging techniques, including MRI advanced sequences as well as nuclear medicine tests, may ultimately improve the prognosis of TBI patients by helping to select patients most likely to benefit from targeted treatments.

Following this short introduction, we aim to highlight the state of the art of some modern functional imaging techniques in the context of TBI. However, we anticipate that no single imaging technique alone is superior over others, as the neuropathologic consequences after head injury vary in etiology, and each method has its intrinsic advantages and limitations. We briefly review some basic technical concepts of each technique, and then we address its current specific contributions in clinical practice or research scenarios related to TBI.

## T2*-Weighted Gradient-Recalled Echo and Susceptibility-Weighted Imaging

The hemorrhagic lesions of TBI are specially conspicuous in MR sequences sensitive to the susceptibility artifacts derived from blood products, namely, T2*-GRE and SWI. The T2*-GRE sequence has been reported to be more sensitive than T2-weighted spin-echo sequence (Fig. 13.2) to the magnetic susceptibility induced by static field inhomogeneities arising from paramagnetic blood breakdown products, such as deoxyhemoglobin, methemoglobin, and hemosiderin [18]. Fazekas et al. [19] demonstrated that focal areas of signal intensity loss on T2*-GRE correspond histopathologically to areas with previous extravasation of blood, in the absence of other possibly related morphologically abnormalities, such as focal calcifications or small vascular malformations.

Interestingly, one study demonstrated that the number of lesions detected by T2*-GRE correlated with the degree of intracranial hypertension and outcome in DAI [20]. It has been demonstrated that 3 Tesla MRI examination using standard GRE sequences is twice as sensitive as 1.5 Tesla MRI in terms of lesion number and volume in patients with DAI [21].

SWI is even more sensitive to hemosiderin deposition and is superior to conventional MRI for detecting microbleeds after TBI (Fig. 13.2). More microhemorrhages were detected in amateur boxes with SWI in comparison with T2 fast spin-echo or T2*-GRE sequences [22].

SWI is best obtained at higher field strengths and is also very sensitive for hemorrhagic lesions in the brain stem and cerebellum [11, 23]. The SWI method has higher spatial resolution as it uses a tridimensional gradient-echo technique, with thin slices and flow compensation. It plays an important role to categorize clinical injury severity and to predict long-term neurocognitive outcomes [23–25].

A work demonstrated the prognostic use of regional SWI-lesion quantification with regard to neuropsychological outcomes at 6 months to 1 year following pediatric head injury [26].

## Diffusion-Weighted Imaging and Diffusion Tensor Imaging

The water molecules tend to move freely and randomly in homogeneous solutions, a phenomenon known as the Brownian movement. The probability of water diffusion in these solutions is the same in all directions, the so-called isotropic diffusion [27]. In the brain, several components hinder the water diffusion in all directions, making the diffusion anisotropic. This anisotropic diffusion depends on the geometry and composition of natural barriers, such as neurofilaments, microtubules, and axonal membranes, and especially due to myelin, which is abundant in the brain white matter (WM) [28].

Increases in water concentration in the brain tissues (such as observed in vasogenic edema or gliosis) cause nonspecific hyperintensity on FLAIR and other T2-weighted images, but the abnormal cellular uptake of water (cytotoxic edema) or restricted water between myelin membranes (intramyelinic edema) reduces its molecular diffusion, showing high signal intensity on diffusion-weighted imaging (DWI) with decreased apparent diffusion coefficient (ADC) [29].

In the acute setting of TBI, it is possible to detect multifocal areas with restricted diffusion, which appear bright on DWI and dark on ADC maps (Fig. 13.3) [11]. This is com-

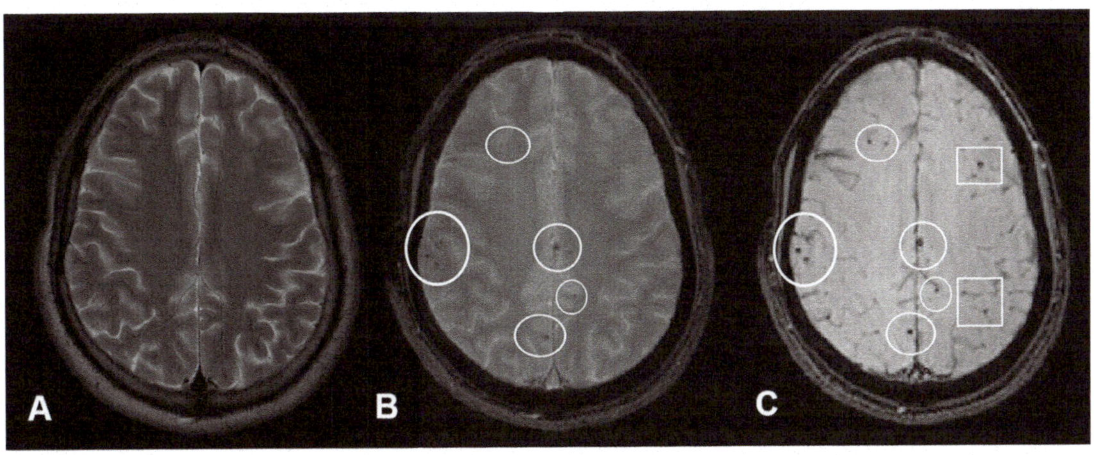


**Fig. 13.2** A 19-year-old male patient with DAI and GCS of 8 after a motorcycle accident. While T2 conventional sequences (**a**) are rather insensitive for hemorrhagic lesions, T2*-GRE (**b**) shows numerous foci of signal loss (circles) in the subcortical white matter corresponding to areas of extravascular blood. SWI (**c**) is even more sensitive than the previous two sequences, exhibiting more conspicuous (circles) and numerous lesions (squares) on both cerebral hemispheres. The images were performed sequentially during the same examination at a 3 Tesla scanner

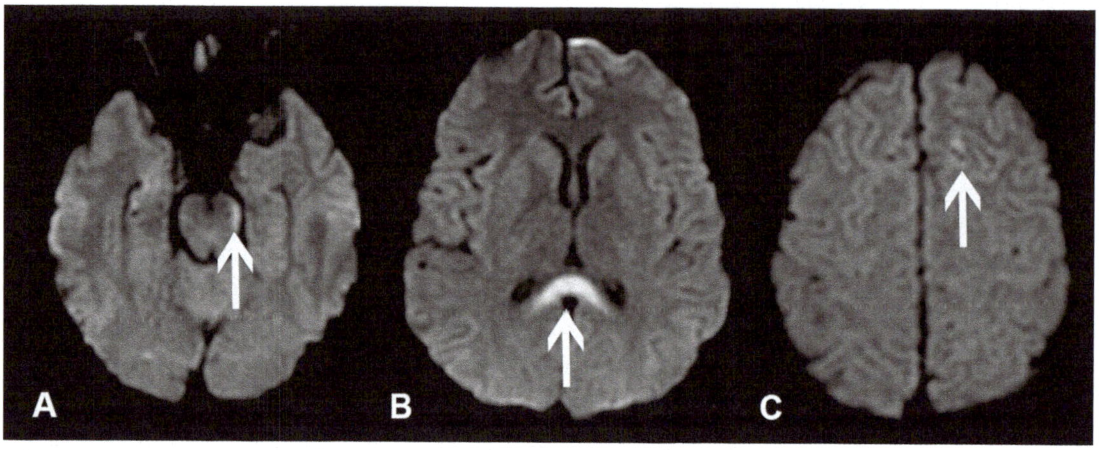


**Fig. 13.3** Diffusion-weighted images in the axial plane of a young patient 4 days after a head trauma demonstrate bright lesions (arrows) in areas typically affected in DAI: left cerebral peduncle (**a**), splenium of the corpus callosum (**b**), and subcortical frontal white matter (**c**). The lesions were dark on ADC maps (not shown)

mon in DAI, as pathological studies show axonal swelling and stretching, impaired axoplasmic flow, cytoskeletal disruption, and accumulation of structural protein fragments and organelles [11–15]. This restricted water diffusion may vanish in a few days or may evolve into residual lesions with persistent high signal intensity on FLAIR and T2-weighted images [11].

The diffusion tensor imaging (DTI) takes advantage of the intrinsic property of anisotropic diffusion of water molecules in neural tissues to estimate the structural organization and integrity of the brain. If at least six diffusion-encoded image sets are acquired along noncollinear directions, the diffusion tensor can be calculated [30]. The fractional anisotropy (FA) represents the degree of anisotropy, or strength of diffusion direction, and is notably high (close to 1) in the normal WM, but it is usually lower in the damaged white matter and close to zero in the cerebrospinal fluid. The mean diffusivity (MD) reflects the overall degree of water diffusion in all directions, regardless its orientation dependence. Other DTI-derived indices are radial (RD) and axial diffusivities (AD), which represent diffusion perpendicular and parallel to the diffusion's tensor principal direction. Studies with animal models suggest that while the RD correlates with demyelination, the AD seems to be associated with more profound tissue damage and axonal loss [31, 32]. The combined quantification of such DTI metrics is recommended to better understand any putative changes in brain structural integrity.

These information can be represented graphically as cross-sectional images, such as FA colormaps, in which each color represents the main direction of WM tracts (conventionally, red is used for left-right, green for anteroposterior, and blue for superior-inferior directions), and the degree of brightness is proportional to the anisotropy [30].

There are several distinct approaches to analyze DTI datasets. The most straightforward and practical one is the analysis of region of interest (ROI). However, some shortcomings of the ROI technique are that placement of ROIs is user dependent and it yields examination of only a limited part of the cerebral structure or WM tract. Tractography overcomes some of these limitations and can be acquired through semiautomatic or automatic processing, based on a priori knowledge or anatomical atlas. Because WM tracts are linked to specific cognitive, motor, or behavioral functions, this technique is of particular interest in clinical or research studies (Fig. 13.4). Still, tractography may be limited by the inability to deal with the presence of crossing or fanning fibers and also to differentiate afferent from efferent fibers [27, 30, 33].

Voxel-wise approaches, such as tract-based spatial statistics (TBSS), offer operator-independent global analyses of brain parenchyma and are particularly useful for group comparisons. The voxel-wise approach may be problematic, however, because it may be prone to multiple comparison errors. It also requires smoothing, alignment, and registrations of brain volumes to a common space with its inherent imprecisions [34].

The advent of DTI favored a wide window of opportunities for the noninvasive study of the brain in several physiologic and pathologic conditions. It is also possible to investigate the natural history of diseases, biomarkers of severity and prognosis, and the effect of treatment [35, 36].

One study revealed that, despite normal CT imaging and GCS of 15, adolescents with mild TBI were found to have altered FA, ADC, and RD values in the corpus callosum within 6 days after injury [37]. Other works indicated that the presence of WM changes (as detected with ROI analyses

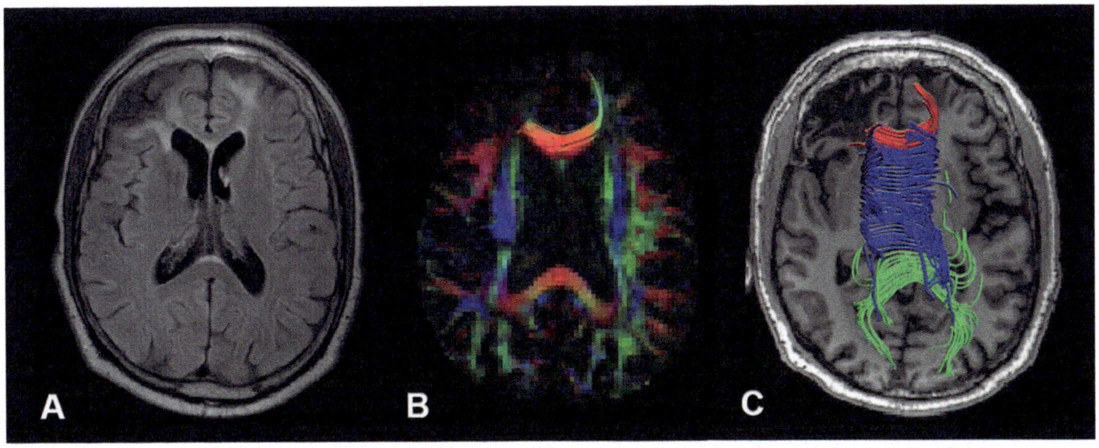


**Fig. 13.4** Axial FLAIR image (**a**) of an adult male patient with chronic post-traumatic sequelae shows gliosis in the frontal lobes, mainly in the right side. (**b**) FA colormap demonstrates paucity of WM fibers and reduction of brightness due to reduction of FA values in the frontal lobes, more pronounced in the right side. (**c**) DTI-based tractography of the splenium, body, and genu of the corpus callosum (represented in green, blue, and red colors, respectively) shows premature termination of streamlines of peripheral fibers of the genu projecting to or from the prefrontal regions coincidental to the areas of low signal intensity on the axial T1-weighted image

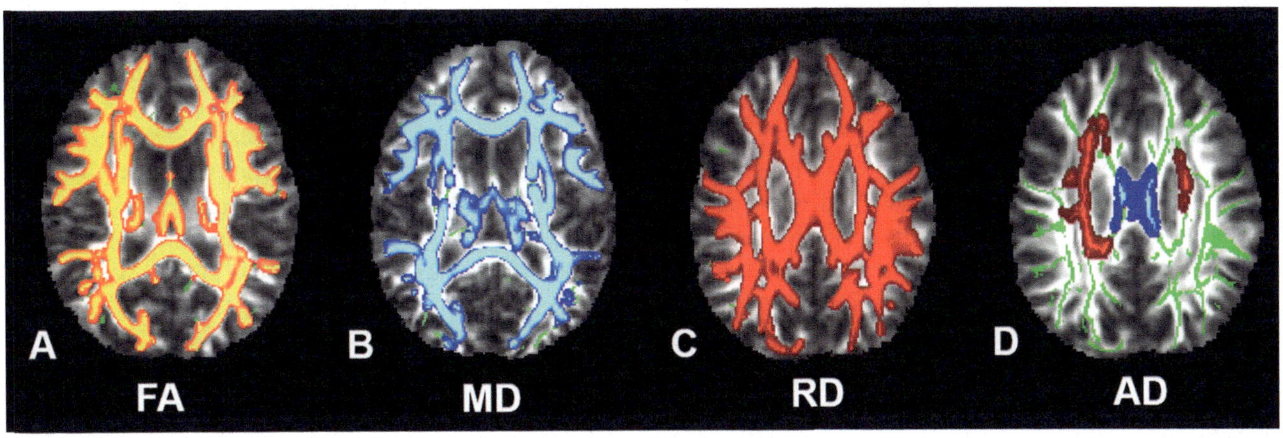


**Fig. 13.5** A study comparison with tract-based spatial statistics (TBSS) between 20 healthy controls and 20 patients with moderate to severe TBI 1 month after the event. Patients exhibited one large cluster with statistically significant lower FA values (**a**). TBI patients also demonstrated significant increases in MD (**b**) and RD (**c**) in extensive areas of the brain, as well as increased AD in a less extensive area (shown in red), except for the corpus callosum that showed increased AD (depicted in blue) (**d**). All comparisons were statistically significant ($p < 0.001$) with threshold-free cluster enhancement in the colored areas in each figure

in several brain areas and tractography) during the early stage of DAI predicts long-term cognitive impairments [38, 39]. Some authors demonstrated that DTI shows WM changes on a spectrum, from mild to severe TBI, and that greater WM pathology predicted greater cognitive deficits in chronic head injury survivors [40–42].

Twenty adults with moderate to severe TBI were evaluated with a 3.0 T MRI in the acute ($t_1 < 3$ months), subacute ($6 < t_2 < 9$ months), and chronic stages ($12 < t_3 < 15$ months) following trauma. By using TBSS analysis, patients exhibited one large cluster with statistically significant lower FA values ($p < 0.001$) at all times ($t_1$, $t_2$, $t_3$) in comparison to controls, but the number of affected voxels decreased over time by 2% at $t_2$ and by 7.3% at $t_3$. The results from group comparisons in the acute phase of all DTI scalar indices are shown in Fig. 13.5. At the chronic stage ($t_3$), patients recovered from WM damage in comparison with the acute stage ($t_1$) with significant increases of FA in the bilateral anterior thalamic radiations, forceps major and minor, corticospinal tracts, cingulum, uncinate, inferior fronto-occipital, and superior and inferior longitudinal fasciculi. Patients' performances on cognitive measures were suboptimal in all three stages but also improved over time in the same fashion as WM recovery [43].

## Functional Magnetic Resonance Imaging

Functional MRI (fMRI) is an advanced technique used to noninvasively assess brain function. Neuronal function is inferred from a blood-oxygen-level-dependent (BOLD) signal that reflects magnetic field inhomogeneity brought about by changes in the state of oxygenation of hemoglobin. This molecule has distinct magnetic properties depending on the concentration of oxygen: oxyhemoglobin behaves as a diamagnetic substance, while removal of some oxygen atoms makes deoxyhemoglobin to become paramagnetic. Within any particular brain volume, the proportion between these two molecules determines how the MR signal will behave in a BOLD image: areas with high concentration of oxyhemoglobin give a higher signal than areas with low concentration. As neuronal activity increases, cerebral blood flow overcompensates such that blood oxygenation actually increases, thereby causing an increase in BOLD signal [44, 45]. Higher field strengths are also generally preferred for fMRI [11].

On task-based fMRI, the images are usually acquired while the patient performs a neurocognitive, behavioral, or motor task (or, in this context, a paradigm) to probe one specific brain function, and differences in local perfusion are measured in real time [11]. In turn, the resting-state fMRI (RS-fMRI) analyzes BOLD fluctuations without imposing an external task by using data-driven types of analysis techniques, such as the independent component analysis (ICA), which decompose the functional MR datasets into spatial patterns with temporal correspondence. The resting-state networks are remarkably consistent across subjects and time. RS-fMRI can be performed in patients incapable of performing specific tasks (such as individuals with reduced consciousness or severely injured), and this is not limited to just one specific domain and its related networks [46, 47].

Although still scant in literature, there is growing evidence that fMRI is sensitive to brain function following TBI and holds promise for understanding its pathophysiology and investigating mechanisms of function recovery [48]. One study using RS-fMRI showed that whole-brain connectivity is altered early (within 1 month) after mild TBI, suggesting that abnormalities in functional networks underlie the cognitive deficits and post-concussive complaints reported by patients with TBI, such as headache, sonophobia, photophobia, and excessive fatigue [49].

A work that evaluated 24 patients with mild TBI and 17 healthy controls revealed abnormal thalamic resting-state networks that point to subtle thalamic injury and abnormal thalamocortical connectivity that may help to explain the complex persistent post-concussive syndrome in head injury survivors [50].

## Perfusion Magnetic Resonance Imaging

Perfusion MRI may be acquired with distinct types of specialized MR acquisition techniques: dynamic susceptibility contrast imaging (DSC) and arterial spin labeling (ASL) [51]. The former uses the passage of intravenous gadolinium-based contrast to extract information on time to peak, mean transit time (MTT), cerebral blood flow (CBF), and cerebral blood volume (CBV). DSC studies in TBI are limited and indicate a rapid decrease in CBF early after the insult in experimental models [52]. One study showed reduced CBV both in normal-appearing and contused brain in patients with TBI and that regional hypoperfusion correlated with a worse clinical outcome [53].

ASL is a quantitative MR-based method, which provides regional and global CBF measurements without exogenous contrast. It uses an endogenous contrast mechanism in which blood cells flowing into the brain are labeled by the MR signal, making this technique completely noninvasive and repeatable [54, 55]. ASL demonstrated decrease of thalamic CBF in patients with mild TBI, and the degree of this hemodynamic impairment correlated with neurocognitive dysfunction during the extended course of the disease, in several domains including processing and response speed, verbal fluency, and executive function [56].

Another ASL study quantified the CBF in 27 individuals with moderate to severe TBI in the chronic stage and in 22 matched healthy controls. The authors found global CBF reductions in the TBI subjects, as well as more prominent regional hypoperfusion in the posterior cingulate cortices, the thalami, and multiple locations in the frontal cortices [57].

## Proton Magnetic Resonance Spectroscopy

Proton magnetic resonance spectroscopy ($^1$H-MRS) noninvasively probes the molecular content in brain parenchyma. Protons are ubiquitously present in metabolites within neural tissues, and resonate at slightly different frequencies based on their chemical environment, resulting in characteristic spectra for distinct compounds. Typical spectra allow identification of N-acetyl aspartate (NAA), creatine (Cr), choline (Cho), glutamate/glutamine (GLx), lactate (Lac), and myo-inositol (Ins) [58].

In short, NAA is synthesized in the mitochondria and is a marker of neuronal integrity, Cr is involved in cellular energy metabolism and is assumed to be nearly constant, Cho is a marker of membrane turnover, Glx are excitatory neurotransmitters, Lac is a marker of anaerobic metabolism (and so on may reflect ischemia and hypoxia), and GLx are excitatory neurotransmitters [58]. $^{1}$H-MRS thus provides a metabolic profile complementary to structural information obtained with conventional MRI. It has found wide clinical use, aiding in diagnosis and treatment monitoring in a variety of diseases [59]. It is a particularly useful tool for repeated research studies in survivors of TBI.

A large body of evidence indicates that NAA levels and NAA/creatine ratios are consistently decreased in TBI, including otherwise normal-appearing brain parenchyma. Moreover, reduced NAA/creatine ratios are predictive of functional outcomes following head injury [60–63]. One study evaluating brain-injured comatose patients demonstrated that combined reductions in FA and in NAA/creatine ratio clearly differentiated patients with an unfavorable outcome from those with a better prognosis and from control groups. The sensitivity and specificity of DTI and MRS together were higher than that with either method alone [64].

## Functional and Molecular Neuroimaging

Recently, a new definition of TBI has been proposed by the Brain Injury Association of America (BIAA): "TBI is defined as an alteration in brain function, or other evidence of brain pathology, caused by an external force" [65]. Therefore, it is presumed that functional neuroimaging methods and even molecular imaging tools would add a significant incremental diagnostic value in addition to the information provided by the functional and conventional MRI sequences, described in the previous sections in this chapter.

In this section we divided the pure functional neuroimaging tests in conventional nuclear SPECT scan and positron-emission tomography (PET) scan. The first is considered a wider available technique, considering the lower costs of instruments and the higher availability of laboratories and radiopharmaceuticals commonly used in this technique. However, PET-CT technology bears higher sensitivity and molecular flexibility, although it is considered a more expensive and consequently a lesser available technique, since it requires a cyclotron installed close or nearby the laboratory.

SPECT imaging explores the determination of regional cerebral blood flow (rCBF), either by qualitative or even by semiquantitative analysis. The use of lipophilic probes labeled preferentially with technetium-99 m (HMPAO or ECD) allows visualizing the gray matter according to the rCBF pattern, with decreasing levels from gray matter to the white matter regions [66]. The information obtained reflects the functional status of the brain at the moment of the intravenous injection of the radiotracer, and this brings many advantages while considering acute neurological injuries.

The exact mechanisms under the cognitive impairment caused by TBI are not yet fully understood considering the level of evidence in the literature. The use of brain SPECT has been investigated by different groups, with a variety of functional results reported. A recent systematic review done by Raji et al. (2014) evaluated 19 longitudinal and 52 cross-sectional studies meeting inclusion criteria. Three longitudinal studies investigated the diagnostic predictive value and showed the increased predictive value shortly after the injury (59%) to 1 year after the trauma (95%). The studies showed localization of brain defects not detected by CT or even MRI, even in the mild and chronic TBI. The most common regions detected by SPECT are in the frontal (94%) and temporal (77%) lobes. Therefore this systematic review can be considered a level IIa class of evidence regarding the clinical value of brain SPECT in traumatic brain injury [67]. Other studies have evaluated the clinical value of SPECT in predicting the cognitive performance after mild TBI. By applying a battery of cognitive tests, it was possible to show that perfusion status in frontal regions was capable to predict poorer performance in the Stroop test (executive function) [68]. However, one strong limitation is that abnormalities seen on SPECT in patients with TBI not always reflect effects of the trauma itself, since those findings are far from specific. A normal study also does not exclude the functional impairment caused by TBI [69]. An example of functional finding in a patient that suffered TBI is shown in the Fig. 13.6.

Other modality is the positron-emission tomography (PET) that provides higher-resolution images compared to SPECT. Normally the hybrid scanners are equipped with computerized tomography or magnetic resonance imaging (PET-CT or PET-MR). PET uses short-lived radioisotopes such as fluoride-18, carbon-11, nitrogen-13, and oxygen-15. In order to obtain these radioisotopes, a cyclotron has to be installed close or nearby a hospital or laboratory, especially when molecular probes labeled with carbon-11 and oxygen-15 are used to test the cerebral functionality. This is one of the reasons that PET technology is less available compared to SPECT.

The most common and highly available molecular probe is the [18F]fluorodeoxyglucose (FDG) that measures the cerebral metabolic glucose rate either regionally or globally. FDG-PET has been investigated in mild, moderate, and severe TBI, either in experimental small animal models or in humans. Selwyn et al. by comparing sham-injured and naïve controls with brain-injured rats were capable of identifying deficits in regional cerebral glucose metabolism related to the induced mild TBI as early as 3–5 days after the injury [70]. Figure 13.7 shows an example of FDG-PET finding in a patient that suffered a vehicle accident.

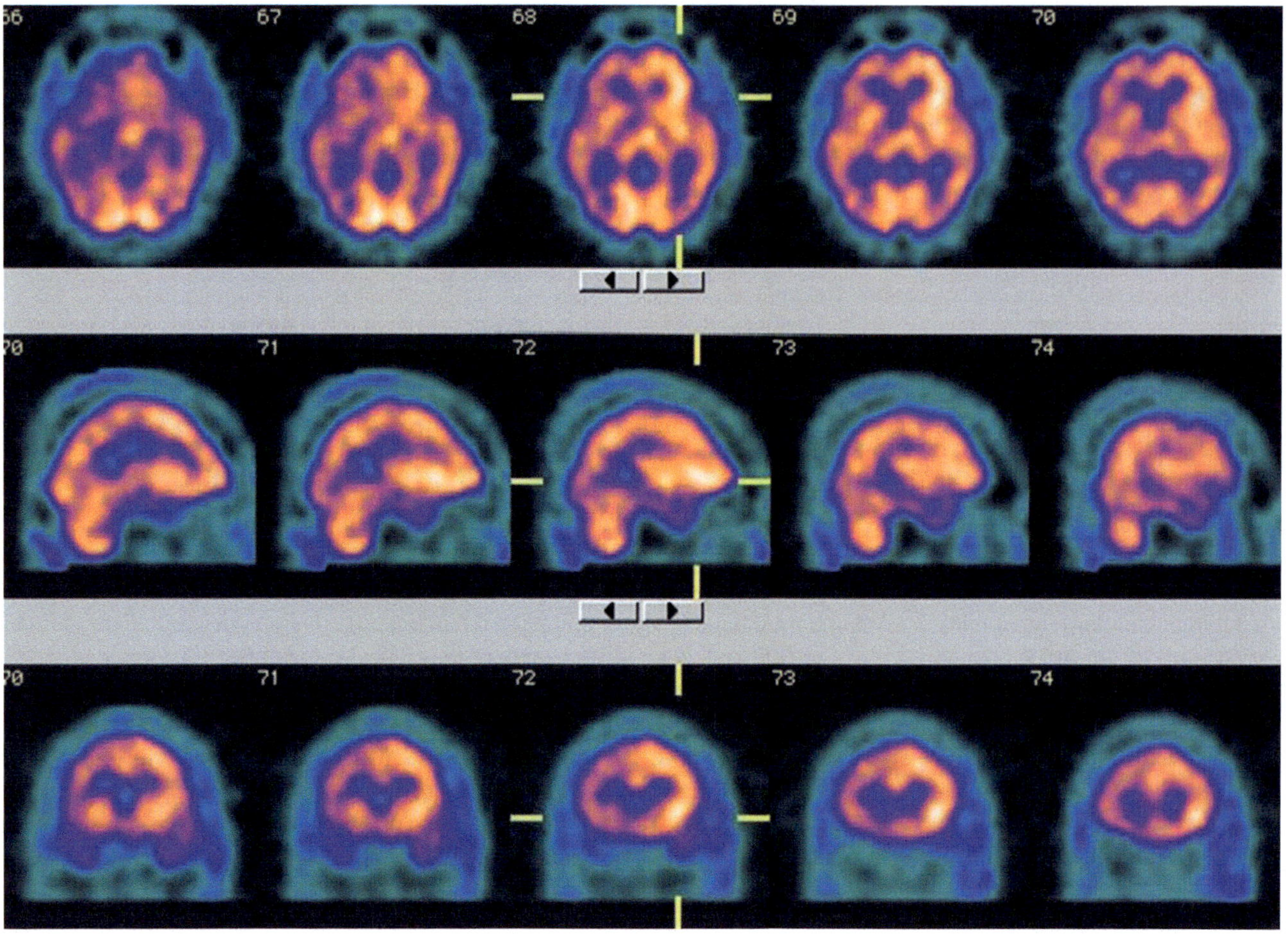


**Fig. 13.6** A SPECT study of a patient 12 months after a severe head trauma showing diffuse reduced regional cerebral flow (rCBF) in the right frontal, temporal, and parietal lobes, explaining the patient cognitive symptoms

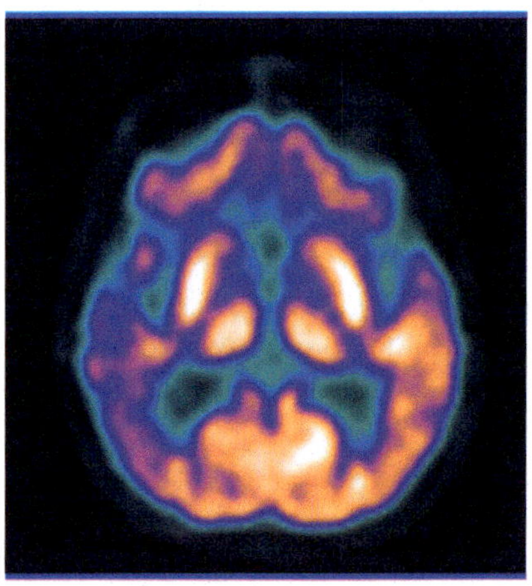

**Fig. 13.7** PET transverse-reconstructed image of a patient that suffered a motor vehicle accident. Note a marked focal hypometabolism in the right temporal lobe compared to the contralateral temporal region

In humans, there has been growing interest in using functional PET imaging in mild TBI, especially when CT and MRI are structurally normal. The first study using FDG-PET was published by Humayun et al. (1989). By evaluating three patients that suffered a recent vehicle accident, the authors were able to detect decreased glucose uptake in posterior temporal and frontal lobes, including the caudate nucleus 3–12 months after injury [71].

Even though we can see a few studies published in the literature, the majority lack in statistical power since the number of patients is consistently small and limited. Other studies evaluate brain metabolic impairments after blast injuries in war veterans. The majority of papers investigating around 20–30 veterans per study showed hypometabolism in different regions of the brains and related to chronic cognitive symptoms raised after the blast injuries [72–74].

Again, the numbers of patients and the different forms of processing and quantifying the images have limited the scientific impact of such evidence in the literature. However, the findings apparently suggest that FDG-PET could be a very sensitive tool to detect functional brain impairments after TBI.

Recently different groups have defended the use of other molecular probes to be used with PET in TBI. Amyloid pathology has been shown in patients diagnosed with

TBI. Preliminary studies showed increased uptake of amyloid plaque agent 11C-Pittsburgh compound B (PIB) in the posterior cingulate cortex and cerebellum of 28 patients evaluated 11 months to 17 years after moderate to severe TBI [75].

The encephalopathy caused by TBI (chronic traumatic encephalopathy (CTE)) is consisted of an acquired primary tauopathy; some authors have showed increased uptake of [F-18]FDDNP, an imaging agent for fibrillar insoluble protein aggregates, in retired professional American football players with suspected CTE. Other more modern agents that link to neurofibrillary bundles caused by disrupted TAU proteins bring new clinical perspectives for the potential use of PET in TBI [76].

Another potential role for PET is the detection of microglia activation. Using special probes for detection of inflammation into the nervous cell raises new potential use of PET in TBI [77].

## Conclusion

In conclusion, MRI, SPECT, and PET are sensitive tests that allow the identification of cerebral abnormalities in patients with symptoms related to different degrees of TBI. However, their exact clinical role remains undetermined since it needed larger prospective studies investigating in what situations to apply those tests and their exact importance in the management of the disease.

## References


1. Corrigan JD, Selassie AW, Orman JA. The epidemiology of traumatic brain injury. J Head Trauma Rehabil. 2010;25(2):72–80.
2. Corso P, Finkelstein E, Miller T, Fiebelkorn I, Zaloshnja E. Incidence and lifetime costs of injuries in the United States. Inj Prev. 2006;12(4):212–8.
3. Shively S, Scher AI, Perl DP, Diaz-Arrastia R. Dementia resulting from traumatic brain injury: what is the pathology? Arch Neurol. 2012;69(10):1245–51.
4. Little DM, Kraus MF, Joseph J, Geary EK, Susmaras T, Zhou XJ, et al. Thalamic integrity underlies executive dysfunction in traumatic brain injury. Neurology. 2010;74(7):558–64.
5. Caeyenberghs K, Leemans A, Leunissen I, Michiels K, Swinnen SP. Topological correlations of structural and functional networks in patients with traumatic brain injury. Front Hum Neurosci. 2013;7.
6. Silver JM, McAllister TW, Arciniegas DB. Depression and cognitive complaints following mild traumatic brain injury. Am J Psychiatr. 2009;166(6):653–61.
7. Bruns TJ, Hauser WA. The epidemiology of traumatic brain injury: a review. Epilepsia. 2003;44:2–10.
8. Saatman KE, Duhaime A-C, Bullock R, Maas AIR, Valadka A, Manley GT, et al. Classification of traumatic brain injury for targeted therapies. J Neurotrauma. 2008;25(7):719–38.
9. Currie S, Saleem N, Straiton JA, Macmullen-Price J, Warren DJ, Craven IJ. Imaging assessment of traumatic brain injury. Postgrad Med J. 2016;92(1083):41–50.
10. Rosa CM, Luigi B, Antonio D, Nicoletta A, Gloria L, Marco G. Early prognosis after severe traumatic brain injury with minor or absent computed tomography scan lesions. Journal of Trauma-Injury Infection and Critical Care. 2011;70(2):447–51.
11. Mechtler LL, Shastri KK, Crutchfield KE. Advanced neuroimaging of mild traumatic brain injury. Neurol Clin. 2014;32(1):31.
12. DiLeonardi AM, Huh JW, Rahupathi R. Impaired axonal transport and neurofilament compaction occur in separate populations of injured axons following diffuse brain injury in the immature rat. Brain Res. 2009;1263:174–82.
13. Yang XF, Wang H, Wen L. From myelin debris to inflammatory responses: a vicious circle in diffuse axonal injury. Med Hypotheses. 2011;77(1):60–2.
14. Jia Li X-Y, Dong-FuPan D-C. Biomarkers associated with diffuse traumatic axonal injury: exploring pathogenesis, early diagnosis, and prognosis. Journal of Trauma-Injury Infection and Critical Care. 2010;69(6):1610–8.
15. Ng HK, Mahaliyana RD, Poon WS. The pathological spectrum of diffuse axonal injury in blunt head trauma - assessment with axon and myelin stains. Clin Neurol Neurosurg. 1994;96(1):24–31.
16. Mathias JL, Beall JA, Bigler ED. Neuropsychological and information processing deficits following mild traumatic brain injury. J Int Neuropsychol Soc. 2004;10(2):286–97.
17. Nakayama N, Okumura A, Shinoda J, Yasokawa YT, Miwa K, Yoshimura SI, et al. Evidence for white matter disruption in traumatic brain injury without macroscopic lesions. Journal of Neurology Neurosurgery and Psychiatry. 2006;77(7):850.
18. Giugni E, Sabatini U, Hagberg GE, Formisano R, Castriota-Scanderbeg A. Fast detection of diffuse axonal damage in severe traumatic brain injury: comparison of gradient-recalled echo and turbo proton echo planar spectroscopic imaging MRI sequences. Am J Neuroradiol. 2005;26(5):1140–8.
19. Fazekas F, Kleinert R, Roob G, Kleinert G, Kapeller P, Schmidt R, et al. Histopathologic analysis of foci of signal loss on gradient-echo T2*-weighted MR images in patients with spontaneous intracerebral hemorrhage: evidence of microangiopathy-related microbleeds. Am J Neuroradiol. 1999;20(4):637–42.
20. Yanagawa Y, Sakamoto T, Takasu A, Okada Y. Relationship between maximum intracranial pressure and traumatic lesions detected by T2*-weighted imaging in diffuse axonal injury. J Trauma-Injury Infection Critical Care. 2009;66(1):162–5.
21. Lucchichenti G, Giugni E, Peran P, Cherubini A, Barba C, Bivona U, et al. 3 Tesla is twice as sensitive as 1.5 Tesla magnetic resonance imaging in the assessment of diffuse axonal injury in traumatic brain injury patients. Funct Neurol. 2010;25(2):109–14.
22. Hasiloglu ZI, Albayram S, Selcuk H, Ceyhan E, Delil S, Arkan B, et al. Cerebral microhemorrhages detected by susceptibility-weighted imaging in amateur boxers. Am J Neuroradiol. 2011;32(1):99–102.
23. Liu J, Kou Z, Tian Y. Diffuse axonal injury after traumatic cerebral microbleeds: an evaluation of imaging techniques. Neural Regen Res. 2014;9(12):1222–30.
24. Chastain CA, Oyoyo UE, Zipperman M, Joo E, Ashwal S, Shutter LA, et al. Predicting outcomes of traumatic brain injury by imaging modality and injury distribution. J Neurotrauma. 2009;26(8):1183–96.
25. Sigmund GA, Tong KA, Nickerson JP, Wall CJ, Oyoyo U, Ashwal S. Multimodality comparison of neuroimaging in pediatric traumatic brain injury. Pediatr Neurol. 2007;36(4):217–26.
26. Babikian T, Freier MC, Tong KA, Nickerson JP, Wall CJ, Holshouser BA, et al. Susceptibility weighted imaging: Neuropsychologic outcome and pediatric head injury. Pediatr Neurol. 2005;33(3):184–94.
27. Mukherjee P, Berman JI, Chung SW, Hess CP, Henry RG. Diffusion tensor MR imaging and fiber tractography: theoretic underpinnings. Am J Neuroradiol. 2008;29(4):632–41.

28. Beaulieu C. The basis of anisotropic water diffusion in the nervous system – a technical review. NMR Biomed. 2002;15(7–8):435–55.
29. Karaarslan E, Arslan A. Diffusion weighted MR imaging in non-infarct lesions of the brain. Eur J Radiol. 2008;65(3):402–16.
30. Mukherjee P, Chung SW, Berman JI, Hess CP, Henry RG. Diffusion tensor MR imaging and fiber tractography: technical considerations. Am J Neuroradiol. 2008;29(5):843–52.
31. Song SK, Sun SW, Ramsbottom MJ, Chang C, Russell J, Cross AH. Dysmyelination revealed through MRI as increased radial (but unchanged axial) diffusion of water. NeuroImage. 2002;17(3):1429–36.
32. Song SK, Sun SW, Ju WK, Lin SJ, Cross AH, Neufeld AH. Diffusion tensor imaging detects and differentiates axon and myelin degeneration in mouse optic nerve after retinal ischemia. NeuroImage. 2003;20(3):1714–22.
33. Farquharson S, Tournier JD, Calamante F, Fabinyi G, Schneider-Kolsky M, Jackson GD, et al. White matter fiber tractography: why we need to move beyond DTI. J Neurosurg. 2013;118(6):1367–77.
34. Smith SM, Jenkinson M, Johansen-Berg H, Rueckert D, Nichols TE, Mackay CE, et al. Tract-based spatial statistics: Voxelwise analysis of multi-subject diffusion data. NeuroImage. 2006;31(4):1487–505.
35. Pierpaoli C, Jezzard P, Basser PJ, Barnett A, DiChiro G. Diffusion tensor MR imaging of the human brain. Radiology. 1996;201(3):637–48.
36. Spalice A, Nicita F, Papetti L, Ursitti F, Di Biasi C, Parisi P, et al. Usefulness of diffusion tensor imaging and fiber tractography in neurological and neurosurgical pediatric diseases. Childs Nerv Syst. 2010;26(8):995–1002.
37. Wilde EA, McCauley SR, Hunter JV, Bigler ED, Chu Z, Wang ZJ, et al. Diffusion tensor imaging of acute mild traumatic brain injury in adolescents. Neurology. 2008;70(12):948–55.
38. Gu L, Li J, Feng D-F, Cheng E-T, Li D-C, Yang X-Q, et al. Detection of white matter lesions in the acute stage of diffuse axonal injury predicts long-term cognitive impairments: a clinical diffusion tensor imaging study. J Trauma Acute Care Surg. 2013;74(1):242–7.
39. Wang JY, Bakhadirov K, Devous MD, Sr., , Abdi H, McColl R, Moore C, et al. Diffusion tensor tractography of traumatic diffuse axonal injury. Arch Neurol 2008;65(5):619–626.
40. Kraus MF, Susmaras T, Caughlin BP, Walker CJ, Sweeney JA, Little DM. White matter integrity and cognition in chronic traumatic brain injury: a diffusion tensor imaging study. Brain. 2007;130:2508–19.
41. Huisman T, Schwamm LH, Schaefer PW, Koroshetz WJ, Shetty-Alva N, Ozsunar Y, et al. Diffusion tensor imaging as potential biomarker of white matter injury in diffuse axonal injury. Am J Neuroradiol. 2004;25(3):370–6.
42. Spitz G, Maller JJ, O'Sullivan R, Ponsford JL. White matter integrity following traumatic brain injury: the association with severity of injury and cognitive functioning. Brain Topogr. 2013;26(4):648–60.
43. Andrade CSZA, Conceição DM, Figueiredo KG, Macruz FBC, Feltrin FS, Otaduy MCG, Leite CC, editors. Longitudinal assessment of diffusion tensor imaging metrics with voxelwise analysis in patients with traumatic brain injury. Chicago: American Society of Neuroradiology; 2015.
44. Amaro E. Applications and design issues in fMRI. Brain Cogn. 2005;57(3):290.
45. Amaro E, Barker GJ. Study design in functional MRI: basic principles. Brain Cogn. 2006;60(3):220–32.
46. Lee MH, Smyser CD, Shimony JS. Resting-state fMRI: a review of methods and clinical applications. Am J Neuroradiol. 2013; 34(10):1866–72.
47. Barkhof F, Haller S, Rombouts SARB. Resting-state functional MR imaging: a new window to the brain. Radiology. 2014;272(1):28–48.
48. McDonald BC, Saykin AJ, McAllister TW. Functional MRI of mild traumatic brain injury (mTBI): progress and perspectives from the first decade of studies. Brain Imaging Behav. 2012;6(2):193–207.
49. Shumskaya E, Andriessen TMJC, Norris DG, Vos PE. Abnormal whole-brain functional networks in homogeneous acute mild traumatic brain injury. Neurology. 2012;79(2):175–82.
50. Tang L, Ge Y, Sodickson DK, Miles L, Zhou Y, Reaume J, et al. Thalamic resting-state functional networks: disruption in patients with mild traumatic brain injury. Radiology. 2011;260(3):831–40.
51. McGehee BE, Pollock JM, Maldjian JA. Brain perfusion imaging: how does it work and what should i use? J Magn Reson Imaging. 2012;36(6):1257.
52. Pasco A, Lemaire L, Franconi F, Lefur Y, Noury F, Saint-Andre J-P, et al. Perfusional deficit and the dynamics of cerebral edemas in experimental traumatic brain injury using perfusion and diffusion-weighted magnetic resonance imaging. J Neurotrauma. 2007;24(8):1321–30.
53. Garnett MR, Blamire AM, Corkill RG, Rajagopalan B, Young JD, Cadoux-Hudson TAD, et al. Abnormal cerebral blood volume in regions of contused and normal appearing brain following traumatic brain injury using perfusion magnetic resonance imaging. J Neurotrauma. 2001;18(6):585–93.
54. Detre JA, Rao HY, Wang DJJ, Chen YF, Wang Z. Applications of arterial spin labeled MRI in the brain. J Magn Reson Imaging. 2012;35(5):1026–37.
55. Telischak NA, Detre JA, Zaharchuk G. Arterial spin labeling MRI: clinical applications in the brain. J Magn Reson Imaging. 2015;41(5):1165–80.
56. Ge Y, Patel MB, Chen Q, Grossman EJ, Zhang K, Miles L, et al. Assessment of thalamic perfusion in patients with mild traumatic brain injury by true FISP arterial spin labelling MR imaging at 3T. Brain Inj. 2009;23(7–8):666–74.
57. Kim J, Whyte J, Patel S, Avants B, Europa E, Wang J, et al. Resting cerebral blood flow alterations in chronic traumatic brain injury: an arterial spin labeling perfusion fMRI study. J Neurotrauma. 2010;27(8):1399–411.
58. Maheshwari SR, Fatterpekar GM, Castillo M, Mukherji SK. Proton MR spectroscopy of the brain. Semin Ultrasound CT MRI. 2000;21(6):434–51.
59. Castillo M, Kwock L, Mukherji SK. Clinical applications of proton MR spectroscopy. Am J Neuroradiol. 1996;17(1):1–15.
60. Brooks WM, Friedman SD, Gasparovic C. Magnetic resonance spectroscopy in traumatic brain injury. J Head Trauma Rehabil. 2001;16(2):149–64.
61. Duckworth JL, Stevens RD. Imaging brain trauma. Curr Opin Crit Care. 2010;16(2):92–7.
62. Vagnozzi R, Signoretti S, Cristofori L, Alessandrini F, Floris R, Isgro E, et al. Assessment of metabolic brain damage and recovery following mild traumatic brain injury: a multicentre, proton magnetic resonance spectroscopic study in concussed patients. Brain. 2010;133:3232–42.
63. Cecil KM, Hills EC, Sandel E, Smith DH, McIntosh TK, Mannon LJ, et al. Proton magnetic resonance spectroscopy for detection of axonal injury in the splenium of the corpus callosum of brain-injured patients. J Neurosurg. 1998;88(5):795–801.
64. Tollard E, Galanaud D, Perlbarg V, Sanchez-Pena P, Le Fur Y, Abdennour L, et al. Experience of diffusion tensor imaging and H-1 spectroscopy for outcome prediction in severe traumatic brain injury: preliminary results. Crit Care Med. 2009;37(4):1448–55.
65. Hayes JP, Bigler ED, Verfaellie M. Traumatic brain injury as a disorder of brain connectivity. J Int Neuropsychol Soc. 2016;22(2):120–37.
66. Léveillé J, Demonceau G, De Roo M, Rigo P, Taillefer R, Morgan RA, et al. Characterization of technetium-99m-L,L-ECD for brain perfusion imaging, part 2: biodistribution and brain imaging in humans. J Nucl Med. 1989;30(11):1902–10.
67. Raji CA, Tarzwell R, Pavel D, Schneider H, Uszler M, Thornton J, et al. Clinical utility of SPECT neuroimaging in the diagnosis and

treatment of traumatic brain injury: a systematic review. PLoS One. 2014;9(3):e91088.
68. Pavel D, Jobe T, Devore-Best S, Davis G, Epstein P, Sinha S, et al. Viewing the functional consequences of traumatic brain injury by using brain SPECT. Brain Cogn. 2006;60(2):211–3.
69. Romero K, Lobaugh NJ, Black SE, Ehrlich L, Feinstein A. Old wine in new bottles: validating the clinical utility of SPECT in predicting cognitive performance in mild traumatic brain injury. Psychiatry Res. 2015;231(1):15–24.
70. Selwyn R, Hockenbury N, Jaiswal S, Mathur S, Armstrong RC, Byrnes KR. Mild traumatic brain injury results in depressed cerebral glucose uptake: an (18)FDG PET study. J Neurotrauma. 2013;30(23):1943–53.
71. Humayun MS, Presty SK, Lafrance ND, Holcomb HH, Loats H, Long DM, et al. Local cerebral glucose abnormalities in mild closed head injured patients with cognitive impairments. Nucl Med Commun. 1989;10:335–44.
72. Wilde EA, Bouix S, Tate DF, Lin AP, Newsome MR, Taylor BA, et al. Advanced neuroimaging applied to veterans and service personnel with traumatic brain injury: state of the art and potential benefits. Brain Imaging Behav. 2015;9(3):367–402.
73. Buchsbaum MS, Simmons AN, DeCastro A, Farid N, Matthews SC. Clusters of low (18)F-Fluorodeoxyglucose uptake voxels in combat veterans with traumatic brain injury and post-traumatic stress disorder. J Neurotrauma. 2015;32(22):1736–50.
74. Byrnes KR, Wilson CM, Brabazon F, von Leden R, Jurgens JS, Oakes TR, et al. FDG-PET imaging in mild traumatic brain injury: a critical review. Front Neuroenerg. 2014;5:13.
75. Scott G, Ramlackhansingh AF, Edison P, Hellyer P, Cole J, Veronese M, et al. Amyloid pathology and axonal injury after brain trauma. Neurology. 2016;86(9):821–8.
76. Barrio JR, Small GW, Wong KP, Huang SC, Liu J, Merrill DA, et al. In vivo characterization of chronic traumatic encephalopathy using [F-18]FDDNP PET brain imaging. Proc Natl Acad Sci U S A. 2015;112(16):E2039–47.
77. Velázquez A, Ortega M, Rojas S, González-Oliván FJ, Rodríguez-Baeza A. Widespread microglial activation in patients deceased from traumatic brain injury. Brain Inj. 2015;29(9):1126–33.

# Neuropsychological Rehabilitation After Traumatic Brain Injury

14

Fabio Rios Freire, Fernanda Coelho, Patricia De Lucia Nadruz, Jéssica Natuline Ianof, and Renato Anghinah

## Introduction

TBI is an important public health problem worldwide. Data from Brazil indicates that approximately 700,000 people suffer a traumatic brain injury (TBI) annually, of whom 20–30% have moderate or severe TBI. About 80% of those who suffer mild TBI are able to return to work, only 20% of moderate and 10% of severe TBI cases can return to their daily routine [1, 2]. TBI is a nondegenerative, noncongenital insult to the brain from an external mechanical force, potentially leading to permanent or temporary impairment of cognitive, physical, and psychosocial functions, with an associated diminished or altered state of consciousness [3].

Cognitive rehabilitation is a clinical area with interdisciplinary action focused on recovery as well as compensation of cognitive functions altered as a result of a head injury [4]. The aim of a cognitive rehabilitation program is to recover an individual's ability to process, interpret, and respond appropriately to environmental inputs and also to create strategies and procedures to compensate for lost functions that are necessary in familial, social, educational, and occupational relationships [5].

The programs of cognitive rehabilitation tend to focus on specific cognitive domains, such as attention, memory, language, and executive functions. By contrast, the focus of compensatory training procedures is generally on making environmental adaptations and changes to provide greater autonomy for patients. A successful cognitive rehabilitation program is the one whose aim is both recovery and compensation based on an integrated and interdisciplinary approach [6].

F. R. Freire · F. Coelho · P. De Lucia Nadruz · J. N. Ianof
Department of Neurology – Cognitive Rehabilitation after TBI, Clinics Hospital – School of Medicine – University of São Paulo, São Paulo, Brazil

R. Anghinah (✉)
Department of Neurology – Cognitive Rehabilitation after TBI, Clinics Hospital – School of Medicine – University of São Paulo, São Paulo, Brazil

Center of Excellence in Neurology – Americas Serviços Médicos, São Paulo, Brazil

## Cognitive Impairments Following TBI

Depending on the severity and site of injury, the type and degree of cognitive impairment following TBI may vary widely. If a focal brain injury occurs, the consequence may be similar to the injury caused by a stroke, such as aphasia, apraxia, unilateral neglect, or visuospatial dysfunction. Nevertheless, these are not the typical findings following TBI. Due to the mechanisms of acceleration-deceleration that often damage the ventral and lateral regions of the frontal and temporal lobes, the most frequently found sequelae are attention and memory deficit, difficulty learning new information, resolving problems, planning, as well as problems associated with impulsivity and self-control. Some "subclinical" findings such as changes in naming, verbal fluency, and auditory discrimination are also reported. Initially, attention deficits are the most common and severe in the residual stage, usually involving difficulty maintaining divided attention. The long-term memory is generally restored, but some individuals continue having difficulties in learning new things and retaining new information. Working memory is frequently affected including the stages of encoding, storage, and retrieval of information. Such changes have a significant impact on social and vocational reintegration [7, 8].

Some individuals are left with amnesic syndrome, which is more common in those who have gone through periods of hypoxia and anoxia. Executive functions may be affected, being related to frontal lobe damage. When the frontal injury is severe, the patient may be inert or lack initiative (medial or lateral frontal injury) or display inappropriate and impulsive behavior. Many individuals with frontal lobe injury in post-TBI retain much of their skills but are unable to initiate, sequence, organize, or monitor their actions so as to meet the targets or goals set. The language disorders most commonly observed occur in the discursive (tendency to produce irrelevant information and omit important information), pragmatic (loss in production of inferences, difficulty in formulating arguments), and conversation levels (loss of initiative and maintenance of topics with inconsistent switching without signaling). These


R. Anghinah et al. (eds.), *Topics in Cognitive Rehabilitation in the TBI Post-Hospital Phase*,
https://doi.org/10.1007/978-3-319-95376-2_14

changes correlate with cognitive impairments in attention, memory, and slow mental processing [6].

## Long-Term Neuropsychiatric Deficits

The most common syndromes post-TBI are behavioral disinhibition, depression, anxiety, psychosis, substance abuse, and attention/cognitive disorders. Post-traumatic stress disorder (PTSD) occurs in up to 27% of cases, including patients with no clear recall of the event. Depression has an incidence of 15–33% and prevalence of 18–42%. Mania occurs in <10% of patients with TBI [9]. Aggression occurs in variable frequencies (ranging from 20% to 49%), and psychosis occurs in <10% of the TBI population [10].

## After the Hospital: Post-acute/Chronic Phase

The cognitive stimulation from the interdisciplinary team (several professionals attending the patient in a holistic manner to enhance operations) at this stage is fundamental because the patient is only able to embark on motor training if a minimum attentional state can be maintained which allows the patient to execute and repeat the tasks proposed [11].

At this stage, temporal-spatial orientation and attention call for redoubled efforts to maximize the communication with the patient so as to improve strategies that use motor and cognitive training. In terms of speech, intervention should promote the structuring of activity, with a highly predictable distraction-free environment and also activities that induce self-monitoring. The biggest hurdle at this stage stems from the fact that most patients have significant attentional deficit that limits the role of comprehensive rehabilitation [12].

After the most critical phase of hospital management, most patients return home. Although some patients manage to regain some degree of independence in their self-care, they are still incapable of applying critical thinking to decision-making processes, providing for the needs of their families, or continuing work, school, or social activities, which can cause difficulties in family relationships and result in a poor quality of life for patients and their relatives. Moreover, patients may manifest mood alteration and depression.

The rehabilitation of these patients after hospital discharge is aimed at a community integration program that provide continuity of patient care with vocational and professional training integrated into the rehabilitation process [12].

The Rancho Los Amigos Levels of Cognitive Functioning Scale is a widely used scale that systematically standardizes the functional level of post-TBI patients in order to establish the possibility of their rehabilitation management [13]. It is considered that a patient is able to enter a rehabilitation program when he is at least at level V, which means that he can pay attention for a few minutes – what is crucial for rehabilitation.

## Rancho Los Amigos Scale (Los Amigos Research and Education Institute)

### No Response

A person at this level will:

Not respond to sounds, sights, touch, or movement.

### Generalized Response

A person at this level will:

Begin to respond to sounds, sights, touch, or movement.
Respond slowly, inconsistently, or after a delay.
Respond in the same way to what they hear, see, or feel. Responses may include chewing, sweating, breathing faster, moaning, moving, and/or increasing blood pressure.

### Localized Response

A person at this level will:

Be awake on and off during the day.
Make more movements than before.
React more specifically to what they see, hear, or feel. For example, patient may turn toward a sound, withdraw from pain, and attempt to watch a person move around the room.
React slowly and inconsistently.
Begin to recognize family and friends.
Follow some simple directions such as "look at me" or "squeeze my hand."
Begin to respond inconsistently to simple questions with "yes" or "no" head nods.

### Confused-Agitated

A person at this level will:

Be very confused and frightened.
Not understand what they feel or what is happening around them.
Overreact to what they see, hear, or feel by hitting, screaming, using abusive language, or thrashing about. This is because of the confusion.
Be restrained so they do not hurt themselves.

Be highly focused on their basic needs, i.e., eating, relieving pain, going back to bed, going to the bathroom, or going home.
May not understand that people are trying to help them.
Not pay attention or be able to concentrate for only a few seconds.
Have difficulty following directions.
Recognize family/friends some of the time.
With help, be able to do simple routine activities such as feeding themselves, dressing, or talking.

## Confused-Inappropriate, Non-agitated

A person at this level will:

Be able to pay attention for only a few minutes.
Be confused and have difficulty making sense of things around them.
Not know the date, where they are, or why they are in hospital.
Not be able to start or complete everyday activities, such as brushing their teeth, even when physically able. They may need step-by-step instructions.
Become overloaded and restless when tired or when there are too many people around, have a very poor memory, and remembering past events from before the accident better than their daily routine or information they have been given since the injury.
Try to fill in gaps in memory by making things up (confabulation).
May get stuck on an idea or activity (perseveration) and need help switching to the next part of the activity.
Focus on basic needs such as eating, relieving pain, going back to bed, going to the bathroom, or going home.

## Confused-Appropriate

A person at this level will:

Be somewhat confused because of memory and thinking problems, remembering the main points from a conversation but forgetting and being confused about the details. For example, they may remember having visitors in the morning but forget what they talked about.
Follow a schedule with some assistance but becomes confused by changes in the routine.
Know the month and year, except when they have a serious memory problem.
Pay attention for about 30 min but has trouble concentrating when it is noisy or when the activity involves many steps. For example, at an intersection, they may be unable to step off the curb, watch for cars, watch the traffic light, walk, and talk all at the same time and brush their teeth, get dressed, feed themselves, etc., with help.
Know when they need to use the bathroom.
Do or say things too fast, without thinking first.
Know that they are hospitalized because of an injury but will not understand all the problems they are having.
Be more aware of physical problems than thinking problems.
Associate their problems with being in the hospital and think they will be fine as soon as they go home.

## Automatic-Appropriate

A person at this level will:

Follow a set schedule.
Be able to carry out routine self-care without help, if physically able. For example, they can dress or feed themselves independently, have problems in new situations, and may become frustrated or act without thinking first.
Have problems planning, starting, and following through with activities.
Have trouble paying attention in distracting or stressful situations. For example, family gatherings, work, school, church, or sports events.
Not realize how their thinking and memory problems may affect future plans and goals. Therefore, they may expect to return to their previous lifestyle or work.
Continue to need supervision because of decreased safety awareness and judgment. They still do not fully understand the impact of their physical or thinking problems.
Think slower in stressful situations.
Be inflexible or rigid and may be stubborn. However, their behaviors are related to their brain injury.
Be able to talk about doing something but will have problems actually doing it.

## Purposeful-Appropriate

A person at this level will:

Realize that they have a problem with their thinking and memory.
Begin to compensate for their problems.

Be more flexible and less rigid in their thinking. For example, they may be able to come up with several solutions to a problem.
Be ready for driving or job training evaluation.
Be able to learn new things at a slower rate.
Still become overloaded with difficult, stressful, or emergency situations.
Show poor judgment in new situations and may require assistance.
Need some guidance making decisions.
Have thinking problems that may not be noticeable to people who did not know the person before the injury.

## Strategies to Manage Post-TBI Patients

### Cognitive Function Evaluation

First of all, patients will be subjected to a reading test, which consists of reading simple children's books to evaluate how long they focus on the book. According to the performance and education of each individual, slightly more complex texts will be presented.

After this first test, each patient will be classified according to the Rancho Los Amigos Scale, and only those who score greater than or equal to 5 (on the scale of 8) will be referred for cognitive rehabilitation. This is necessary because to be rehabilitated, the individual must maintain a minimum time set for the task of greater than 10 min [12].

The next intervention will be to conduct a neuropsychological evaluation, including the Mini-Mental State Examination [14, 15] and clock drawing. The neuropsychological assessment includes the evaluation of affective/emotional state, functional activity questionnaire, batteries of tests of executive functions (Wisconsin Card Sorting Test [16] and Stroop Interference Test [17]), as well as other tests including the Rey Auditory-Verbal Learning Test [18]; WAIS III attention, digit-symbol, and visuo-constructive tests [19]; Trail Making Test parts A and B [20]; verbal fluency tests [21]; and Rey-Osterrieth complex figure [22]. All tests have been previously validated in Brazil with scores for different levels of education. After the neuropsychological evaluation, individual rehabilitation strategies are developed in conjunction with the interdisciplinary team.

### Tools Used in Cognitive Rehabilitation

#### Attention

The treatment is usually based on patient engagement in performing repetitive exercises including sustained, alternating, selective, and divided attention.

**Sustained Attention Training**

1. Listen to a word sequence and identify when you see a word stimulus, which was the one previously presented.
2. Understanding of spoken text of a paragraph (originally short and simple) that has progressively increasing difficulty throughout the course of training.
3. Sequencing of numbers in ascending order and/or decreasing verbally.
4. Math activities – mentally.

**Alternating Attention Training**

1. Exercise in which the patient must identify a previously defined word and word sequence, identifying when it appears in a text or string of words they will listen to, replacing the first word, when identified, with the previously given sequence
2. Tasks with pen and paper, where the patient has to write a number and a letter that complete a sequence written with gaps to be filled
3. Activities that start with a number, which must be sequentially added or subtracted by the other items that are being presented

**Selective Attention Training**

1. Any test which has been reported for sustained attention, with a distractor sound or motion associated
2. Tasks with visual distractors – such as tasks involving drawing with paper and pen (pencil) on a sheet full of tracings and background designs

**Divided Attention Training**

1. The patient reads a few paragraphs paying attention to their content while looking up the proposed word in advance.
2. The patient completes a test battery of sustained attention training, in which the patient has to respond to verbal or parallel visual stimuli (which can be accomplished by including computerized tests) [12].

#### Memory

In order to rehabilitate memory, the first aspect is to verify whether the patient maintains sufficient attention on the stimulus or task given (as seen in the previous topic). The second aspect is to assess whether the patient is able to "decipher" the stimulus given or if the patient knows the word or object (verbal or visual stimulus) or can categorize them (words or objects) into any semantic grouping.

The exercise used for this type of injury consists of repetition of words. Concurrently, it involves categorization of words such as by asking if a cat is an animal seen at the zoo or by eliciting the rhyme of a given word.

Naturally, a team of speech therapists will evaluate losses involving comprehension and language.

**Memory Storage** This involves learning new tasks or old skills that were lost. When there are bilateral hippocampal lesions, the retention mechanism of long-term learning memory is lost. Processes of verbal repetition and writing are important for this training.

**Evocation of Old Memories** This entails training with pictures or words that are subsequently presented and evoked several times. Repetition, writing, drawing, and verbal processes are important in this training. Individuals sustaining frontal lobe injury can remember facts, but not associate them with a context or time of occurrence. Generally, they confabulate based on a preexisting fact. In order to rekindle the old memory, a strategy is to repeat the known facts which the patient is unable to remember, using pictures, or by repeating stories until they are remembered. This differs from the bi-hippocampal lesion, which preserves old memories (except the period of posttraumatic amnesia) but renders the individual incapable of retaining new learning [12].

## Training Strategies Outside the Outpatient Unit

Initially, the patient undergoes neurological, neuropsychological, speech, and occupational therapy evaluation. Once the evaluation is finished, the interdisciplinary team defines the treatment strategy.

The sequence below lists possible training strategies to be developed concurrently with the behavioral training at home:

1. Remember events during the current day (at the end of the day) or for the previous day (in the morning).
2. After recalling the events, write them in a notebook whenever possible.
3. Receive new information – summaries of news about some event or family – and read a short informational text.
4. Plan the morning, day, or week's (whenever possible) activity.
5. Talk about past events that have been forgotten or are not well contextualized after the accident.
6. Follow the primer of daily activities with attention, executive functions, language, and memory activities as well as activities of daily living.
7. Medication approach when neurologist/psychiatrist thinks it is appropriate [12].

## Conclusion

TBI is a major public health problem with neurobehavioral sequelae contributing to the long-term disability that is often associated with moderate to severe levels of injury. Rehabilitation of cognitive skills is fundamental to encouraging the full participation of the individual in home, vocational, and social roles. Cognitive rehabilitation begins with a neuropsychological evaluation to identify cognitive strengths and weaknesses and the degree of change in cognitive ability following a TBI. The conclusions of the assessment are used to formulate appropriate and individualized rehabilitation plans. Attention process training and tasks for attention deficits, compensatory strategies, learning training for memory deficits, social behavior guidance for cognitive-communication disorder, and problem-solving training for executive disorder are the focus of therapy.

**Conflict of Interest** There is no conflict of interest to declare.

## References


1. Schewinsky SR. Reabilitação neuropsicológica da memória no TCE. 1st ed. São Paulo: Livraria Médica Paulista; 2008.
2. Harmon RL, Lawrence JH. Traumatic brain injury. In: Bryan J, Mark A, Steven A, editors. Physical medicine and rehabilitation secrets. 2nd ed. Philadelphia: Mosby; 2001. 2008: xvii.
3. Jang SH. Review of motor recovery in patients with traumatic brain injury. NeuroRehabilitation. 2009;24:349–53.
4. Cappa SF, Benke T, Clarke S, Rossi B, Stemmer B, van Heugten CM. Task force on cognitive rehabilitation: European Federation of Neurological Societies. EFNS guidelines on cognitive rehabilitation: report of an EFNS task force. Eur J Neurol. 2005;12:665–80.
5. Cattelani R, Zettin M, Zoccolotti P. Rehabilitation treatments for adults with behavioral and psychosocial disorders following acquired brain injury: a systematic review. Neuropsychol Rev. 2010;20:52–85.
6. Thornton KE, Carmody DP. Efficacy of traumatic brain injury rehabilitation: interventions of QEEG-guided biofeedback, computers, strategies, and medications. Appl Psychophysiol Biofeedback. 2008;33:101–24.
7. Mansur LL, Radanovic M. Neurolinguistica: princípios para a prática clínica. São Paulo: Edições Inteligentes; 2004.
8. Braakman R, Jennett WB, Minderhoud JM. Prognosis of the post-traumatic vegetative state. Acta Neurochir. 1988;95:49–52.

9. Tuel SM, Presty SK, Meythaler JM, Heinemann AW, Katz RT. Functional improvement in severe head injury after readmission for rehabilitation. Brain Inj. 1992;6:363–72.
10. Nicholl J, LaFrance WC Jr. Neuropsychiatric sequelae of traumatic brain injury. Semin Neurol. 2009;29:247–55.
11. Sohlberg MM, Mateer CA. Cognitive rehabilitation. London: The Guilford Press; 2001.
12. Freire FR, Coelho F, Lacerda JR, Silva MF, Gonçalves VT, Machado S, et al. Cognitive rehabilitation following traumatic brain injury. Dementia & Neuropsychologia. 2011;5(1):17–25.
13. Hagen C. The rancho levels of cognitive functioning, vol. 9. 3rd ed. Downey: Rancho Los Amigos Medical Center; 2008.
14. Folstein MH, Folstein SM, McHugh PR. "Mini-Mental State": a practical method for grading the cognitive state of patients for clinicians. J Psychiat Res. 1975;12:189–98.
15. Bertolucci PHF, Mathias SC, Brucki SMD, Carrilho PEM, Okamoto IH, Nitrini R. Proposta de padronização do Mini-Exame do Estado Mental (MEEM): estudo piloto cooperativo (FMUSP/EPM). Arq Neuropsiquiatr. 1994;52:225.
16. Wisconsin Card Sorting Test. Psychological Assessment Resources. Inc-Odessa; 1993.
17. Spreen O, Strauss E. Compendium of neuropsychological tests: administration, norms, and commentary. 2nd ed. New York: Oxford University Press; 1998a.
18. Rey A. L'examen psychologique dans les cas d'encephalopathie traumatique. Arch Psychol. 1941;28:286–340.
19. Wechsler D. Wechsler Adult Intelligence Scale, vol. 3. New York: Psychological Corporation; 1997.
20. Trail Making Test. In: Spreen O, Strauss E, editors. A compendium of neuropsychological tests: administration, norms, and commentary. 2nd ed. New York: Oxford University Press; 1998. p. 533–46.
21. Brucki SM, Rocha MS. Category fluency test: effects of age, gender and education on total scores, clustering and switching in Brazilian Portuguese-speaking subjects. Braz J Med Biol Res. 2004;37(12):1771–7.
22. Spreen O, Strauss E. A compendium of neuropsychological tests: administration, norms, and commentary. 2nd ed. New York: Oxford University Press; 1998b. Rey-Osterrieth complex figure test (SFT). p. 341–63.

# "Come Back to Community and Work After Traumatic Brain Injury"

# 15

Selma Lancman, Andrea Toshye Sato, Tatiana de Andrade Jardim Rodriguez, and Juliana de Oliveira Barros

## Traumatic Brain Injury in Brazil

In Brazil, the largest country in Latin America in terms of territorial extension, population, and gross domestic product (GDP) [1], an estimated annual number of 700 thousand to 1.1 million new cases of traumatic brain injury emerge (TBI). Of these, approximately 20% are characterized as moderate or severe [2].

The consequences of TBI are high rates of mortality and morbidity, mainly affecting young adults at a productive age. This may be verified when considering that in Brazil, the highest prevalence of TBI is in men in the age range of 15 to 24 years, with the main cause being automobile accidents [2, 3]. According to Brazilian Social Security data [4], in the year 2015, in total 4.654 benefits of the social security type for assistance with illness were granted to persons who suffered fractures of the skull and facial bones – the classification in which TBI is included.

Furthermore, around 500 thousand per year are hospitalized with brain injuries acquired after TBI, and from 70 to 90 thousand persons who suffered TBI evolve to irreversible loss of some neurological function [2]. Between January 2005 and September 2006, in São Paulo alone – the most populated city in the country – 48,872 persons were observed to be hospitalized because of TBI, and for these cases, a 9.63% mortality rate was verified [5].

These data are relevant on showing the individual and social burden of the problem: the first is directly related to the loss of functional and financial independence of the individuals and the impact on the capacity to reconstruct their social and work life. The second refers, above all, to the impact of expenditure on health assistance offered by the Brazilian Public Health System (SUS), and the benefits granted, under the responsibility of Assistance and Social Security [6].

Therefore, public expenditure on those who suffer TBI is significant and extrapolates to the field of health. These expenses involve not only the processes of treatment and motor and cognitive rehabilitation but also possible difficulties with inclusion in the work market, being laid off from work, sick leave, early retirement, and unemployment. This being so, these impacts result in the question being considered not only a serious public health problem but a social security and social problem as well [7].

## TBI, Social Inclusion, and Work

Depending on the area affected, TBI may generate motor, cognitive, sensory, and behavioral sequelae. Cases of slight injuries may be completely asymptomatic with normal physical exam and without neurological changes. Of these, around 3% present worsening of the condition, with sever neurological dysfunction [8]. In cases in which the injuries are moderate, these sequelae may be reversible in up to 15% of cases; however, in the remainder, these are of a permanent nature [9].

The temporary or permanent incapacities resulting from TBI may interfere in the performance of daily life activities, work, and in living with other people, limiting social participation in a more far-reaching way and having drastic impact on the individuals' quality of life [10, 11].

Quite often, even if those who suffered TBI manage to achieve independence for daily life activities[1], [12], they

S. Lancman (✉) · A. T. Sato · T. de Andrade Jardim Rodriguez
J. de Oliveira Barros
Department of Physical Therapy, Speech Therapy and Occupational Therapy – School of Medicine – University of São Paulo, São Paulo, Brazil
e-mail: lancman@usp.br; andrea.sato@usp.br; tati.ajardim@usp.br; juliana.obarros@usp.br

[1] They refer to activities that demand more basic skills, such as self-care (personal hygiene, eating, dressing, etc.), mobility (mobility in bed, transfers, locomotion, etc.), and communication (oral language, written, use of amplification devices for communication, etc.) [13].


R. Anghinah et al. (eds.), *Topics in Cognitive Rehabilitation in the TBI Post-Hospital Phase*,
https://doi.org/10.1007/978-3-319-95376-2_15

come up against difficulties relative to social and/or inclusion in work [11]. The latter are considered complex activities because they involve skills that are more advanced: problem solving, social problems, and different environmental interactions [13].

Inclusion in work is important to the extent that in addition to being a source of income, it is a central element in people's lives and a significant space for social integration and self-fulfillment. Participating in the community is also considered to take place through work, as it generally involves living together with other people, the need to frequent certain spaces, and the possibility of coping with and resolving challenges and contributing to the society [10, 11, 14].

One study observed that 2 and 7 years, respectively, after the trauma, severe TBI victims who had made some type of social adjustment were mainly those that continued to work. At the same time, those who did not work demonstrated loss of structured daily life routine and a group of friends and lack of objectives to attain or opportunities to show competence [6].

Burt [10] affirmed that incapacity to work may generate difficulties with performing other social roles, such as roles played within the family circle. In addition to change in lifestyle resulting from financial problems, forced inactivity and dependence led to depression, a little psychosocial adaptation.

It is important to point out that the types of capacity of individuals and the way they are affected by illness, traumatisms, or even aging differ. The term intrinsic capacity is used to deal with the set of physical and mental capacities, while functional capacity refers to the capacity for performing activities, considering intrinsic capacity added to the possibilities the environment provides and/or access to the use of auxiliary devices [15], whereas the term capacity for work is related to the type of work the person does; that is, it concerns the person's intrinsic capacity to interact with the organization (content, division of labor, hierarchical levels, rules and production procedures, rhythm and goals, etc.) and working conditions (materials and physical installations with reference to the work) available for performing the professional activities foreseen [16–20].

Therefore, although a subject has sequelae resulting from TBI (whether they are motor, cognitive, sensory, and/or behavioral), it is considered possible to maintain the capacity for work if the respective conditions and organization enable the development of activities that consider the individual's limitations.

However, in Brazil it is observed that the capacity for work is still seen as the subject's individual responsibility, with focus on his/her intrinsic capacity. Thus, the major portion of companies do not have an organization that allows the working participation of persons who have intrinsic difficulties. This reality affects a significant number of persons who suffered TBI, reconsidered incapable of working, according to the intrinsic criteria only [21, 22].

This may be observed when it is noted that the probability of returning to work after a TBI is related to the degree of compromise of the traumatism: the greater the extent of compromise, the lower the chance of returning to work. Studies have indicated that of the subjects who suffered a slight TBI (or, i.e., possibly present little or no sequela), around 80% usually return to work, whereas only 20% of persons who had suffered a moderate TBI and 10% of those who suffered a severe TBI return to their work activities [23].

O'Brien and Wolf [24] conducted a study in which they interviewed 98 men between 30 and 65 years of age, who suffered a cerebral vascular accident (CVA), another problem with the possibility of leading to significant neurological impairment. From the interviews, they were able to note that of the total number of participants, 63% returned to work without having gone through the professional/vocational rehabilitation program. Of these, 90% immediately returned to the jobs they held before the CVA. Of those who returned to work, 56% considered that they did not have their full capacity for work, but nevertheless, the majority felt that they were doing their work with the same quality as they had done it before the CVA and felt satisfied with their work performance. Therefore, once again it emphasizes that the degree of incapacity resulting from the CVA may have influenced their return to work, favoring those who have light to moderate compromised functions. Moreover, it should be considered that, among the interviewees, the accidents were recent (they had occurred 6 months previously) and that, before the CVAs, the subjects had worked full time, in different fields of activity.

In this context, an overall rehabilitation program that involves professional/vocational rehabilitation gains importance in the daily lives of those who suffer neurological disturbances, because it allows the individuals to completely or partially return to the activities they previously performed (such as work, studies, and/or daily life activities) in addition to assuring their engagement in significant activities that promoted their independence and personal growth [11].

## Professional/Vocational Rehabilitation and Return to Work

At present, overall post-TBI rehabilitation involves three main stages, according to the period of occurrence of the trauma:

1. Acute stage (right after the trauma, in which the individual generally finds himself/herself hospitalized with the purpose of guaranteeing his/her survival and avoiding greater complications).

2. Subacute stage (still during hospitalization, with the aim of reducing the sequelae of TBI; increasing his/her physical, cognitive, and psychosocial independence; compensating for the deficiency; and minimizing suffering).
3. Outpatient stage (occurs in an extra-hospital context to provide continuity of the objectives established in the subacute stage, with focus on social participation, including reintegration into significant activities and maintenance of quality of life) [25].

Although professional/vocational rehabilitation should be understood as a constituent and undissociable element of the overall rehabilitation process, bearing in mind (as previously pointed out) the importance of work in people's lives, access to it is still limited. This is due to the little importance attached to this aspect, which results in few offers of jobs that offer this type of attention [11, 30].

Professional/vocational rehabilitation seeks to make the means possible to find a job that is compatible with and healthy for subject, in addition to making it easy to reduce or overcome his/her intrinsic, emotional, and social limitations, thereby enabling an increase in his/her capacity for work. By these means, this modality of intervention seeks to articulate the actions developed in the overall therapeutic process with those that are focused on the organization and working conditions that must receive the worker, with the end purpose of not only to return to work but above all to remain in the job [12, 26].

Maeno and Vilela [26] pointed out that this is a complex approach and demands that the person being rehabilitated, professional rehabilitation team, and the company assume their responsibility in the process. As this involves changes in the work itself, diverse aspects must always be considered, such as the context of the work, its organizational characteristics, and the various actors of which this scenario is composed.

Therefore, the professional/vocational rehabilitation must help the individual recover or develop skills, to maintain and encourage social relations and encourage the development of new ties, promoting the return to daily life activities, to daily life activities, and to work. Moreover, follow-up and mediate the return to work, including proposing adaptations when necessary.

Foy [27], for example, observed that over half of the young adults with TBI who participated in the long term, in a neurological program integrated into a professional/vocational rehabilitation in England, managed to insert/reinsert themselves into remunerated or voluntary full-time or part-time work.

However, other studies have affirmed that a large proportion of individuals with brain injuries are unemployed and underemployed and have low rates of returning to work after sustaining the injury [21, 22]. O'Neill and Wolf [28] affirmed that the programs of rehabilitation for work are designed mainly to help persons with musculoskeletal disabilities, and there is a need to adapt the theoretical models for the return to work of persons with cognitive deficiencies. In this context, those who have studied this field have made an effort to contribute with methodologies that promoted the inclusion/reinsertion of persons who had suffered a TBI or any other neurological problem [12, 21, 24, 27–31].

The authors affirmed the need for the interventions directed to the return to work to be instituted early, because the longer the time off work, the lower the probability of returning to work or remaining in the job [31–35]. Moreover, they pointed out that although the actions in this sphere have a general flow of referral and attendance, they must be molded according to each patient's demand [31].

With the purpose of determining the capacity for work and subsidizing recommendations to make their development feasible, Kita et al. [21] presented the following guidelines for professional evaluation of persons with TBI:

1. Identification of who made the request for the evaluation and the subject to be evaluated (obtain the consent of the person evaluated and collect demographic and health data, educational and work history, and information about present social situation of the person evaluated).
2. Evaluation of the individual perspective of the subject (interests, objectives, and meaning attributed to pre- and post-lesion work; individual self-perception of the capacity for work, considering strong and weak points and compensatory strategies; evaluation of the costs and benefits of working).
3. Evaluation of the domains (physical, neuropsychological/cognitive, psychosocial, communication, functional state/level of independence, general behaviors, skills/behaviors related to work).
4. Evaluation of the working conditions and organizations.
5. Analysis and synthesis of the information to draw the conclusion and recommendations of the evaluation.

These guidelines may be used by health professionals, those in the area of human resources, and employers and other individuals involved in planning and decision-making related to work, with a view to facilitating return to work, particularly of persons who had suffered TBI at an economically active age [21].

Another study by Kita et al. [30] discourses about identifying the main factors that must be considered in the professional evaluation of the individual who suffered TBI to return to work, with findings similar to the previously cited study. In this study, seven key points were identified as relevant to the professional evaluation:

1. Identification of the purpose and rationality of the evaluation.
2. Processing of the admission (demographic data, pre-lesion history, educational and work history, compromise resulting from the lesion).

3. Evaluation of the person (evaluation using the following domains: Physical, neuropsychological/cognitive, psychosocial, communication, functional state/level of independence, general behaviors, and individual perspectives).
4. Evaluation of the working conditions and organization.
5. Evaluation of the occupation/work requisites.
6. Analysis and synthesis of the results of the evaluation.
7. Development of recommendations.

Culler et al. [29] conducted a study to identify the factors that facilitated the return to work of persons who had suffered CVA, or made it difficult for them to do so. From the point of view of the subjects affected, the following are considered factors that made it difficult to return to work: intrinsic (motor, perceptive, psychological, cognitive, and communication) and extrinsic difficulties (lack of social and environmental support). Professional/vocational rehabilitation professionals have described the following barriers to return to work: lack of knowledge about the deficiencies by the subject who suffered the CVA, the need for follow-up surgeries, prolonged time elapsed since the last job, lack of support from the spouse/family, lack of motivation, unrealistic expectations, and lack of professional experience, whereas facilitators cited flexibility, motivation to work, having a realistic work objective, and being aware of one's limitations. The employers mentioned that the deficiency had no impact on the hiring process, but the characteristics of the subject did have impact, and they described the facilitator aspects as follows: having the support of professional/vocational rehabilitation specialists and the ability to interact with these specialists during the hiring process.

Although studies in the field of return to work and remaining in the job were not specifically focused on persons with TBI, they found that success or failure in this process would depend on diverse aspects: working conditions and organization, interpersonal relations (e.g., the resistance of colleagues to receiving a worker with deficiencies), and professional training (the presence or absence of training and education for the development of a new function, if necessary) among others. This would also depend on the way the return is conducted by the various actors involved: health services, professional rehabilitation team, employers, and the workers themselves. All of these aspects show that success in action in this sphere is related to the involvement of diverse bodies, fields, professionals, and social actors that must direct their actions toward a common and collectively predefined objective.

## Brazilian Context

Brazil has legal particularities that may influence the processes of professional/vocational rehabilitation of those who suffered TBI and need to be elucidated for greater understanding by the reader.

In Brazil, the Federal Constitution of 1988 established the concept of social security that integrated the actions that assure the rights relative to health, care, and social security. Health care, provided by the Brazilian Public Health System (SUS), is free with universal and full access to cover. Social security refers to a social insurance, of a contributory nature by and mandatory affiliation of workers in the formal work market, assuring cover for medical leave of absence due to illness and retirement by age, time of work, and invalidity, whereas social assistance (Lei Orgânica da Assistência Social – LOAS) is provided for whoever may need it, whether the subject is a contributor to social security or not [12, 36, 37].

In this context, there are some benefits directed to persons that are considered "inept" to work; these benefits, however, cease if the individual goes back to work. One of these is the continuous provision of this benefit ("Benefício de Prestação Continuada (BPC)) by social assistance, destined for persons with deficiencies who are unable to insert themselves into the work market and who prove that they have no means of providing their own subsistence or that of their family [38].

Another benefit is the *aid in cases of illness* ("Auxílio-Doença"), destined for individuals who contribute to social security, who were affected by some disease or accident, and who are temporarily unable to perform their work activities. This benefit is provided by the National Social Security Institute ("Instituto Nacional do Seguro Social (INSS)), which is the Federal agency belonging to the Ministry of Social Security. When the INSS evaluates an individual as being permanently incapable of exercising any labor activity and unable to be rehabilitated in another profession, the person receives an invalidity pension [38].

In addition to these benefits, there is the law of quotas: Companies are obliged to hire a percentage of persons with deficiency, according to the number of employees they have [39].

## Professional/Vocational Rehabilitation in Brazil

Some Brazilian studies have revealed that persons who suffered TBI and had a job before the trauma returned to productive activity in up to 1 year after the accident, even without having gone through a professional/vocational rehabilitation program. However, a portion of these persons do not or did not return with changes in their work activities and/or with a feeling of worse performance in these, demonstrating the difficulty of transforming the work situation to receive the individual in conditions differing from those of the period before the accident [6, 40].

In Brazil, professional/vocational rehabilitation is still a challenge, both with reference to integrating affected persons to work and to the question of the burden that falls on the state, either through the Brazilian public health system (SUS) or social assistance [26].

There are few initiatives related to professional/vocational rehabilitation, especially those directed toward specific pathologies. The existent programs are generally destined to the return to work of individuals with osteomuscular and mental health diseases resulting from the work itself. Therefore, the rehabilitation is frequently directed only to the pathology and does not involve the possibility of access to work, for example, of individuals who had not worked previously.

Moreover, it must be considered that in Brazil there is a lack of articulation between the areas of health and social security and between these and companies, an aspect that configures as a barrier to the effectiveness of professional/vocational rehabilitation programs [26, 41].

Based on the foregoing presentation, a lack of effective professional/vocational rehabilitation programs in Brazil was verified, considering the complexity of the process and the need for integration among the various stages of treatment (post-trauma assistance and physical, cognitive, psychosocial, and professional rehabilitation).

## The Pilot Professional/Vocational Rehabilitation Program (PPVRP)

The "Hospital das Clinicas" of the University of São Paulo Medical School (HCFMUSP) is one of the main hospitals with highly complex facilities, directed toward care, teaching, and research in the State of São Paulo, Brazil. The cognitive rehabilitation outpatient clinic ("Ambulatório de Reabilitação Cognitiva" (ARCO)), linked to the Neurological Department of HCFMUSP, provides pioneering services directed specifically toward patients who have suffered TBI and have reached a stable health condition, that is, a chronic stage as far as the sequelae left by the trauma are concerned.

The patients attended in this service have gone through the physical rehabilitation process, and the main focus of attention in this stage of treatment is cognitive rehabilitation with emphasis on functional independence. The outpatient clinic team is composed of doctors, neurologists, ophthalmologists, speech therapists, psychologists, neuropsychologists, nurses, and occupational therapists.

Over the years of operation of ARCO, the team has observed that the patients who attended brought demands, desires, and needs related to work: return, inclusion, and remaining in jobs. Having detected the need to add a professional/vocational rehabilitation program to the services already offered, the coordinators of ARCO sought the investigation and intervention in health and work laboratory ("Laboratório de Investigação e Intervenção em Saúde e Trabalho (LIIST))"[2] of the occupational therapy course of FMUSP, in 2014, requesting partnership for the development of a professional/vocational rehabilitation program. LIIST has a wide experience in the development of programs of return to work and remaining in the job, particularly with workers who suffered work-related accidents or illnesses. In view of the demand put forward by ARCO, LIIST accepted the challenge and broadened the scope of action of the occupational therapy area present in the outpatient clinic which, up until then, had focused its actions on cognitive rehabilitation, to include a pilot project of professional/vocational rehabilitation, during the period from August 2014 to November 2015.

In view of the entire abovementioned context, the purpose of the present chapter was to present and discuss the experience of this pilot project with regard to an axis of action of the overall rehabilitation plan for individuals who had suffered TBI, in addition to analyzing the potentialities, limitations, and challenges based on the experience of the program.

## Process of Education and Initial Proposal of PPVRP

In Brazil, occupational therapy is recognized as one of the main professions that develop professional/vocational rehabilitation programs [41–44]. This is because, on the one hand, the aim of the study of these professionals is to evaluate the work the subjects effectively do, by means of analyzing the activities and listening to accounts of the patients' professional experience. On the other hand, it is to evaluate the working capacities (fundamental for subsiding the possibility of remaining in a job) and to help with intermediating the return and/or inclusion in the work, by providing bosses and peers with guidance, favoring the reception of the worker and processes of cooperation. Thus, the occupational therapists are educated to favor dialog and achieve compatibility between the demands of the work activity from the physical, cognitive, and psychic point of view and the subject's health conditions, with a view to making possible adaptations and providing guidance in the work environment [14, 24, 41–45].

The PPVRP must attend the patients referred to it by members of the outpatient clinic's multiprofessional team, according to the following eligibility criteria: the patients' interest in working, the team identifying that the patients have the motor

[2]LIIST, existent for over 15 years, is responsible for research, extension, and teaching activities of the occupational therapy course of FMUSP. It is composed of professors and occupational therapists who are specialists in the field of "health and work," with wide experience in the specific area of "return to work," mainly with workers with reduced working capacity and/or work-related diseases.

and/or cognitive capacity for this purpose, and whether or not the patients have any ties to previous work situations – in this case, return or entry into the work market.

The authors point out that a professional/vocational rehabilitation with this population is unprecedented in Brazil and was developed to be of an experimental nature. Other professional rehabilitation and internal readaptation programs, which were developed in other services directed toward workers affected by work-related illnesses or accidents, were taken as reference.

The program was also based on experiments conducted in other countries, with emphasis on Canada. Part of these experiments were focused on the process of return to work, directed toward persons with musculoskeletal disturbances [46, 47] and part directed toward persons with mental health problems [48, 49]. In both cases, it was shown to be a program in which the return to work occurred gradually and progressively, with adequacy of the workplace, workload, and activities of the worker. In addition, as key points to its success, there were notes to provide the bosses, peers, and management of the company with support.

Initially, the program was conceived by means of the following actions:

1. Anamnesis, that is, an interview with the purpose of finding out and understanding the patients' possibilities, their activities of interest, their educational and occupational history, and their possibilities of returning to work and employability.
2. Preparation of individuals for returning to work, discussing their limitations to work and fears, understanding the dynamics of the work, and relating it to the patients' health possibilities.
3. Moreover, whenever it was the case, expect to make contact with the company of origin to facilitate the return and professional accessibility, intermediate the relationships with bosses and peers, analyze the content of work activities and proposals for suiting these to the patients' needs, and, in addition, periodically follow up the individuals in the process of return to work.

## Characterization of the Population Attended

In the PPRVP, nine patients were attended, of whom four were women and five men, in the age range between 17 and 61 years. They studied from 8 to 11 years and the time of injury of TBI was of at least 9 months and maximum of 5 years. There were no data about the etiology of the TBI of all the patients, but many of them were known to have resulted from being run over or automobile accidents.

Furthermore, of the total number of patients attended, the majority had cognitive sequelae, although there were those who also had motor sequelae. Relative to work, one of the patients was a student and two had never worked before. The remainder used to work formally before the TBI, performing activities in the service sector (civil construction, transport, education, among others). However, after the trauma occurred, these patients were dismissed or resigned from their jobs because of the difficulties resulting from the sequelae of the traumatism.

## Implementation and Development of the PPRVP

Throughout the implementation and development of the PPVRP, the patients attended presented different demands. Therefore, although the initial proposal of the program concerned the return to work, the attendances varied according to the demand of each individual. Anamnesis was an important time to learn of these demands and thus define the patients' follow-up in the program.

Three subjects presented demands that were mainly directed toward clearing up doubts related to labor and social security legislation in a broader manner. Therefore, some attendances were conducted to provide information and explanations about vacancies for disabled persons in the public and private work market, support and incentive to enter the work market, retirement due to invalidity, and social security benefits. In these cases, attendances were made by appointment, without follow-up afterward, and by choice of the patient and/or family member, without the presence of family members at the attendances.

The program also performed follow-up directed toward the patient in higher education. This follow-up covered the following: attendances at the outpatient clinic with the patients and family member who accompanied them, to understand their desires and difficulties; follow-up in one of the classes to observe the context and day-to-day study dynamics; discussion with the board of the teaching institution about the question of including the patient; and the ways in which the professionals of the educational institution dealt with the difficulties that arose.

Two of the patients demanded actions with the purpose of inclusion in the work market, as they had no previous work experience. In their case, anamnesis was performed, their résumés' were prepared, and the possibilities of their inclusion in the work market were jointly evaluated.

With the three patients that had work experience before the TBI, anamnesis was performed to understand their demands and make a joint evaluation of the possibilities of reinsertion into the work market. In addition, attendances were held to deal with the emotional and motivational questions pertaining to their return to work. Furthermore, the program created a partnership with an institution that maintained a database of employment vacancies for disabled persons. Some of these patients were referred to seek a vacancy by intermediary of this institution.

## Difficulties Found and Outcome of Cases Attended

Through implementation of the PPRVP, the professionals identified the difficulties present in the process of including the patients attended in the work market. Some of these difficulties were perceived through the understanding of the occupational therapists who were members of the program team, some were mentioned by the subjects themselves, and others were related to the return to work itself of persons who had suffered TBI.

The difficulties mentioned by the patients during the process of inclusion in work were insecurity and functional limitations resulting from the sequelae of the TBI (motor, visual, behavioral, and cognitive), difficulty in dealing with and accepting these limitations, mistakenly associating them with the incapacity to do the work, family problems not related to the patients, scarcity of work vacancies, and the fact that they resided far from the city center, an aspect that limited traveling to places that offered most employment vacancies. Apart from this, although they showed interest in returning to work, some patients reported lack of motivation: they felt "discouraged about everything."

The difficulties observed by the occupational therapists who were members of the program team were Brazilian legislation, low educational level and professional inexperience of the patients, absence of support or family protectiveness, and lack of independence for performing daily life activities. Brazilian legislation was considered a barrier because in acquiring an employment tie, the patients would lose their financial benefits assured by the social security system, which generated worry in the patients, and frequently, they desisted from returning to work. The low educational level and professional inexperience determined a smaller range of possibilities of employment vacancies, because for many of these, some education or experience was demanded. The absence of support or excessive protectiveness and the lack of independence to perform daily life activities were also considered difficulties, because these difficulties limited patients' self-confidence in relation to work and their mobility to go to possible places of work.

Up to November 2015, only one patient continued in the program in search of a work vacancy. Three patients were considered concluded cases, because they mentioned that the attendances were for the purpose of obtaining information and clearing up doubts. The other five patients abandoned the program before conclusion of the process for the following reasons: loss of interest, lack of family support, fear related to returning to work, and loss of the continuous benefit provided ("Benefício de Prestação Continuada").

## Limitations, Potentialities, and Adequacy of the PPVRP

Because it concerned a pilot program, the authors verified potentialities and limitations that needed to be better developed and overcome. One of the limitations was related to the incompatibility between the objectives previously elaborated by the program (return to professional activity developed before occurrence of the trauma) and the demands of some of the patients attended. This mainly resulted from the fact that the majority of the patients attended had no work ties before the TBI and their demands were directed toward explanations about access to social security benefits and the inclusion of disabled persons in the work market.

Thus, with development of the program, the authors noted that this should change the scope initially foreseen to a practice more related to the concept of professional/vocational rehabilitation because, in many cases, there was more concern about thinking of a program of professional development than of rehabilitation.

From this aspect, it was necessary to seek new areas of interest, compatible with the new health condition presented by each of the patients attended. For this purpose, when discussing inclusion in work, it was important to consider aspects such as professional history, educational level, interests, limitations, competences and skill, as well as the possibility of changing the work activity.

The profile of patients attended, Brazilian legislation, the lack of family support, and dismotivation (cited by patients in the program) led to the occupational therapists reflecting about the scope of the program and seeking to readjust it to the reality found.

The fact that many patients did not have a job before the TBI probably made it even more difficult for them to find a job after the trauma. Moreover, the lack of previous work experience related to the age of patients and low educational level possibly restricted the possibilities of working [29]. Another important aspect was the mean time after the TBI to being with the program, since it is known that the earlier this began, the better would be the results [31–35]; that is, the program must be part of the early attendance of TBI victims.

With further regard to the patients' profile, the authors point out that the presence of motor and particularly cognitive deficiencies has been pointed out in the literature as being a factor that limited the engagement in work of persons who have suffered neurological pathologies. These studies affirmed that these limitations could be attenuated by means of other points, such as awareness and emotional acceptance of the deficiencies and the existence of a realistic work objective [29, 45].

The Brazilian legislation, created to protect disabled persons financially, was shown to be a barrier to the process of inclusion in work, because, as previously mentioned, it generated fear of replacing the guarantee of receiving the social security benefit with the possible instability of a job. Another aspect verified was the patients' feeling of being unprepared for work activity, due to the difficulty of coping with the competitive work market and the work relations that involved processes of evaluation and relationship with peers and bosses, among other factors [50].

The TBI also had impact on the patients' families and respective financial situation, frequently leading to other members of the family experiencing depression, social isolation, stress, anxiety, and consequent reduction in quality of life [51]. For this reason, the family must not be left out during the professional/vocational rehabilitation process. Studies have shown that the acceptance and support of the family for the work are considered essential factors for the process of inclusion and reinsertion in work [29, 45, 52]. Therefore, the authors considered involvement of the family members in the support for work to be another important point that must be inserted in the development of the program.

Frequently, the dismotivation, cited by patients, was a reflection of the difficulties they found. These were mainly related to family questions, the sequelae of TBI, and difficulties of resuming the projects of life, including insertion in the work market. However, professional/vocational rehabilitation specialists have affirmed that the lack of motivation is considered an important barrier to the process of return to work of persons who have neurological pathologies. In addition to the abovementioned barrier, they mentioned the lack of knowledge about the deficiencies, need for surgeries and follow-up, time elapsed since the last job, the spouse/family, unrealistic expectations, and the lack of professional experience [28, 29].

This demonstrated the need for attendance by a multidisciplinary team and integration between the program of inclusion in work in conjunction with the overall rehabilitation treatment (conventional neurological and educational, etc.) of patients with TBI [27].

The awareness of the importance of work in a cognitive rehabilitation outpatient clinic was one of the major gains of the program. However, the authors perceived that this awareness attained the multiprofessional team to a greater extent that it did attended the patients and their families. As potential aspect of the program, we also have discussion with the outpatient team about the criteria for referral for professional/vocational rehabilitation, creation of an individual space (OT and patient) for receiving the questions related to work, and creation of partnerships with institutions that could help with seeking work vacancies.

From the pilot program, on the one hand, the intention is to improve it, suiting it better to the profile of patients attended. On the other hand, by means of demonstrating the possibility of the patients acting in concrete work situations, the purpose would be to make them and their respective family members aware of this possibility, so that they would be more active and participate in the process of return to work.

The following were among the changes required in the program:

1. Broadening its scope: Return to work, professional/vocational training, and rehabilitation.
2. By the multiprofessional team performing more adequate triage to include patients with interest in the proposal offered by the program.
3. The need for forming a group of patients (and family members) with the purpose of raising awareness of the importance of work as a strong element of participation in society and sharing fears, insecurities, and solutions of problems.
4. Raising awareness and explanation about the program, the Brazilian laws, and the quota laws.
5. Providing the family with guidance about the benefits linked to work and encouraging adhesion to and participation in the process of including patients in work.
6. Raising the awareness of companies for effectuation of follow-up of workers in the place of work, including guidance for bosses and peers.
7. Increasing partnerships with institutions that work with supported employment programs, training and education, and government (state and municipal) programs.

## Conclusion

When considering that the subjects who suffered TBI commonly have difficulty in being included in the community and that work may be a way to make this inclusion possible, the authors understood that the development of professional/vocational rehabilitations directed toward persons who have suffered TBI was of utmost importance.

Post-TBI inclusion in work was a complex process, since it did not depend only on the health (physical, emotional, and/or cognitive) conditions of subjects but also on other factors, such as sociodemographic characteristics (age, educational level, type of previous occupation exercised, level of income before the trauma), work market, and social support that the individuals receive, in addition to participation in an overall rehabilitation program that involves professional/vocational rehabilitation [53, 54].

To illustrate a model that could be one of these professional/vocational rehabilitation programs, in this chapter, the authors presented the process of development of the PPRVP performed in Brazil in a pioneering manner. The authors considered that it presented limitations and potentialities that could guide the respective improvement and help with the construction of other programs of this nature.

The proposal of insertion/reinsertion of patients into the work market after TBI was recent in the cognitive rehabilitation outpatient clinic of HCFMUSP; however, it represented significant advancement with reference to the integral care of persons who experienced a situation of TBI and had potentially incapacitating sequelae. Therefore, receiving the demands that transcended the original scope of the program proposal became a challenge and has been understood to be a qualitative gain in the actions developed.

**Acknowledgments** The authors thank Dr. Renato Anguinah and Dr. Silvia Veitzman for the opportunity to develop this program.

## References

1. Instituto Brasileiro de Geografia e Estatística – IBGE. Geociências. Disponível em: <http://www.ibge.gov.br/home/mapa_site/mapa_site.php#geociencias>. Acesso em: 13 de junho de 2017.
2. Freire FR, Coelho F, Lacerda JR, Silva MF, Gonçalves VT, Machado S, Velasques B, Ribeiro P, Basile LFH, Oliveira AMP, Paiva WS, Kanda PAM, Anghinah R. Cognitive rehabilitation following traumatic brain injury. Dement neuropsychol. 2011;5(1):17–25.
3. Gaudêncio TG, Leão GM. A epidemiologia do traumatismo crânio encefálico: um levantamento bibliográfico no Brasil. Rev Neurocienc. 2013;21(3):427–34.
4. Ministério da Previdência Social. Tabelas – CID – Ano 2015. Disponível em: <http://www.previdencia.gov.br/dados-abertos/estatsticas/tabelas-cid-10/>. Acesso em: 13 de junho de 2017.
5. Malloy-Diniz LF, Mattos P, Abreu N, Fuentes D. Neuropsicologia – Aplicações clínicas. Editora Artmed. 2016;
6. Sousa RMC, Koizumi MS. Vítimas de trauma crânio-encefálico e seu retorno a produtividade após 6 meses e 1 ano. Rev Esc Enf USP. 1999;33(3):313–22.
7. Cassidy JD, Carroll LJ, Peloso PM, Borg J, Von Holst H, Holm L, Kraus J, Coronado VG, WHO Collaborating Centre Task Force on Mild Traumatic Brain Injury. Incidence, risk factors and prevention of mild traumatic brain injury: results of the WHO Collaborating Centre Task Force on mild traumatic brain injury. J Rehabil Med. 2004;(43 Suppl):28–60.
8. Gentile JKA, Himuro HS, Rojas SSO, Veiga VC, Amaya LEC, Carvalho JC. Condutas no paciente com trauma crânioencefálico. Rev Bras Clin Med. 2011;9(1):74–82.
9. DePalma RG. Combat TBI: History, Epidemiology, and Injury Modes. In: Kobeissy FH, editor. Brain Neurotrauma: Molecular, Neuropsychological, and Rehabilitation Aspects. Boca Raton (FL: CRC Press; 2015.
10. Burt CM. Avaliação do Trabalho e Preparação para o Retorno ao Trabalho. In: Pedretti LW, Early MB, editors. Terapia Ocupacional: capacidades práticas para disfunções físicas. São Paulo: ROCA. p. 2005.
11. Silva CB, Brasil ABS, Bonilha DB, Masson L, Ferreira MS. Retorno à produtividade após reabilitação de pacientes deambuladores vítimas de trauma cranioencefálico. Fisioterapia e Pesquisa. 2008;15(1):6–11.
12. Maeno M, Takahashi MAC, Lima MAG. Reabilitação profissional como política de inclusão social. Acta Fisiatr. 2009;16(2):53–8.
13. Foti D. Atividades da Vida Diária. In: Pedretti LW, Early MB, editors. Terapia Ocupacional: capacidades práticas para disfunções físicas. São Paulo: ROCA. p. 2005.
14. Lancman S, Ghirardi MIG. Pensando novas práticas em terapia ocupacional, saúde e trabalho. Rev Ter Ocup Univ São Paulo. 2002;13(2):44–50.
15. Organização Mundial da Saúde - OMS (2015). Relatório mundial de envelhecimento e saúde. Disponível em: <http://sbgg.org.br/wp-content/uploads/2015/10/OMS-ENVELHECIMENTO-2015-port.pdf>. Acesso em: 8 de junho de 2017.
16. Hilleshein EF, Souza LM, Lautert L, Paz AA, Catalan VM, Teixeira MG, Mello DB. Capacidade para o trabalho de enfermeiros de um hospital universitário. Rev Gaúcha Enf. 2011;32(3):509–15.
17. Berger W, Hakkarainen O, Ikonen J, Karjalainen P, Sokura S, Sorsa S. Ageing in working life. Pertti Laitinen editors. Joensuu: North Karelia University of Applied Sciences; 2012.
18. Hilleshein EF, Lautert L. Capacidade para o trabalho, características sociodemográficas e laborais de enfermeiros de um hospital universitário. Rev Latino-Am Enfermagem 2012; 20(3).
19. Martinez MC, Latorre MRDO, Fischer FM. Capacidade para o trabalho: revisão de literatura. Ciência & Saúde Col. 2010;15(1):1553–61.
20. Abrahão J, Sznelwar LI, Silvino A, Sarmet M, Pinho D. Introdução à Ergonomia: da prática à teoria. São Paulo: Blucher; 2009.
21. Kita MS, Dawson D, Rappolt S. Inter-professional clinical practice guideline for vocational evaluation following traumatic brain injury: a systematic and evidence-based approach. J Occup Rehabil. 2012;22:166–81.
22. Mills AL, Kreutzer JS. Theoretical applications of positive psychology to vocational rehabilitation after traumatic brain injury. J Occup Rehabil. 2016 Mar;26(1):20–31.
23. Ianof JN. Análise comparativa do eletroencefalograma em pacientes com doença de Alzheimer e lesão axonial difusa. 2017. Dissertação (Mestrado em Neurologia) - Universidade de São Paulo, São Paulo; 2017.
24. O'Brien AN, Wolf TJ. Determining work outcomes in mild to moderate stroke survivors. Work. 2010;36(4):441–7.
25. Ministério da Saúde. Secretaria de Atenção à Saúde. Diretrizes de atenção à reabilitação da pessoa com traumatismo cranioencefálico / Ministério da Saúde. Secretaria de Atenção à Saúde. Departamento de Ações Programáticas Estratégicas. – Brasília: Ministério da Saúde; 2013.
26. Maeno M, Vilela RAG. Reabilitação profissional no Brasil: elementos para a construção de uma política pública. Rev Bras Saúde Ocup. 2010;35(121):87–99.
27. Foy CM. Long term efficacy of an integrated neurological and vocational rehabilitation programme for young adults with acquired brain injury. J Occup Rehabil. 2014;24(3):533–42.
28. O'Neill K, Wolf TJ. Development and pilot testing of a work readiness assessment battery. Work. 2010;36(4):423–30.
29. Culler KH, Wang YC, Byers K, Trierweiler R. Barriers and facilitators of return to work for individuals with strokes: perspectives of the stroke survivor, vocational specialist, and employer. Top Stroke Rehabil. 2011;18(4):325–40.
30. Kita MS, Dawson DR, Rappolt SG. An integrated review of the processes and factors relevant to vocational evaluation following traumatic brain injury. J Occup Rehabil. 2011;21:374–94.
31. Donker-Cools BH, Daams JG, Wind H, Frings-Dresen MH. Effective return-to-work interventions after acquired brain injury: a systematic review. Brain Inj. 2015;8:1–19.
32. Toldrá RC, Daldon MB, Santos MC, Lancman S. Facilitadores e barreiras para o retorno ao trabalho: a experiência de trabalhadores

atendidos em Centro de Referência em Saúde do Trabalhador – SP, Brasil. Rev Bras Saúde Ocupac. 2010;35(121):10–22.
33. Loisel P, Durand P, Abenhaim L, Gosselin L, Simard R, Turcotte J, Esdaile JM. Management of occupational back pain: the Sherbrooke model. Results of a pilot and feasibility study. Occup Environ Med. 1994;51(9):597–602.
34. Arnetz BB, Sjögren B, Rydéhn B, Meisel R. Early workplace intervention for employees with musculoskeletal-related absenteeism: a prospective controlled intervention study. J Occup Environ Med. 2003;45(5):499–506.
35. Scopel MJ. Retorno ao trabalho: trajetória de trabalhadores metalúrgicos portadores de LER/DORT. 2005. Dissertação (Mestrado em Psicologia Social e Institucional) – Universidade Federal do Rio Grande do Sul, Porto Alegre; 2005.
36. Ministério da Previdência Social. Previdência Social. Disponível em: <http://www.previdencia.gov.br/perguntas-frequentes/previdencia-social/>. Acesso em: 04 de julho de 2017.
37. Secretaria de Desenvolvimento Social. Sistema Único de Assistência Social – SUAS. Disponível em: <http://www.desenvolvimentosocial.sp.gov.br/portal.php/assistencia_sistema>. Acesso em: 20 de junho de 2017.
38. Ministério da Previdência Social. Benefícios do INSS. Disponível em: <http://www.previdencia.gov.br/servicos-ao-cidadao/beneficios-do-inss/>. Acesso em: 20 de junho de 2017.
39. Ministério do Trabalho. Lei de Cotas (Lei 8.213 de 24 de julho 1991). Disponível em: <http://trabalho.gov.br/portal-mte/>. Acesso em: 24 de maio de 2017.
40. Oliveira NLB, Sousa RMC. Retorno à atividade produtiva de motociclistas vítimas de acidentes de trânsito. Acta Paul Enferm. 2006;19(3):284–9.
41. Lancman S, Toldrá RC, Santos MC. Reabilitação profissional e saúde mental no trabalho. In: DMR G, Rocha LE, editors. Saúde mental no trabalho: da teoria à prática. São Paulo: ROCA. p. 2010.
42. Lancman S, Daldon MT, Barros J, Gonçalves R, Jardim T. Processos de retorno e permanência no trabalho: elementos estruturantes para a construção de um modelo de ação. In: Simonelli AP, Rodrigues DS, editors. Saúde e trabalho em debate: velhas questões, novas perspectivas. Brasília: Paralelo 15; 2013.
43. Rodrigues DS, Simonelli AP, Lima J. A atuação da terapia ocupacional na saúde do trabalhador. In: Simonelli AP, Rodrigues DS, editors. Saúde e trabalho em debate: velhas questões, novas perspectivas, vol. 115. Brasília; 2013.
44. Lancman S. Construção de novas teorias e práticas em Terapia Ocupacional, Saúde e Trabalho. In: Lancman S. Saúde, Trabalho e Terapia Ocupacional. São Paulo: Roca; 2004.
45. Leng CM. Description of a return-to-work occupational therapy programme for stroke rehabilitation in Singapore. Occup Ther Int. 2008;15(2):87–99.
46. Durand MJ, Loisel P. Therapeutic return to work: rehabilitation in the workplace. Work. 2001;17(1):57–63.
47. Loisel P, Durand MJ, Berthelette D, Vezina N, Baril R, Gagnon D, Larivière C, Tremblay C. Disability prevention: The new paradigm of management of occupational back pain. Dis Manag Health Out. 2001;9(7):351–60.
48. St-Arnaud L, St-Jean M, Damasse J. Towards an enhanced understanding of factors involved in the return-to-work process of employees absent due to mental health problems. Can J Commun Ment Health. 2006;25(2):303–15.
49. St-Arnaud L, Bourbonnais R, St-Jean M, Rhéaume J. Determinants of return-to-work among employees absent due to mental health problems. Indust Relat J. 2007;62(4):690–713.
50. Matsushima AM, Sato AT, Conti J, Barros JO, Lancman S, Jardim TA. Retorno ao trabalho de pacientes pós-traumatismo cranioencefálico: relato de experiência da atuação da Terapia Ocupacional. In: XII Jornada Acadêmica de Terapia Ocupacional da USP "Este mundo está grávido de outros mundos: terapia ocupacional e as lutas na atualidade", 2015, São Paulo. Anais (on-line). Disponível em: <http://files.jornadadetousp.webnode.com/200001061-f41b000f01/Anais%20-%20XII%20Jornada%20Acad%C3%AAmica%20de%20Terapia%20Ocupacional%20da%20USP%20-%202015.pdf>. Acesso em: 14 de junho de 2017.
51. Moriarty H, Winter L, Robinson K, Piersol CV, Vause-Earland T, Iacovone DB, Newhart B, True G, Fishman D, Hodgson N, Gitlin LN. A randomized controlled trial to evaluate the Veterans' Inhome program for military veterans with TraumaticBrain injury andTheir families: report on impact for family members. PMR. 2016;8(6):495–509.
52. Gravina MER, Nogueira DP, Rocha LE. Reabilitação profissional em um banco: facilitadores e dificultadores no retorno ao trabalho. Rev de Ter Ocup USP. 2003;14(1):19–26.
53. Corrigam JD, Bogner JA, Mysiw WJ, Clinchot D, Fugate L. Life satisfaction after traumatic brain injury. J Head Trauma Rehabil. 2001;16(6):543–55.
54. Morris JA, Sanchez AA, Bass SM, Mackenzie EJ. Trauma patients return to productivity. J Trauma. 1991;31(6):827–34.

# Index




R. Anghinah et al. (eds.), *Topics in Cognitive Rehabilitation in the TBI Post-Hospital Phase*,
https://doi.org/10.1007/978-3-319-95376-2

Printed by Printforce, the Netherlands